Understanding Figures in Neuroscience Research

This innovative text introduces neuroscience students to the visual language of scientific publications, teaching scientific literacy, research methods, and graphical literacy in an engaging way. Employing a "pictures first" pedagogical approach, it walks the reader step by step through the interpretation of neuroscience figures and explains the principles of experimental design. The text explores the major research techniques – from neuroimaging, to behavioral methods, to genetics and comparative approaches – and illuminates how they are represented graphically in journal articles, and their strengths and limitations as research tools. More than 120 example figures provide experimental paradigms for the more difficult-to-visualize methods, and depict actual results taken from the recently published scientific literature. Data from several study designs are discussed, including clinical case studies, meta-analyses, and experiments from behavior to molecular genetics. Concrete examples of experiments are provided along with each method, helping students with the design of their own research questions.

Austin Lim is the lead author on the *Open Neuroscience Initiative*, a free to access and adopt textbook for students of introductory neuroscience. In 2023, he was the recipient of the Excellence in Teaching Award from DePaul University. He published an educational board game, NeuroNavigator, designed to teach students about neuroanatomy. He has also published two children's books about brain science: *Cellular Neurobiology for Babies!* and *Neuroscience from A to Z for Babies!*

"Lim's text shines a light on an often overlooked aspect of neuroscience education, covering a range of concepts in an accessible manner. An excellent resource for those seeking to deepen their grasp of neuroscience research, and a fabulous teaching tool."

Shona McQuilken, University of Glasgow

"This book is about more than just figures – it is an ambitious tour through the experiments and methodology that generate them."

Ashley Juavinett, University of California, San Diego

"Creating and reading empirical data figures is truly an art form, and one that is not often explicitly taught in the classroom. This text provides a diverse range of examples pulled from the literature to contextualize commonly used methods and analyses, culminating in a key resource for promoting student learning, application, and interpretation of data across neuroscience and related fields."

Jennifer Honeycutt, Bowdoin College

Understanding Figures in Neuroscience Research

A Guide to Interpreting Graphs and Methods

Austin Lim

DePaul University

CAMBRIDGE
UNIVERSITY PRESS

CAMBRIDGE
UNIVERSITY PRESS

Shaftesbury Road, Cambridge CB2 8EA, United Kingdom

One Liberty Plaza, 20th Floor, New York, NY 10006, USA

477 Williamstown Road, Port Melbourne, VIC 3207, Australia

314–321, 3rd Floor, Plot 3, Splendor Forum, Jasola District Centre, New Delhi – 110025, India

103 Penang Road, #05–06/07, Visioncrest Commercial, Singapore 238467

Cambridge University Press is part of Cambridge University Press & Assessment, a department of the University of Cambridge.

We share the University's mission to contribute to society through the pursuit of education, learning and research at the highest international levels of excellence.

Information on this title: www.cambridge.org/highereducation/isbn/9781009344227

DOI: 10.1017/9781009344241

When citing this work, please include a reference to the DOI 10.1017/9781009344241

First published 2024

A catalogue record for this publication is available from the British Library.

Library of Congress Cataloging-in-Publication Data
Names: Lim, Austin, 1985– author.
Title: Understanding figures in neuroscience research : a guide to interpreting graphs and methods / Austin Lim.
Description: Cambridge, United Kingdom ; New York, NY : Cambridge University Press, 2025. | Includes bibliographical references and index.
Identifiers: LCCN 2024005662 | ISBN 9781009344227 (hardback) | ISBN 9781009344265 (paperback) | ISBN 9781009344241 (ebook)
Subjects: LCSH: Neurosciences – Research – Methodology. | Neurosciences – Graphic methods.
Classification: LCC RC337 .L56 2025 | DDC 616.890072–dc23/eng/20240301
LC record available at https://lccn.loc.gov/2024005662

ISBN 978-1-009-34422-7 Hardback
ISBN 978-1-009-34426-5 Paperback

Additional resources for this publication available at www.cambridge.org/lim

Contents

Detailed Contents

Preface

As the saying goes, a picture is worth a thousand hours of literature searches, carefully planned experiments, and meticulous data analysis. *Understanding Figures in Neuroscience Research* was born out of the way I gain information from academic publications: pictures first. To me, a good figure conveys results as convincingly as numbers do, and an elegant summary figure shows results in a fraction of the time needed to digest an entire publication. Pictures not only provide a visual respite from blocks of text, but also engage additional circuits in the brain, helping to enhance learning.

This "pictures first" strategy is also my pedagogical approach, whether the course is in research methods, cellular neurobiology, or neuropsychopharmacology. My undergraduate and graduate students know that my approach to working through the results of a publication is to focus on what is being presented in the images, then using these data as a guide to understanding the methodology. This approach is also helpful when interpreting figures in scientific presentations and poster sessions, where the time and space needed for completely explaining background concepts are often limited.

Inspiration for this text came from supplemental documents I made for my upper-level neuroscience majors in laboratory research methods and reading-heavy seminar courses. In previous years, students have found that the interpretation of some elements of the primary literature, such as electrophysiological evidence of long-term potentiation, can be challenging. Some figures require a deep comprehension of several basic elements of neuroscience to understand what is being displayed, and my supplemental documents functioned as a reminder of those elements. This book is here to unwrap and demystify that implicit, unexplained information.

Unlike similar books that function as a catalog of the methods used in neuroscience research, this book has a special emphasis on

- describing the figures that are used to represent data, explaining the variables that are plotted, and interpreting what differences between groups may mean in a bigger context
- giving concrete examples of the types of neuroscience questions that each experimental method is suited for, which provides the reader with ideas about developing their own research questions
- explaining the results of real data from the published scientific literature, which the reader can compare with data they encounter elsewhere.

Through this approach to research methods, readers are immersed in questions of a higher order in Bloom's taxonomy of learning objectives, such as applying knowledge and designing experiments.

I have made efforts to maintain the key pedagogical elements of many other textbooks, such as defining terminology, explaining the "how-to"s, outlining the advantages and limitations of each method, and providing a list of select key terms at the end of each chapter. I also dedicate time to explaining statistics, with an emphasis on the measures that often appear in graphs.

The textbook is organized as a tool for teaching neuroscience research methods, with the general flow of the chapters moving “from big to small”: starting from behavior and brain imaging, through cells and molecules, down to electrophysiology and genetics. Introductory material from each section may build on previous chapters, but the chapters are largely usable in any order. The accompanying Online Resources provide both multiple-choice and essay questions for students looking to test their understanding of the material, and the instructor’s manual offers a chapter-by-chapter outline including key points and vocabulary. Lecture slides containing the images used in this book are also available for download.

The book also functions as a reference guide, useful for undergraduate students who are taking courses with a heavy focus on reading and understanding the primary literature, graduate students who are navigating the vast neuroscience literature, and neuroscience researchers of all backgrounds who are looking to add more techniques to their experimental toolbox. Finally, I wrote this textbook for past me, who would’ve benefited tremendously from a guide like this.

Acknowledgments

This book wouldn't have been possible without my editors, Stephen Acerra and Emma Collison. I am grateful to my advisors, Tony West, Dan McGehee, and Jim Surmeier, who all took a chance on me and shaped me into the scientist and educator I am. I thank my parents for their never-ending love and support. And I thank the ones who complete my life: Allie, Polo-bear, Little-bear, and Peanut.

CHAPTER ONE

Introduction to Data in Research

Figures are everywhere in the sciences, especially in the field of neuroscience. They take up most of the space on slides during academic talks, feature prominently on scientific posters, and are a central focus of attention in publications. Figures are so useful because they can summarize large amounts of information in an easily digestible manner. A good figure can show information that would otherwise take hundreds of words to explain.

This textbook is a guide to understanding the data contained in some of the commonly used types of figures in neuroscience. But to fully appreciate those data, it is also critical to understand the techniques that are used to generate the figures. In other words, this book helps you answer the questions "what did the researchers do, and how have their results been represented as an image?"

Learning Objectives

By the end of this chapter, you will be able to:

- Describe different types of figures and study designs and explain the purpose and limitations of each
- Define different types of variables
- Describe different types of control experiments
- Describe some elements of statistical methods used to explain data
- Understand and interpret the different types of graphs that may be used to represent data

1.1 Types of Figures

In neuroscience publications, figures are usually depictions of major ideas or conclusions. Figures often contain several **panels**, which may show different experiments that all support the same conclusion. Figures are usually identified by number, and panels by letter.

Different types of figures are used for showing different types of information:

- **Experimental protocol figures** are a graphical representation of the methods section of a research report, showing how experiments were done. For example, an experimental protocol figure may be a flow chart of how groups were treated differently or a timeline of which experiments were performed when. It may show the order in which stimuli were presented to a person during a brain scan. It may be a picture or diagram of the apparatus used for collecting data, especially when describing a new technique for the first time.

Experimental protocol figures are not always present, but they tend to appear earlier in a publication.

- **Data** or **results figures** show what each set of experiments has taught us. In a typical primary research paper, most figures will show data. These images may be **representative data figures**, which show the results from only a single subject. This might be one neuron's spontaneous action potential firing pattern, one animal's movement in a maze, or one person's brain scan results. Ideally, the representative data are selected because they are most similar to the average of the combined data. Alternatively, data may be shown in **combined data figures**, which show the results from several subjects, often represented as a graph. Most graphs are made to show comparisons between groups, such as if one treatment led to an increase in protein levels.
- **Summary figures** are used to illustrate big-picture ideas and serve as a visual representation of the abstract. These figures combine the results of several experiments. They are commonly found in review papers but are not always present in primary research papers. They often appear at the beginning or at the end of the publication. Summary figures may propose a mechanism explaining some phenomenon (such as cartoon representations of the molecules involved in vesicle fusion), or they may show how the results of the experiments answer a small part of a bigger question (such as a novel connection between two brain areas in the context of reward behavior).

Figure 1.1 shows examples of four types of figure that are often used in the presentation of neuroscience research. The experimental protocol shows a timeline of when different manipulations were performed on mice. In this experiment, pain induction was initiated at postnatal day 1 (P1), treatment with fentanyl was delivered from days P1 through P8, BrdU labeling was performed from P9 through P11, weaning and sexing at P21, and perfusion at P39.

The representative data in Figure 1.1 is from a different experiment and shows slices taken of the pons, a region of the brain stem. Oligodendrocyte cells have been labeled in green using genetic manipulation. Here, a normal mouse (known as 'wild type', here called WT/WT) is compared with a mouse model for the neurodegenerative disease spinocerebellar ataxia type 3 (a mutant, here called Q84/Q84). Each image is from a different animal under different conditions (either 4 weeks old or 16 weeks old, either WT or mutant). Only in the condition on the far right (16 weeks old, Q84/Q84) are there visibly fewer oligodendrocytes.

The combined data show bar graphs of the results from the same experiment. Multiple animals have been included for each group, and the percentages of green cells are plotted on the *y*-axis. Data from each animal are represented as shapes. The group data confirm what was observed in the representative data: the Q84/Q84 mice at 16 weeks old have fewer oligodendrocytes. The Q84/WT mice, which are heterozygous for the mutation, only present an intermediate phenotype at 16 weeks.

The summary figure, from a different experiment again, presents a schematic diagram outlining a proposed hypothesis from a Parkinson's disease experiment. In this example, researchers argue that cells of the substantia nigra are vulnerable to loss in Parkinson's disease because of three key factors: DA handling and release, axonal trafficking, and pacemaking.

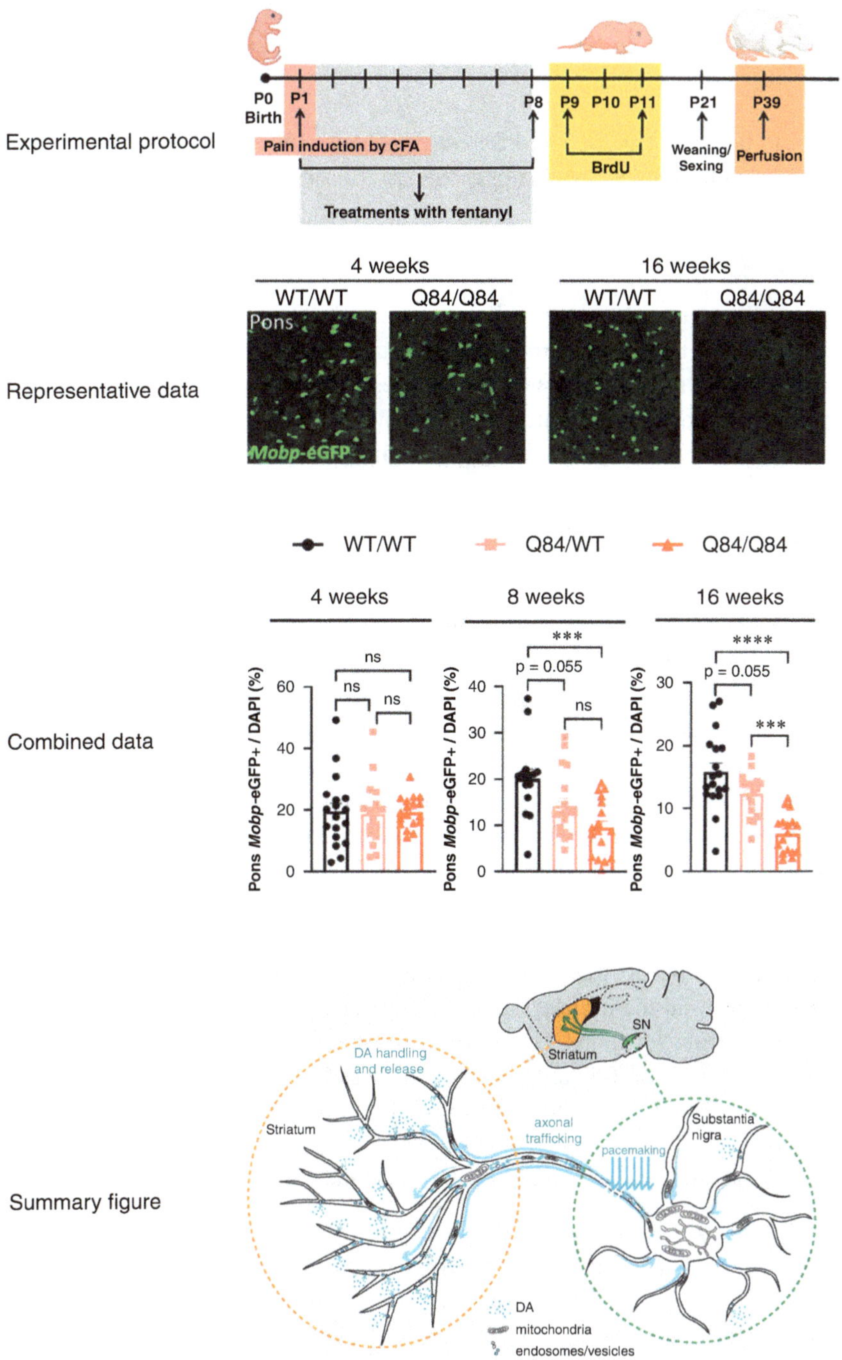

Figure 1.1 Examples of commonly occurring figure types. Sources: Rêgo DSB, Silva CS, Mello LEAM, Leslie ATFS. Early life nociceptive stimulus and fentanyl exposure increase hippocampal neurogenesis and anxiety but do not affect spatial learning and memory. *Front Neurosci.* 2022; 16:988096. Schuster KH, DiFranco DM, Putka AF, Mato JP, Jarrah SI, Stec NR, Sundararajan VO, McLoughlin HS. Disease-associated oligodendrocyte signatures are spatiotemporally dysregulated in spinocerebellar ataxia type 3. *Front Neurosci.* 2023; 17:1118429. Zampese E, Surmeier DJ. Calcium, bioenergetics, and Parkinson's disease. *Cells.* 2020; 9:2045. http://creativecommons.org/licenses/by/4.0/. Figures cropped and rearranged.

1.2 Study Designs

Research can be done using many different possible study designs. Most study designs in neuroscience are divided into two major categories: **observational studies** and **experiments**.

1.2.1 Observational Studies

Observational studies are reports where the manipulation, exposure, or treatment has not been assigned by the researcher. These studies are often cheaper and simpler to conduct than experiments, and they involve less interference from a third-party influence and are therefore more naturalistic. Observational studies help to generate hypotheses and can prompt new questions. Many studies examining humans with diseases are observational.

A limitation of observational studies is that they can only demonstrate **correlation**, a relationship where one variable is *associated* with an outcome. They cannot show that the variable *caused* that outcome. There may be a "which comes first" or "chicken-or-the-egg" problem in observational studies. For example, consider a study examining the brain volumes of people with alcohol use disorder (AUD). Observational studies cannot determine if alcohol exposure leads to changes in brain volume, or if differences in brain volume make someone more likely to develop AUD.

Another weakness of observational study design is the possibility of **confounding variables**: unexpected variables that explain both the exposure and the outcome. In the study of brain volume and AUD, it may be possible that adverse childhood experiences, such as famine or war, cause both a decrease in brain volume and an increase in AUD likelihood. In this case, the effect of the confounding variable – early adverse experiences – may not be addressed in the study.

Observational studies are limited in scope due to ethical and practical reasons. Thinking again about the brain volume–AUD study, it would be unethical to randomly assign some people to an AUD group and force them to drink. Instead, it is only acceptable to recruit participants who have already been diagnosed with AUD and others who have not, and then perform observations of their brain volumes for comparison.

Observational studies can be further subdivided into study types.

1. **Case studies** (or **case reports**) are in-depth, thorough explanations of a clinically notable person or a very small group of patients. Typically, the interesting features of a case study are described in text, and many case studies only show a couple representative figures (if even). When they are presented, figures may include structural imaging scans of rare head injuries or **congenital** (meaning "present since birth") abnormalities, or maybe images of cells with unusual pathology. The major limitation of case studies is they often have poor generalizability since the circumstances leading to some outcome of interest may never happen again.

2. **Case–control studies** are used to compare people with some outcome of interest (cases) and those without (controls). In doing so, these studies look to discover risk factors that may have led to the outcome or are protective against the outcome. For example, consider cases with an Alzheimer's disease diagnosis. A study might look to see if occupational exposure to pesticides increases risk or if regular coffee consumption decreases risk. Case–control studies are all **retrospective**, meaning they are looking backwards from the diagnosis.
3. **Cohort studies** are similar, except the researchers separate the population based on exposure first, and then look to the outcomes. In the example above regarding Alzheimer's disease diagnosis, a related cohort study might recruit several people who work with pesticides, then see how many of them develop the diagnosis. Cohort studies may either be retrospective or **prospective**, which is when a group is followed beyond the beginning of the study to determine their outcomes.

Case–control and cohort studies often contain more tables than figures, but sometimes these studies plot their results in a Kaplan–Meier survival curve (which we will cover in Section 2.7).

1.2.2 Experiments

Experiments are studies where the researcher assigns the treatments or manipulations. An experiment might see two groups of genetically identical mice randomly assigned to receive a brain injury or not, and then see how well they perform on a balance task. Alternatively, human participants might be given either a drug or a placebo and then placed into an fMRI scanner.

In the clinical setting, the main type of experimental design is the **randomized controlled trial (RCT)**. Here, the population of participants is divided and randomly assigned to groups that are treated differently, and the comparisons are made between data collected from the groups. For example, an RCT might have a population of patients with a diagnosis of depression. One half, selected at random, will be given transcranial electrical stimulation, while the other half will be exposed to the same apparatus but without the stimulation.

Experiments are the gold standard in science. Through testing hypotheses, they can establish **causation**, the relationship where some variable leads to an outcome.

Additional Resources

Dupépé EB, Kicielinski KP, Gordon AS, Walters BC. What is a case–control study? *Neurosurg*. 2019 Apr; 84(4):819–826. DOI: 10.1093/neuros/nyy590.

1.3 Comparing Group Data

One of the main objectives in a research study is to make comparisons. A comparison between two different populations is a **between-subject design**, where the research question can be distilled down to "does one group differ from another?" A between-subject research question might ask "Do stressed rats have a greater amount of kainate receptor protein?" In this question, the groups being compared are the stressed rats versus the nonstressed rats. In another experiment asking "Do benzodiazepines decrease the duration of REM sleep?", groups being compared would be those taking benzodiazepines versus those not taking the drug.

To make a valid comparison between groups, the subjects or patients should be treated as similarly as possible. This way, any difference between the groups can be attributed to the **experimental manipulation**, the main question of interest (such as stress exposure or drug administration). **Control experiments** must be performed, and the data collected from these control groups serve as the comparison for the data from the experimental group. The reason why control experiments are performed is not usually explained explicitly in the figures, so identifying the control condition is an important step in understanding the results. Using the correct control experiments eliminates or minimizes the influence of confounding variables.

There are many different types of controls that can be performed; here is an overview of some of them.

- A **matched sample** is a population of people who are like the experimental group based on several characteristics, such as demographics. For example, in a study about Alzheimer's disease, an age-related neurodegenerative condition, control participants should be of a similar age to the experimental group to eliminate the effect of healthy aging as a confounding variable.
- A **placebo** is an inert treatment that resembles the experimental treatment without containing the active ingredient. Typically, "placebo" refers to its use in the human literature. A placebo might be a pill made from inert material such as starch. In the REM sleep study described above, for example, one group of patients may receive a benzodiazepine (experimental group) while the other patients receive the placebo (control group).
- Inert control injections are used to control for the effect of the process of injection, which can be inherently stressful and painful. **Saline** is the 0.9% sodium chloride (NaCl) solution that matches the osmolarity of mammalian blood. Saline is often used as an injection control solution. For example, if the researcher is curious about the effect of cocaine on rat movement, the experimental group might receive an injection of cocaine dissolved in saline, while the control group receives an injection of saline alone. This way, both animals are subjected to the injection process and are therefore equally stressed when the movement test is performed.

  Other injection control solutions include **Ringer's solution**, which contains other salts, sugars, and is pH balanced at 7.3 to 7.4, and **DMSO**, which is used when the substance being injected is lipophilic and does not dissolve readily in water.
- **Sham surgery** is a surgery that mimics all the steps of a surgery without the experimental manipulation. For example, imagine we are looking to model neuropathic pain in rats. To do this, we may need to anesthetize the animal to perform an operation. However, this process introduces additional manipulations, such as an effect of anesthesia and the tissue

inflammation produced by the surgery, both of which might influence pain sensation after recovery. A sham surgery controls for these confounding variables, since both groups are exposed to all of the steps of the surgery. Sham surgeries are only done in nonhumans.

- **Wild type (WT)** animals are those that have not been genetically modified. For example, consider if you wanted to examine the role of the TRPV1 receptor. You could compare a genetically modified mouse, one that is lacking the TRPV1 receptor, with a wild type mouse and see how each behaves differently.

All of these examples are **negative controls**, meaning that they are expected to show no difference from the natural state.

Another experimental design that allows comparisons is the **within-subject design**. The difference is the tested population: a within-subject design uses the participant or subject as their own baseline for comparison. In this design, the research question is summarized by "how does an observation change before and after the manipulation?" For example, an experiment using a within-subject design might answer "How does the firing rate of a neuron change after application of a chemical?" or "How does a mouse change their social behavior after exposure to MDMA?"

Keep in mind that the same question can be addressed using either a between- or a within-subject design. For example, consider the question "do benzodiazepines decrease the duration of REM sleep?" A between-subject design would give one group the drug while the other gets the placebo, and both groups would then undergo REM sleep analysis. A within-subject design would give participants the placebo on the first night and the benzodiazepine on the second night, and would perform the REM sleep analysis on both nights. (A well-designed experiment would **counterbalance** the design: a different group of participants would receive the benzodiazepine on the first night, then the placebo on the second.)

Another important type of comparison is a **reversal of effect experiment**. In these experiments, some manipulation produces a predictable response, but that observation is not the main question of interest. Instead, the researchers care more about a further manipulation that blocks or enhances that effect. These experiments are great for understanding mechanisms. For example, it is well described that morphine decreases pain. A reversal of effect experiment might investigate whether coadministration of morphine with an opioid receptor antagonist would show a reversal of effect, hinting at the mechanism through which morphine acts.

Reversal of effect experiments are also good for demonstrating **return to baseline**, a control experiment that eliminates the influence of the variable associated with time, giving clues as to how long an effect lasts.

Figure 1.2: The *y*-axis plots changes in neuron firing rate in rats following exposure to different chemicals. The main observation is that toluene increases the firing rate in a dose-dependent manner – the higher the concentration, the greater the increase (gray bars). A question of interest is: what is the mechanism that leads to the increase? The graph shows that the increase does not depend on certain neurotransmitter systems, as they are not inhibited by the cocktail of antagonists M+A+C+B (red bars). However, adding quinine to that blend

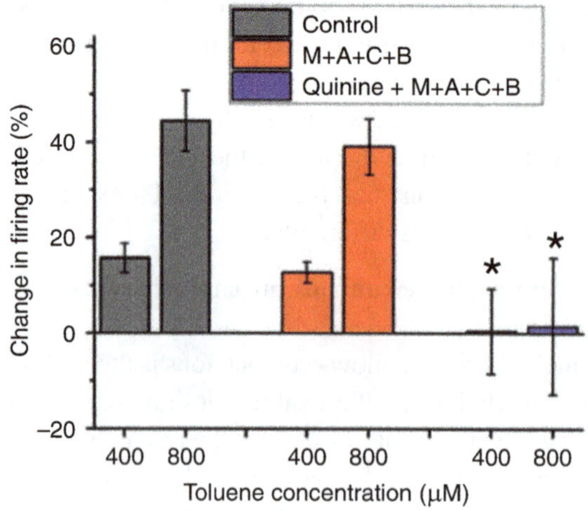

Figure 1.2 A reversal of drug effect experiment. Source: Nimitvilai S, You C, Arora DS, McElvain MA, Vandegrift BJ, Brodie MS, Woodward JJ. Differential effects of toluene and ethanol on dopaminergic neurons of the ventral tegmental area. *Front Neurosci.* 2016; 10:434. https://creativecommons.org/licenses/by/4.0/. Image cropped.

blocks the increase in excitation (blue bars), suggesting that the increase is mediated by quinine's targets. In this experiment, the quinine data show a reversal of effect.

Figure 1.3 is an example of a return to baseline study, with three representative images (left) and group data (right). Here, the time course of a manipulation is illustrated. A mouse was injected with the neuroinflammatory agent LPS, and cell counting analysis was performed at two time points: 24 hours after injection (middle representative image) and 72 hours after (bottom representative image). Cells shown in red are microglia, and increase only at 24 hours after exposure, but not at 72 hours after.

1.4 Variables

In research, variables are characteristics that can be measured. A key element of the scientific method is making careful observations of the variables. There are several types of variables.

1.4.1 Variable Types

- A **categorical variable** is one where the value falls into a category rather than a specific value. For example, a history of schizophrenia diagnosis is a categorical variable, since a person will either have been diagnosed or not. Another categorical variable is whether the shape of a dendritic spine is long and thin, short and stubby, mushroom-shaped, or two-pronged. A common categorical variable in both experimental studies and randomized clinical trials is whether the group received a drug or not.

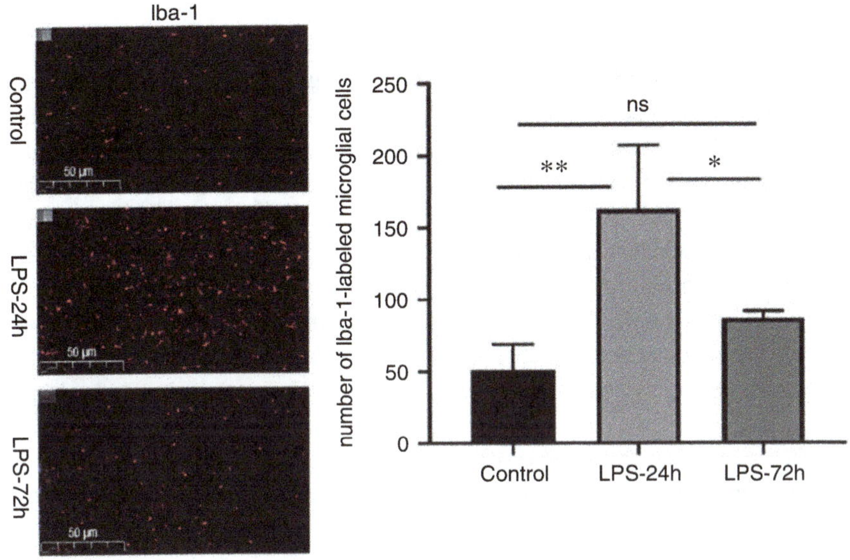

Figure 1.3 A return to baseline experiment. Source: Qiu T, Guo J, Wang L, Shi L, Ai M, Xia Z, Peng Z, Kuang L. Dynamic microglial activation is associated with LPS-induced depressive-like behavior in mice: An [18F] DPA-714 PET imaging study. *Bosn J Basic Med Sci.* 2022 Jul 29; 22(4):649–659. www.bjbms.org/ojs/index.php/bjbms/article/view/6825. Image cropped and panels rearranged.

A categorical variable that can take only one of two states is called a **binary** (or **dichotomous) variable**. Binary variables are essentially "yes" or "no." In addition to the schizophrenia diagnosis example above, other binary variables include whether or not cells in a culture dish were exposed to a chemical, or if exposure to a flash of light does or does not cause a silent neuron to fire an action potential.

- A **numerical variable** is one where a number value can be assigned to the variable. Numerical variables can either be discrete or continuous.
    - **Discrete variables** are "counted" values and are reported as whole numbers (integers). Some examples of discrete variables in neuroscience research include the number of times an animal presses a lever to receive a juice reward, how many action potentials are observed in response to a depolarizing step, or how many neurons express a specific receptor in a brain area.
    - **Continuous variables** are "measured" values, and the values may fall in between two integers (contain a decimal). For example, it is possible to record that a neuron's membrane potential depolarizes by 7.431 millivolts in response to a certain drug, or that a rat spends 133.2 seconds grooming itself.

  Because mathematical operations on continuous numerical variables are meaningful, many dependent variables in neuroscience studies will be reported as numerical continuous variables.

1.4.2 Variables in Research

- The **independent variable** is an element that is being manipulated in the experiment or that changes independently of the experiment. An independent variable might be manipulated by the researcher: for example, the concentration of a chemical that is washed on top of a cell culture, or the intensity of light that is shone into a person's eye. Independent variables may also be characteristics that change on their own, such as time. On a graph, independent variables are usually shown on the x-axis. Because there is no manipulation in observational studies, they do not have independent variables.
- The **dependent variable** is the outcomes that are measured. Dependent variables are essentially the data that are collected by the experimental technique. Dependent variables related to the examples above might be how many action potentials are fired in the cell culture in response to the chemical wash, or how much the pupil constricts in response to the light. On graphs, dependent variables are usually plotted on the y-axis.
- **Confounding variables** are additional factors that may influence the values of the dependent variables. These are present in both observational and experimental studies. They are not explicitly part of the hypothesis. For example, high emotional states and medications both affect baseline pupil diameter, and would be considered confounds for the pupil constriction experiment. Good control experiments eliminate or minimize the influence of confounding variables. A within-subject design tends to introduce fewer confounding variables than a between-subject design, since each participant serves as their own control.
- **Constant variables** are features of the experiment that are left unchanged during the experiment. Variables held constant are generally assumed and are not usually discussed in the reporting of the research.

Additional Resources

Vetter TR. Fundamentals of research data and variables: The devil is in the details. *Anesthesia & Analgesia*. 2017 Oct; 125(4):1375–1380. DOI: 10.1213/ANE.0000000000002370.

1.5 Statistics

In the context of research, statistics refers to tools and techniques used to analyze data. There is tremendous nuance in the application of statistics, and this textbook only provides a broad overview of the statistics that are commonly used in the description of neuroscience data.

1.5.1 Central Tendency (Averages)

The most common method to compare numerical data between groups is to compare averages. An **average** is any numerical measure of central tendency. The average measures most often used in neuroscience are the arithmetic mean and the median. Averages are often shown in graphs that present combined data.

The **arithmetic mean** (or just **mean**) is the sum of all data points divided by the number of data points. While using the word "average" to denote arithmetic mean is technically correct, it is not fully descriptive, akin to someone saying "I love my animal" instead of "I love my dog."

The **median** is the middle value of the data set when it is arranged in rank order – that is, from lowest to highest. In a data set with an even number of points, the median is the mean of the two in the middle of the rank order.

1.5.2 Dispersion and Uncertainty

Dispersion refers to how spread apart the data points are distributed. For example, consider two data sets, both with a mean and median of around 4.5.

A: [2, 3, 4.2, 4, 4.5, 5, 5.5, 5.8, 6, 7]
B: [0.5, 1.3, 1.6, 1, 4.5, 5, 6, 8, 9, 10.1]

The data points in set A are closer to 5, so we say it has less dispersion.

In Figure 1.4 the data from sets A and B are plotted on the *y*-axis, with each data point represented as a red dot. Both data sets have the same mean (4.7) and median (4.75), but they have very different dispersions: data A are more tightly clustered, while data B are more widely distributed.

Uncertainty exists because of fluctuations among what is being measured. These fluctuations may be due to natural biological variability that cannot be predicted based on the measurement tools. For example, if you were to measure how much a rat moves around in an open space (which we'll discuss further in Section 2.2.1), different rats will naturally react to their surroundings differently: some explore out of curiosity, while others hide in the corner out of fear. In another experiment, imagine you are measuring the resting membrane potentials of several neurons using whole cell patch clamp electrophysiology (discussed in Section 6.2.1). There are factors that affect membrane potential, such as Na^+/K^+ pump ATP-ase function and spontaneous neurotransmitter release, which are not considered in taking these measurements.

Uncertainty also happens when the measurement tools are incapable of getting accurate results. For example, one way to observe rat movement is to divide the space into a grid of infrared beams, detecting when those beams are interrupted. The grid can only precisely measure rat position on the order of centimeters, so movements smaller than that are not detected. As another example, when measuring resting membrane potential the equipment cannot detect changes in membrane potentials smaller than hundredths of millivolts because of outside electrical interference.

Both dispersion and uncertainty may be represented in figures, often as **error bars**, which are lines or areas that extend above and below group average data. Measurements of dispersion or uncertainty include the following:

- **Interquartile range (IQR)** is the range within which 50% of all data points fall. If all data points are arranged in rank order (lowest to highest) and then divided into four

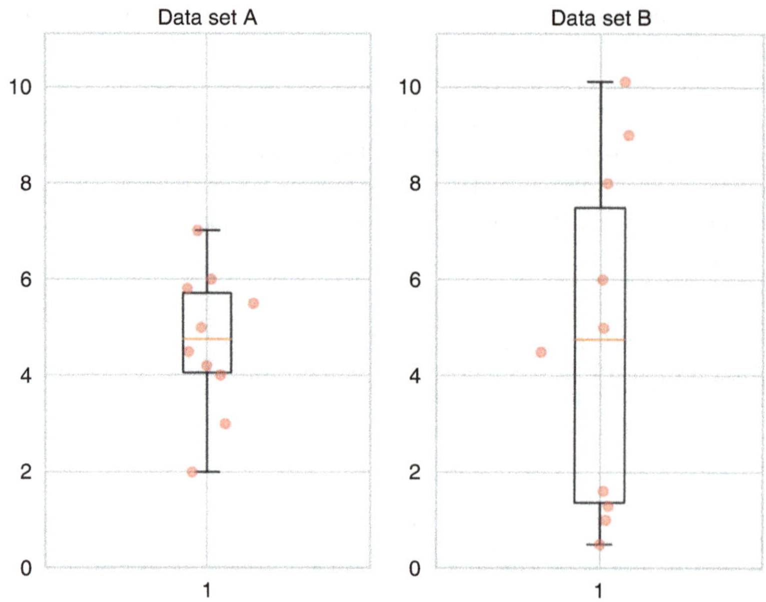

Figure 1.4 The dispersions of data sets A and B

groups (**quartiles**), the IQR represents the two groups in the middle. A larger IQR indicates that the data are more spread apart.

- **Standard deviation** (**SD**) refers roughly to how widely distributed the data of the sample are. A small SD means the data are clustered around the average closely; a large SD means the data are farther spread apart. SDs are used in descriptive statistics. For example, SD may be reported when looking at the volumes of thalamus as measured by a new imaging method, or when summarizing the concentration of cortisol in the blood for a specific clinical population. SD is not appropriate for making comparisons between groups, so many experiments of that type will report a different measure of uncertainty.
- **Standard error of the mean** (**SEM**, or **SE**) is also a measure of how spread apart or clustered together the data are. The formula to calculate the SEM considers sample size, so the SEM allows for generalization to the whole population which is being sampled. As with SD, a small SEM indicates close clustering around the mean, while a large SEM means a wide distribution of points. Most experimental studies in neuroscience report the SEM.
- **95% confidence intervals** (**CI**) are values above and below the sample mean. If the sample mean is collected several times, 95% of the time the true population mean will be contained within that range. The other way to think about the 95% confidence interval is that it corresponds to the data that fall within 1.96 standard errors from the average. Reports of CI are more common among large-population epidemiological data (e.g.

studying the risk of mortality from multiple sclerosis) or in randomized clinical trials (e.g. studying how well a new drug can decrease symptoms of multiple sclerosis).

In written data, an uncertainty measure is sometimes written after the average in parentheses. For example, if a table reports 23.7 (1.8), the data had an average of 23.7 and an uncertainty of 1.8.

In the study represented in Figure 1.5, researchers were curious as to whether an additional spinal surgery on an adult human was more likely to be performed depending on the location of the first surgery, either anterior or posterior. The solid and dotted lines plot the number of follow-up surgeries for both groups and the shaded regions indicate the 95% confidence intervals, with the dark shading corresponding to anterior surgery and the light shading to posterior surgery. In this study, there was a large overlap between the 95% confidence intervals, suggesting no difference in the risk of additional surgery between the two groups.

Additional Resources

Cumming G, Fidler F, Vaux DL. Error bars in experimental biology. *J Cell Biol.* 2007 Apr 9; 177(1):7–11.

O'Brien SF, Yi QL. How do I interpret a confidence interval? *Transfusion.* 2016 Jul; 56(7):1680–1683.

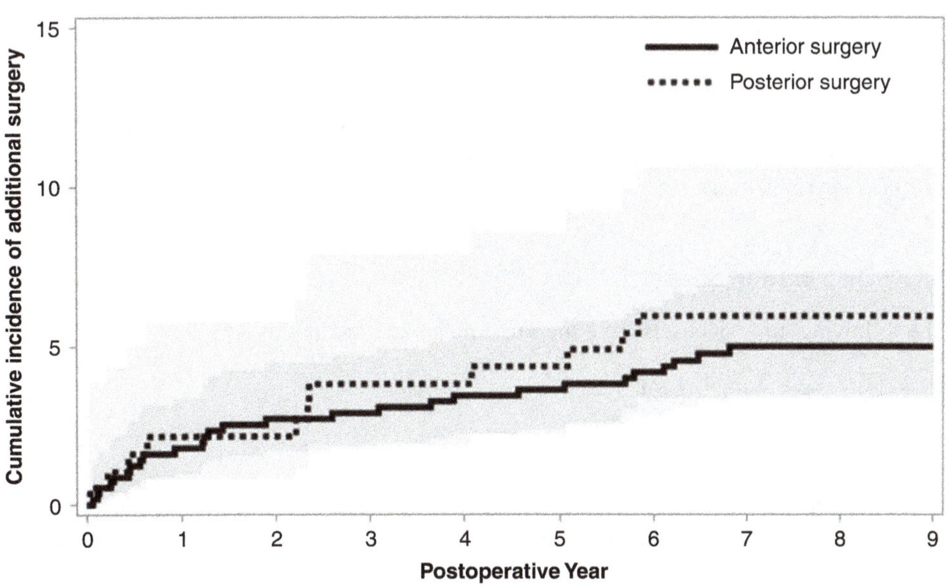

Figure 1.5 Plot of 95% confidence intervals. Source: Yuh WT, Kim M, Choi Y, et al. Nationwide sample data analysis of additional surgery rate after anterior or posterior cervical spinal surgery. *Sci Rep.* 2023; 13:6317.

1.5.3 Outliers

Some data points may be extremely high or low with respect to the other data. These are called **outliers**. Outliers may be mistakes made during measurement due to human or machine error; these should always be excluded from analysis. On the other hand, outliers may also be meaningful biological observations. Whether or not these outliers are excluded from analysis will vary on a case-by-case basis. If outliers are excluded, the rationale should be explained.

Generally, a data point is considered an outlier if it is outside some amount of uncertainty above or below the average. Some common exclusion criteria include:

- Observations that are 1.5 times the interquartile range above the third quartile and below the first quartile. These data points are called **fences**.
- Observations that fall 3 standard deviations above or below the mean, which can be measured by calculating the ***z*-score** for each data point (the *z*-score is simply the number of standard deviations that data point is away from the mean). These measures are only applicable for normally distributed data (described in Section 1.5.4).

The mean is more sensitive to the influence of outliers compared to the median. Consider this data set:

A: [1, 1, 1, 1, 2, 2, 2, 2, 2, 86]

The mean is 10, while the median is 2. The median value of 2 is more representative of the data set as a whole.

Additional Resources

Gress TW, Denvir J, Shapiro JI. Effect of removing outliers on statistical inference: Implications to interpretation of experimental data in medical research. *Marshall J Med.* 2018; 4(2):9.

1.5.4 Distribution Shapes

The following three data sets have the same mean and median of 3:

A: [1, 2, 2, 3, 3, 3, 4, 4, 5]
B: [1, 2, 2, 2, 3, 4, 4, 4, 5]
C: [0, 0, 0, 0, 3, 3, 3, 8, 10]

But it is clear that the data sets have very different distributions. One way to see the distribution of data is to build a **histogram**, a graph that plots ranges of dependent variable measurements on the *x*-axis and number of observations on the *y*-axis.

Distributions of data may have the appearance of one of the following:

- **Normal distributions** are when the data fall onto a **bell curve**, with most data points being centered around the average, and fewer data points as you look farther away from the average. For example, intelligence quotient scores fall on a normal distribution. Normal distributions are symmetric above and below the middle, and may have different degrees of **variance**, which is a measure of how "wide" the bell curve is around its peak. Statistical tests such as Shapiro–Wilk or Kolmogorov–Smirnov tests are used to identify whether a distribution is normal or nonnormal.
- **Bimodal distributions** have data points that center around two points rather than one (a normal distribution is unimodal). A bimodal distribution may suggest that the sample is actually made up of two distinct populations. For example, the distribution of height across a human population is usually a bimodal distribution, with men typically being taller than women. Although there are women who are much taller than most men, and men who are much shorter than most women, these people's heights are on ends of the bell curve for their sex.
- While a bimodal distribution has two peaks, a **multimodal distribution** has several peaks that appear in the histogram. An example of a multimodal distribution is the observation of quantal release of neurotransmitter, where each individual vesicle contains a similar amount of neurotransmitter, and release of neurotransmitter happens one vesicle at a time.
- **Skewed distributions** have data points unevenly distributed around the center. If more points fall to the right of the peak, this may be called a **rightward skew** or a **right tail**. Likewise, having more data points to the left is a **leftward skew** or a **left tail**.
- **Uniform distributions** have an equal likelihood of any given measurement, which will appear flat on a histogram. Uniform distributions are rarely seen in biological data.

Histograms, such as the graphs shown in Figure 1.6, plot number of observations on the y-axis and ranges of measurements on the x-axis. They are useful for illustrating differences in data distribution. On the left are data points from a normal distribution, where most observations fall around a central measure. As the dependent variable becomes larger or smaller, there are fewer observations. In the middle is a bimodal distribution, where observations cluster around two distinct measurements. On the right is a leftward skew, where there are many observations with large values and fewer at small values.

1.5.5 Differences between Groups

Statistical tests are performed on the data to determine whether the group averages differ meaningfully. The results of these tests are a ***p*-value**. Many different statistical tests will produce a p-value. The p-value is a number from 0 to 1, and the lower the p-value, the more confidently you can say there is a meaningful difference between the group averages. When p is less than 0.05, we say the difference is **statistically significant**. Although this cutoff is entirely arbitrary, it is generally accepted in biomedical research.

P-values on figures are often denoted by asterisk symbols. By standard convention, most research will use the following code for presenting statistical significance:

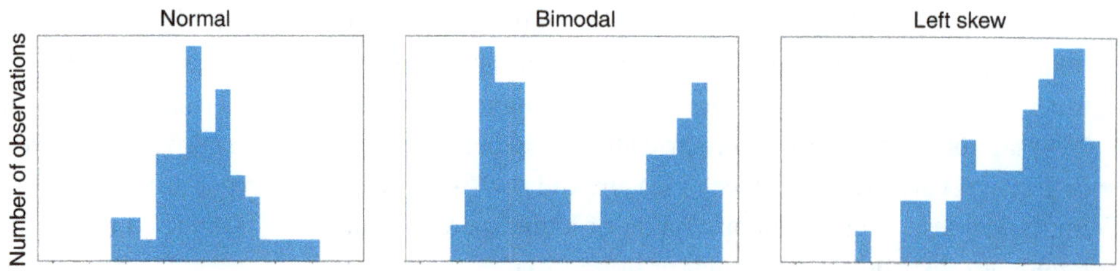

Figure 1.6 Histograms showing different distribution patterns

* *p*-value is between 0.01 and 0.05
** *p*-value is between 0.001 and 0.01
*** *p*-value is between 0.0001 and 0.001

One general exception to the ranges of *p*-values is when very large sets of data are collected, such as in fMRI data or in population genetics research. The larger the data set, the more likely a statistically significant difference will appear, even though none actually exists. These are called false positives, or **type I errors**. To minimize these errors, it is common for one asterisk to indicate a much lower *p*-value in these types of experiments.

Different types of statistical tests are used depending on the type of data collected.

- **Parametric tests** are those that can be used when the data fall along a normal distribution. Parametric tests include t-tests and analysis of variance (ANOVA).
- **Nonparametric tests** are used when data fall along a nonnormal distribution. Nonparametric tests are considered less powerful than parametric tests, offering less confidence in the conclusions. Common nonparametric tests include Mann–Whitney or Kruskal–Wallace tests.
- **Linear regressions** are used when the variables are not classified into groups but exist on a range or spectrum. These are used to look for associations between two continuous variables. For example, researchers might want to know how strongly the amount of a certain protein in the cerebrospinal fluid (CSF) is associated with the volume of the frontal cortex.

1.5.6 Effect Strength

Even if the distribution of data points is statistically different between two groups, it is possible for that difference to be tiny. The magnitude of an effect is calculated using statistical tests such as Cohen's d or Hedges' g.

Cohen's d is the difference between means of groups expressed in standard deviations. Values technically range from 0 to positive infinity, but typically values will fall between 0.2 and 1, and rarely go up to 5. The larger the Cohen's d value, the stronger the observed effect. Cohen's d is appropriate for larger sample sizes (*n* greater than 20).

Hedges' g is a similar measure, except it is more accurate at small sample sizes (n smaller than 20). Hedges' g is interpreted just like Cohen's d: larger Hedges' g values indicate a greater difference between group means.

As a rough guideline for interpreting statistical values of effect strength:

Less than 0.2 = no effect
Between 0.2 and 0.5 = weak effect
Between 0.5 and 0.8 = moderate effect
Higher than 0.8 = strong effect

In linear regressions, the **correlation coefficient**, or ***r*-value**, is a measure of the strength of the correlation between the two variables. R-values fall between −1 and 1, and larger absolute values indicate a stronger correlation.

Cohen's d, Hedges' g, and r-values must be interpreted with respect to the outcome being measured. For example, a new drug treatment that offers even a tiny decrease in the number of human deaths is very impactful.

1.6 Graph Types

There are several ways that group data can be represented graphically. Each of the four types of data visualization graphs described in Sections 1.6.1–1.6.4 provides more information than the previous type of graph.

1.6.1 Bar Graphs

Bar graphs represent data as solid blocks with their bases at zero. The tops of the bars often represent some numerical value, such as averages or counts in a histogram. Colors may be used to indicate different groups. Usually, bar graph data are presented as vertical bars, with different groups across the x-axis. Horizontal bar plots may also be used, with the dependent variables along the x-axis. These are more common when data from several groups are being compared, such as when quantifying the amount of a protein across 25 different brain areas.

Error bars extend above and below the average value; smaller error bars indicate that the data are more tightly clustered around the average. Error bars not overlapping is not a guarantee that the group averages are significantly different. Significance differences between groups are often denoted with an * symbol along with the accompanying p-value.

One of the shortcomings of bar graphs is that they only show two pieces of information: the average and the uncertainty. They also mask the distribution of the data. Different distributions can produce the same bar graph. This limitation can be overcome by plotting individual data points alongside or on top of the bar graph.

1.6.2 Boxplots

Boxplots (or **box and whiskers plots**) represent data using free-floating boxes with lines that extend from the tops and bottoms of each box (whiskers). The box is divided by a line that indicates the average. The borders of the box represent the **upper** and **lower quartiles**, meaning that the highest 25% of points are greater than the upper edge of the box, while the lowest 25% are smaller than the lower edge of the box. The span of the box is the interquartile range (IQR, discussed in Section 1.5.2); 50% of all data points fall within the area of the box. The extent of the whiskers is the range of the data set. Data that fall outside of the whiskers are outliers, and these may be shown as individual points.

Box and whiskers plots provide hints about data distribution. A right skew will have a taller section above the middle of the graph and a longer upper whisker, while a left skew will have a taller section below the middle of the graph and a longer lower whisker. A bimodal distribution will have a large box with short whiskers.

However, different data sets can still produce the same bar graph. Multimodal data can look similar to a normal distribution, for example. As with the bar graph, a good way to overcome this limitation is to present individual data points alongside or overlaying the boxplot.

1.6.3 Violin Plots

Violin plots show all the statistical information of the boxplot (average, range, and interquartile range) along with a **kernel density plot**, which considers some degree of variance and predicts how likely it is that a data point will fall along a distribution. The thicker the "violin" at a certain value, the more likely the data point is to fall in that value. Most of the time, the violins are symmetrical, but a **split violin plot** might be used to compare two closely related variables within an experimental group, such as animal sex or age group.

As an advantage, violin plots are able to represent the distributions of data more meaningfully than boxplots, since data sets with multimodal distributions will be evident in a violin plot.

1.6.4 Raincloud Plots

A **raincloud plot** is essentially a violin plot with individual data points plotted below (the kernel distribution is the cloud, while the data points are the falling raindrops). Raincloud plots are the most complete representation of the data because they can meaningfully represent data maxima and minima and nonstandard distributions, which other plots may not be able to do.

Figure 1.7 shows a bar graph (left), a boxplot (middle), and a violin plot (right) of the same set of data, as below:

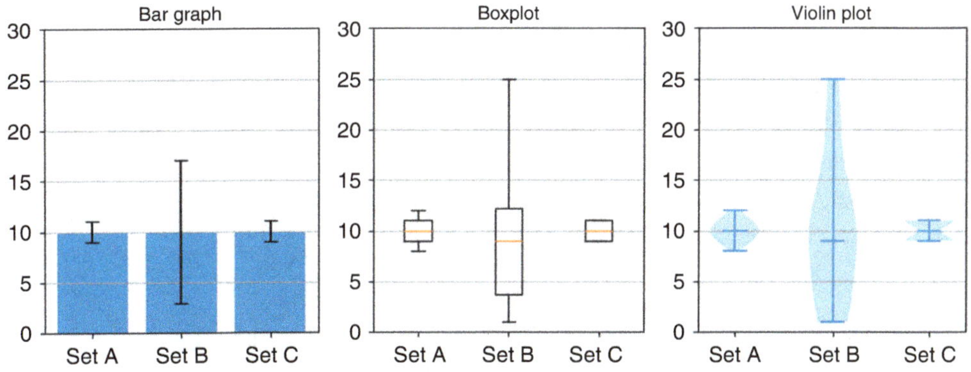

Figure 1.7 Three types of graphs that plot the same data set

Set A: [8, 9, 9, 9, 9, 10, 10, 10, 10, 10, 10, 11, 11, 11, 11, 12]
Set B: [1, 2, 2, 3, 4, 9, 9, 9, 9, 10, 12, 12, 13, 18, 22, 25]
Set C: [9, 9, 9, 9, 9, 9, 9, 9, 11, 11, 11, 11, 11, 11, 11, 11]

All three data sets have the same mean of 10. A bar graph shows differences in dispersion, as sets A and C have small standard deviations and therefore error bars of similar length. The bar graph does not show range information, whereas both boxplots and violin plots can tell us both the maximum and minimum values of the data set. Sets A and C have different distributions, and the violin plot shows these differences: set A has normally distributed data (a convex-shaped violin) while set C has characteristics of a bimodal distribution (a concave-shaped violin).

Figure 1.8 shows raincloud plots for two different data sets (groups 1 and 2), with a half violin plot (filled-in curve) and individual data points.

1.6.5 Scatterplots and Lines of Best Fit

While the four types of graphs described above are useful for visualizing comparisons between groups of data, sometimes it is useful to compare two continuous variables to look for correlations. These data are often presented in a **scatterplot** and analyzed statistically with a linear regression which produces a **line of best fit**.

In scatterplots, the closer the data points are to the line of best fit, the more strongly the two variables are correlated (the greater the absolute value of the r-value). Another meaningful observation of the scatterplot is the slope of the correlation: a positive slope suggests the two are correlated together (positive r-values), while a negative slope suggests an inverse relationship (negative r-values).

In Figure 1.9, three scatterplots show the relationship between two variables, as well as a line of best fit (orange) produced by a linear regression. In the left graph, the values of the variables rise with each other and are close to the line of best fit, so this shows a strong positive correlation ($r = 0.93$). In the middle graph, values do not very obviously rise with

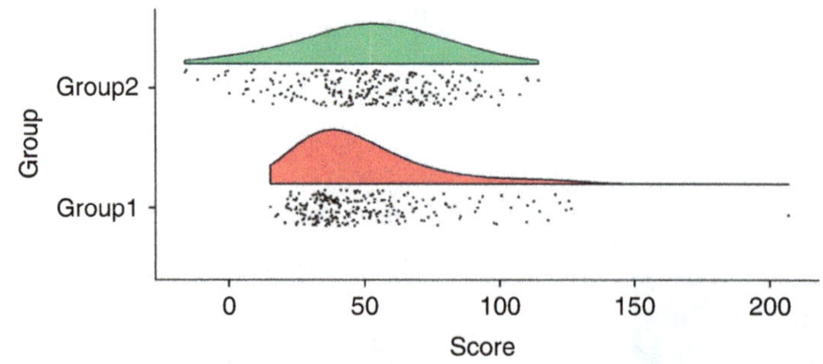

Figure 1.8 Raincloud plots. Source: Allen M, Poggiali D, Whitaker K, Marshall TR, Kievit RA. Raincloud plots: A multi-platform tool for robust data visualization. *Wellcome Open Res.* 2019 Apr 1; 4:63. https://creativecommons.org/licenses/by/4.0/. Image cropped.

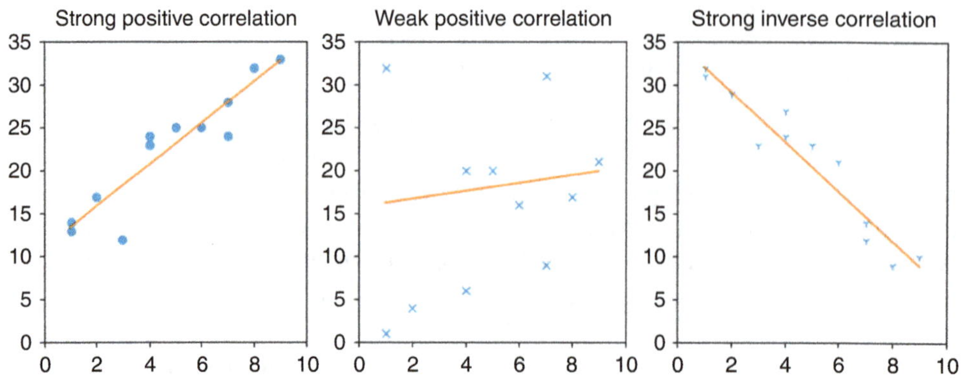

Figure 1.9 Three scatterplots showing lines of best fit

one another; data points may be far from the line of best fit ($r = 0.01$). In the right graph, the values are strongly anticorrelated, and one variable rises as the other variable falls ($r = -0.96$).

Additional Resources

Allen EA, Erhardt EB, Calhoun VD. Data visualization in the neurosciences: Overcoming the curse of dimensionality. *Neuron*. 2012 May 24; 74(4):603–608. DOI: 10.1016/j.neuron.2012.05.001. PMID: 22632718; PMCID: PMC4427844.

Allen M, Poggiali D, Whitaker K, Marshall TR, Kievit RA. Raincloud plots: A multi-platform tool for robust data visualization. *Wellcome Open Res*. 2019; 4:63. https://doi.org/10.12688/wellcomeopenres.15191.1.

Hu K. Become competent within one day in generating boxplots and violin plots for a novice without prior *R* experience. *Methods Protoc.* 2020; 3:64. https://doi.org/10.3390/mps3040064.

1.7 Understanding Graphs at a Glance

Because there are several techniques used to collect neuroscience data and even more ways to present that data, this book cannot possibly explain all of them. Instead, consider following this generic step-by-step guide to understanding graphs (such as those used to show combined data, rather than representative data) at a quick glance.

Step 1. Read the axes and units, starting with the *x*-axis.

On the *x*-axis, the independent variable is usually plotted. Much of the time, the different categorical variables that appear on the *x*-axis are populations or conditions. This is one of the more common ways to present data in a graph. For example, a graph might show two data sets, one from nicotine-exposed animals and the other from saline-exposed animals. Relatedly, it may show data from the same population at two different time points, such as before and after treatment with transcranial magnetic stimulation, for example.

If the *x*-axis plots a continuous variable, such as time, pay attention to the units that are being reported. Some phenomena, such as action potentials or synaptic release, take place on the order of milliseconds. Others, such as behavior or plasticity, happen over seconds or even days.

The *y*-axis usually plots the dependent variable, which are the measured results. Here, the units provide information needed for interpreting the data. Careful, however: if the *y*-axis plots number, check if the graph is a histogram.

Step 2. Identify the control condition.

Every good experiment will have control conditions. Some experiments may have several control experiments plotted on the same graph. Controls are what the experimental results are compared with. Common control labels include pre- (or before) treatment, healthy, placebo, saline, ACSF, sham, DMSO, or wild type (WT), although many other labels for control groups may be used.

First identify what groups are being compared, and which group is an experimental group versus a control group. Identify how the experimental group is treated differently from the control group. There may be several control groups to eliminate the influence of several variables, so make sure to understand these groups and the variables they control for. There may also be several experimental groups, each of which answers a specific research question or controls for a different variable. Identify the specific question that is being asked about each group.

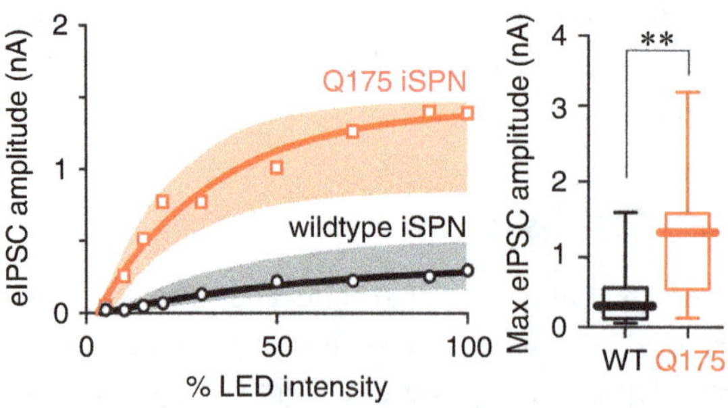

Figure 1.10 Putting it all together. Source: Lim SAO, Surmeier DJ. Enhanced GABAergic inhibition of cholinergic interneurons in the zQ175+/− mouse model of Huntington's disease. *Front Syst Neurosci.* 2021; 14:626412.

Step 3. Look for indicators of statistical significance.

The most common indicators are an asterisk with nearby text reporting the p-value. These are the comparisons the researchers want to highlight. Sometimes, when several groups are being compared, brackets will appear over some data sets to indicate that that comparison shows a statistically significant difference, while others may not. Data without asterisks are not found to have statistical significance and are called **negative data**.

Looking at Figure 1.10, we can put together the steps for reading a graph. Step 1: read the axes. The left figure plots % LED intensity on the x-axis, which suggests this is an optogenetics study. The y-axis shows the dependent variable that is being measured in the experiment, which is an evoked IPSC amplitude, a measure of synaptic connection. Step 2: identify the control condition. Here, wild type mice (black curve and bars) are the control comparison, so this must be a characterization of synaptic connections in a genetic mutant (Q175, red curve and bars). This is a between-groups comparison. Step 3: look for indicators of statistical significance. The box and whiskers graph (right figure) plots the maximum eIPSC amplitude for the wild type compared to the mutant, and two * symbols denote a statistical significance at $p < 0.01$. As for effect strength, the median of the wild type group is around 0.4 nA, while the median for the Q175 mutants is closer to 1.4 nA. The maximum is also greater among the Q175 mutants.

Summary

This chapter contains background information that will help in the interpretation of many different types of figures shown over the following chapters. Knowing what type of study is being described puts some context around the figures and some constraints on the interpretation of results. Understanding control conditions prepares you for comparisons that are made in observational and experimental neuroscience. The brief description of statistics provided here introduces key elements in studies where the main objective is to look for differences.

You inevitably will encounter a new graph type in your reading, and this is when the three-step approach described in Section 1.7, "Understanding Graphs at a Glance," can guide you through those data.

Equipped with this information, you are now prepared to learn about methods used in nonhuman behavioral neuroscience, the subject of Chapter 2.

Key Terms

- 95% confidence interval
- average
- bar graph
- bell curve
- between-subject design
- bimodal distribution
- binary variable
- box and whiskers plot
- boxplot
- case–control study
- case study
- categorial variable
- Cohen's d
- cohort study
- combined data figure
- confounding variable
- constant variable
- continuous variable
- control experiment
- correlation coefficient
- counterbalance
- data figure
- dependent variable
- discrete variable
- dispersion
- DMSO
- error bar
- experimental protocol figure
- experiment, experimental study
- false positive

- fence
- Hedges' g
- histogram
- independent variable
- interquartile range
- kernel density plot
- line of best fit
- linear regression
- matched sample
- mean
- median
- multimodal distribution
- negative control
- negative data
- nonparametric test
- normal distribution
- numerical variable
- observational study
- outlier
- panel
- parametric test
- placebo
- *p*-value
- quartile
- raincloud plot
- randomized control trial (RCT)
- representative data figure
- return to baseline experiment
- reversal of effect experiment
- Ringer's solution
- *r*-value
- saline
- scatterplot
- sham surgery
- skewed distribution
- standard deviation
- standard error of the mean
- statistical significance
- summary figure
- type I error

- uncertainty
- uniform distribution
- violin plot
- wild type (WT)
- within-subject design
- z-score

CHAPTER TWO

Nonhuman Behavioral Methods

2.1 Introduction to Nonhuman Behavioral Methods

Behavioral methods are experimental paradigms that measure what an animal does while interacting with other animals or with their surroundings. Humans can engage in extremely complex behaviors, such as creative storytelling and deception with the intent to harm others. However, this chapter will focus exclusively on studying behavior in nonhuman animals. Even among nonhumans, the range of behaviors is vast and varies tremendously in complexity. On the "simple" end of the spectrum, worms wriggle toward lithium but away from copper, and rats quickly and reflexively pull their paws away from something hot. On the more complex end, female fruit flies exhibit aggression toward pairs of mating fruit flies, and monkeys can learn to play Pac-Man, a video game with highly abstract goals.

The methods used in behavioral neuroscience are all at the macro end of the scale, examining the whole, intact organism as it does various actions. Because behavioral experiments are performed while the animal is alive, they are considered *in vivo* experiments.

Learning Objectives

By the end of this chapter, you will be able to:

- Identify some of the advantages and disadvantages of using different nonhuman species for studying behaviors
- Describe some methods used to observe and quantify nonhuman behavior
- Interpret the figures presented to show behavioral data

2.1.1 Animal Models in Neuroscience

While a wide variety of animals has been studied in the past, a few animal models remain as the standards accepted in the field. Even within a species, there may be behavioral differences based on **strain**, which is a subtype of species resulting from small phylogenetic differences. Some experimental models are **inbred** lines, where each animal is theoretically genetically identical to others; others are **outbred**, where individual animals are genetically unique from the others.

Below is a nonexclusive list of animal models that have been used in the past and present. Each has specific advantages that may make them ideal for studying different types of behaviors, and each also has disadvantages.

Invertebrates:

- Nematode (*Caenorhabitans elegans*, commonly called ***C. elegans*** or informally **worms**). In the lab, they live on petri plates (dishes) or in liquid solution, and are large enough (1 mm in length) to be imaged under a dissecting microscope. If a substance is added onto the petri dishes, this addition is called a **lawn**. The suite of behavioral tests performed are commonly measures of avoidance from, or attractance to, the lawn. Outside of behavior, *C. elegans* are also used to study nervous system development on a molecular level.
- Fruit fly (***Drosophila melanogaster***, just called **Drosophila** or informally **flies**). In the context of research on, for example, vision or decision making, researchers can present Drosophila with stimuli while observing changes in locomotor behavior. They can use these observations to quantify social behaviors such as mating and light-sensitivity. Outside of behavioral paradigms, Drosophila can also be useful for genetics research, studying the development of neural circuits, or electrophysiological activity *in vivo*.
- California sea hare (***Aplysia californica***, sometimes called a **sea slug**). Despite their relatively simple nervous systems, they are capable of learning behaviors such as the **gill withdrawal reflex**, where the animal retracts its gill when a different part of the body is touched. Observing this behavior was the basis for experimentally identifying plasticity at a cellular and molecular level. This animal model became popular in the 1960s, ultimately earning researchers a Nobel Prize in 2000, but they are not commonly used today.

Nonmammalian vertebrates:

- **Zebrafish** (*Danio rerio*). From hatching until about one week of age, zebrafish larvae bodies are completely transparent, which allows for easy visualization. A wide host of behavioral assays can be performed in research areas ranging from social interaction to cognitive impairment. Zebrafish can also be used for studying questions of the effects of toxin exposure on development.
- **Zebra finch** (*Taeniopygia guttata*). Early in life, this species of songbird acquires a language (**birdsong**) which is learned through their parents' vocalization. This learning process shares many traits in common with human speech acquisition, so these animals serve as a model for language learning.

Nonhuman mammals:

- Mouse (*Mus musculus*). The mouse is the most common nonhuman mammal studied in neuroscience research. The most popular strain is the **C57BL/6** mouse (pronounced "**C57 Black 6**," sometimes just called **C57** or **Black 6** mice). Other commonly used mice include the **BALB/c** strain and the **CD-1** stock ("strain" is used in reference to inbred lines; "**stock**" is used for outbred lines). Inbred strains may show decreased variability on behavioral testing compared to outbred lines. There are several genetically modified strains of mice available, which allow for studying the functions of different genes. These are often described as being on a specific **background**, such as when one part of the C57 genome is modified.
- Prairie vole (*Microtus ochrogaster*). Because these voles are socially monogamous after mating, including behaviors such as resources sharing and mutual parenthood of offspring, they can be used as a model for romantic attachment.

- Rat (*Rattus norvegicus domestica*). Rats are the second most commonly used mammal in neuroscience research. They tend to perform more reliably than mice on behavioral tests, but there are typically fewer options for genetically modified rats. The most common stocks are the **Sprague-Dawley**, **Wistar**, and **Long Evans** rats.
- Guinea pig (*Cavia porcellus*). Although one of the earliest mammalian models used in biological research, guinea pigs are rarely used today in neuroscience. Studies using guinea pigs may involve research on stress and on parental rearing.
- House cat (*Felis catus*). Rarely used today in modern studies. Historically, they were used in the early studies demonstrating the developmental organization of the visual system.

Primates:

- **Macaque monkey** (*Macaca mulatta*). Macaques are the most commonly used **nonhuman primate** (or **NHP**) in neuroscience research. Currently, macaques are used for studying **brain–computer interfaces (BCIs)**, devices which include a sensor that allows for control of robotic limbs. Because of ethical limitations on NHP research, it is common to have very low ***n*-values** (small sample sizes) in macaque experiments.
- Human (*Homo sapiens*). Human studies face the strictest regulations regarding the types of studies that can be done. Humans are used for imaging studies, in psychology research for our capacity to self-report and describe experiences, clinical trials with controlled doses of medications, and post-mortem analysis of nervous tissue. Because human behavioral tests belong more in the realm of psychology, they are not covered in depth here.

Additional Resources

Żakowski W. Animal use in neurobiological research. *Neurosci*. 2020 May 1; 433:1–10.

2.1.2 Nonhuman Housing

Housing conditions of vertebrates are standardized per institution, and must be approved by each organization's **Institutional Animal Care and Use Committee (IACUC)**. Part of the conditions involve a regulation of the **home cage**, the place where the animal spends the majority of their time. Good living conditions are not only important for the ethical treatment of experimental animals, but also for good science, since variability in data may be explained by poor living conditions.

Standard housing conditions for mammals may include the following:

- Unlimited (or ***ad libitum***) access to food and water. Food for mammals is often a standard lab **chow** that differs depending on the species. Water is typically either tap water or **deionized (DI) water**. Rats daily eat approximately 5 g per 100 g of their body weight and drink around 10 ml per 100 g of their body weight.

- Regular cycling of lights on and lights off to mimic natural day and night cycles. Typically, this split is 12 hours on and 12 hours off, sometimes written as 12h:12h. Some labs use a 14h:10h division. Rodents are **nocturnal**, and therefore tend to perform more robustly on behavioral tests during their active period (in the dark), so they may be kept on a reverse day-night cycle with the lights off during our daytime (or under red light, which they cannot see and therefore perceive as night). Monkeys are diurnal, so their lights on and off periods approximate our day and night.
- Clean housing, with frequent changes (at the longest, weekly, but usually more frequently) to replace old and soiled bedding. Animals are often provided with additional material to encourage foraging and play behaviors.
- Standardized and controlled temperature (~21°C) and humidity (~40–60%).
- **Weaning**, which is the separation of mammalian young (also called **pups** for rodents) from their parents. With rodents, weaning is performed as the pups reach around 21–28 days. NHPs are usually weaned at a much older age, usually on the order of months. After separation, they are segregated by sex, which in rodents is assessed by measuring the **anogenital distance** (distance between the anus and the genitals), which is roughly twice as long in males compared to females.
- Shared housing for socialization. Depending on the size of the cage, rodents are usually group housed (two per cage for rats, five per cage for mice). Monkeys have historically been singly housed, at least from the 1950s, but recent suggestions from various regulatory agencies in the 1990s have recommended pair housing for nonhuman primates.

However, deviations from standard housing conditions may be implemented depending on the specific research question.

- Deviations from standard lab chow can be useful for studying, for example, the influence of a high-calorie diet, food restriction, or dietary supplements on behavior. Temporary food restriction (to a fraction of expected body weight, typically more than 80%; or a fraction of food intake, typically more than 50%) or water restriction may be implemented as a means to improve learning on **instrumental conditioning tasks** (e.g. lever-pressing or nose-poking) such as **self-administration**.
- Changing the day-night cycle can be helpful for addressing questions about circadian disruption, sleep deprivation, sleep apnea, or other models of sleep disorders.
- Early weaning, prior to 21 days of age, can be a model for studying developmental disorders. Late weaning is not often performed in rodents, since fathers may cannibalize their young.
- Singly housed animals may be a model for social isolation. Singly housed animals are known to engage in **stereotypies** (repetitive, purposeless movements) and self-injurious behavior.

Environmental enrichment (EE) is an intentional manipulation of the animal's home cage that differs from standard housing. The purpose of EE is to improve cognitive, sensory, and social stimulation through allowing more "natural" species-specific behaviors. An environmentally enriched home cage for rodents may include the addition of physical items into their home cage (multiple stories, running wheels, tubes to play in, foraging materials, etc.) or social enrichment (large group housing). These types of enrichment improve several health outcomes, while impoverished housing worsens health outcomes. They also have effects at the cellular and molecular level, which can be seen at the level of receptors, cell morphology, and neural connectivity. Figure 2.1 shows examples of environmental enrichment equipment for mouse cages, which can include exercise equipment, structural enhancements, and objects to interact with in foraging behavior.

Requirements for EE have changed over the past several decades by country and by animal model, a caveat to consider when comparing recent data with older data. For example, the passing of the Animal Welfare Act of 1966, the establishment of the modern IACUC in 1986, and the approval of the European Convention for the Protection of Vertebrate Animals used for Experimental and other Scientific Purposes in 1991 (which not all signatory countries signed at the same time) represent major milestones in how laboratory animals have been treated, sometimes with respect to EE. Typically, animals used in newer studies are given EE by default.

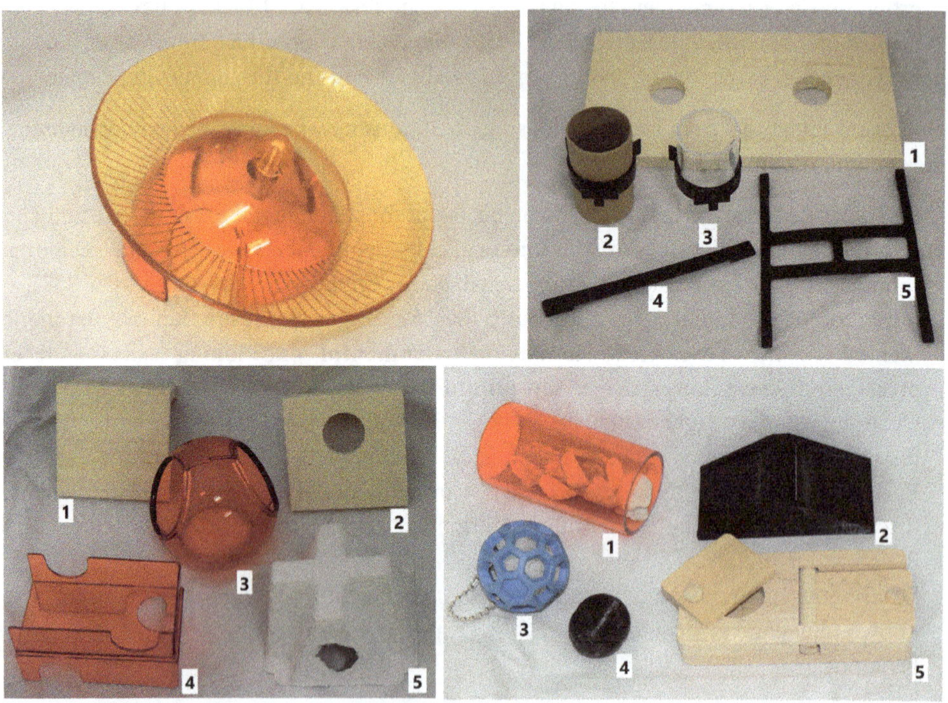

Figure 2.1 Examples of environmental enrichment equipment for mice: a running wheel, structural enhancements, and foraging enrichments. Source: Hobbiesiefken U, Mieske P, Lewejohann L, Diederich K. Evaluation of different types of enrichment – their usage and effect on home cage behavior in female mice. *PLOS ONE*. 2021; 16(12):e0261876. https://creativecommons.org/licenses/by/4.0/.

Despite the researcher's best efforts to standardize housing conditions, many unexpected sources of variation can influence animal performance on behavioral tasks: among these are day-to-day conditions such as ambient noise due to passersby and construction, or researcher-dependent variables such as the introduction of the smell of a researcher's new pet that the lab animal might notice.

Additional Resources

Hutchinson E, Avery A, VandeWoude S. Environmental enrichment for laboratory rodents. *ILAR J.* 2005; 46(2):148–161.

2.1.3 Validity in Behavioral Research

Researchers using behavioral methods often concern themselves with **validity**, which is how well a method actually measures what it is intended to measure. There are different forms of validity to consider.

- **Face validity** is related to the question "How much does the model *look* like the real condition?" For example, a neurotoxic lesion with the chemical 6-OHDA causes rats to change their posture and to move slowly (a symptom called **bradykinesia**). These symptoms are also seen in people with Parkinson's disease, whose posture and movement also change. Therefore, this model has high face validity. A shortcoming of face validity is that it can often be subjective since it requires the observer to make judgment calls, and it is therefore considered a weaker form of validity.
- **Ethological validity** is related to "How naturalistic is the stimulus?" or "How likely is it that the animal will encounter this stimulus outside of the laboratory?" The laboratory environment is very well controlled and does not often mimic the natural environment of the animals in the wild. For example, nowhere in nature is the animal given unlimited food and drink, nor are they restricted to a tiny living area. Many behavioral tests therefore suffer from poor ethological validity.

  At the top of Figure 2.2, the left side of the arena (NEST) is an area that provides a sense of safety, as there are more walls to shelter the animal. The middle area (FORAGING AREA) is a space for the animal to roam where they may find food (Pellet). A tone may also be played to alert the animal that the test session is beginning. Exploring beyond the dotted line (Trigger zone) may cause a shock to be delivered to the animal or the presentation of an artificial owl emerging from the right (as shown in the bottom image), which mimics one of the rat's natural predators.
- **Predictive validity** answers the question "Does a treatment that works for humans also work for nonhumans?" For example, opioid drugs such as morphine are very effective at reducing acute pain in humans. If the behavioral test attempts to model acute pain in rats, and opioids decrease the pain response in that rat, then the test exhibits good predictive validity.

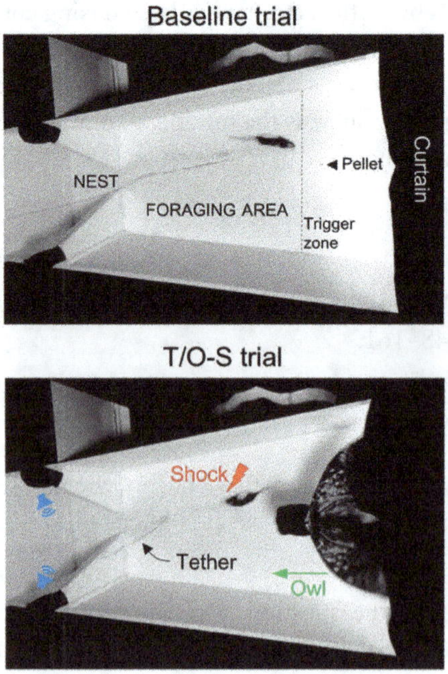

Figure 2.2 A model for fear learning with high ethological validity. Source: Zambetti PR, Schuessler BP, Lecamp BE, et al. Ecological analysis of Pavlovian fear conditioning in rats. *Commun Biol.* 2022; 5:830. https://creativecommons.org/licenses/by/4.0/. Text label has been removed.

Additional Resources

Homberg JR. Measuring behaviour in rodents: Towards translational neuropsychiatric research. *Behav Brain Res*. 2013 Jan 1; 236(1):295–306.

2.2 Motor Behaviors

Motor behaviors refer to actions involving muscle movement. Motor activity consists of several different behaviors, including:

- **Locomotion**, which refers to moving the entire body from place to place. Typically, locomotion includes muscle movement involved in **quadrupedal** (on four legs, like rodents most of the time) and **bipedal** (on two legs, like humans) walking, but also many other movement patterns such as crawling, running, bounding, swimming, or galloping. **Gait analysis** provides an objective way to quantify locomotion, recording variables such as stride length or swing time. Alternatively, the **Basso, Beattie, and Bresnahan (BBB) locomotor rating scale** is a subjective scoring system for rats that provides a measure of locomotor success on a 21-point ordinal scale.

- **Posture**, which refers to whole body position as determined by the degree of muscle flexion and joint position. Posture is an important element for maintaining balance. Atypical postures can be detected with gait analysis.
- **Fine motor skills**, which includes complex tasks involving the hands or paws, such as engaging with tools, gripping or pinching small objects, twisting, and properly applying the correct amount of force depending on the object being grasped. These skills are largely assessed in primates, who perform these tasks more reliably than other animals. Fine motor skills can be measured in rodents by observing paw pronation and supination, or with a **Montoya staircase test**.

  Figure 2.3 represents the Montoya staircase test, which puts half of the animal's body on an even platform while the opposite paw is assessed for how well it can grasp food pellets placed on the staircase, measuring number of pellets or success rate.
- **Orofacial muscle activity**, including behaviors such as jaw, tongue, and throat muscle coordination used in chewing and swallowing, showing expressions associated with emotions, moving the eyes in a specific direction (called **oculomotor** activity), and vocalization.
- **Reflexes**, which are motor activities that happen before conscious engagement. Famously in humans, the **knee-jerk** (or **patellar**) **reflex** is muscle movement (a kick of the lower leg) following a tendon stretch induced by a light hammer tap just below the knee. Other reflexes include the acoustic startle response, the suckle reflex in mammals, and the gill and siphon withdrawal reflex in *Aplysia*.

Successfully combining these motor behaviors improves the survival of animals in the wild. For example, a hungry rodent might need to coordinate both forepaws (fine motor) to pluck a berry from a bush before eating (facial muscle movement) the fruit. When a predator lunges, it might need to run (reflexive locomotion) and adjust its body rapidly to uneven terrain (posture).

Additional Resources

Larson SG. Nonhuman primate locomotion. *Am J Phys Anthropol.* 2018; 165:705–725.

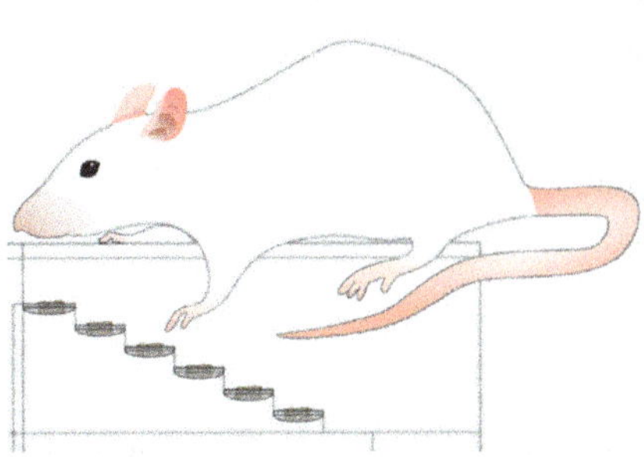

Figure 2.3 The Montoya staircase test. Source: Patricio F, Morales Dávila E, Patricio-Martínez A, et al. Intrapallidal injection of cannabidiol or a selective GPR55 antagonist decreases motor asymmetry and improves fine motor skills in hemiparkinsonian rats. *Front Pharmacol.* 2022; 13:945836. https://creativecommons.org/licenses/by/4.0/.

2.2.1 Open Field Test (OFT)

Background Information

In the **open field test**, an animal is placed into a square or circular walled chamber with a flat floor. The chamber is equipped with some means to measure the position of the animal, such as an overhead camera. Older open field systems use a series of infrared beams parallel to the floor that criss-cross the arena like a grid, and the position and duration of **beam breaking** is recorded.

The open field test is a fairly common behavioral paradigm because it is relatively low cost and can be used to measure several different behaviors, including:

- **Horizontal activity**, a measure of how much the animal moves around the field – the most common measure of locomotor activity.
- **Vertical activity** (called **rearing** in rodents), the measure of how often the animal comes off of their forepaws. An infrared beam system may not capture these behaviors as accurately as cameras can. Both vertical and horizontal activity are signs of **exploratory behavior**, which is expected whenever an animal is exposed to a new environment.
- Time spent in different predefined zones. Rodents have a natural propensity to prefer corners and walls while avoiding open spaces where they are more exposed to potential predators. Dividing the field into predefined zones, such as a **center** area and a **surround** (or sometimes **wall** or **border**; possibly further subdivided into **wall** versus **corner**), allows the researchers to approximate the animal's preference for the potentially dangerous area in the center compared to the safer areas along the periphery of the testing chamber. This is used as a proxy measure for anxiety-like behaviors. A similar test has been adapted for zebrafishes, where the top part of the tank closer to the surface of the water is riskier for them, and is therefore roughly analogous to the center area of the open field.
- Velocity. Rodents achieve speeds on the order of centimeters per second. Animal speed cannot be accurately measured by an infrared system.
- Rotations, the measure of how frequently and in which direction the animal turns, which may be reported in studies about movement disorders or animals with unilateral manipulations. These behaviors cannot be measured with an infrared beam system.

The OFT is usually performed with rodents, but the test has been modified for Drosophila in petri dishes and fish in tanks.

Reading the Graphs

Data figures from OFT experiments often represent horizontal activity. When data are collected by an overhead camera, the representative images show a trail of where the animal had been over the course of the session (also called a **trace diagram**). These graphs condense time down into a single snapshot. A higher density of lines indicates more movement.

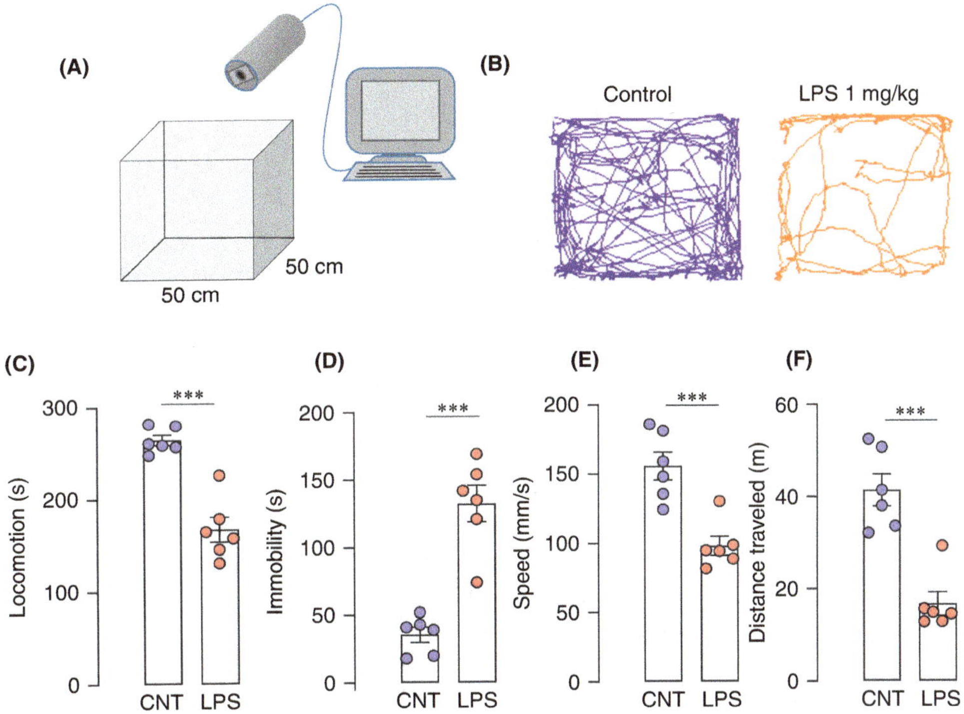

Figure 2.4 Locomotor activity on an open field test. Source: Hasriadi H, Wasana PWD, Vajragupta O, Rojsitthisak P, Towiwat P. Automated home-cage monitoring as a potential measure of sickness behaviors and pain-like behaviors in LPS-treated mice. *PLOS ONE*. 2021; 16(8):e0256706. https://creativecommons.org/licenses/by/4.0/.

Figure 2.4 reflects data from an open field test in which injection with lipopolysaccharide (LPS) decreased overall locomotor activity. Panel A shows the experimental apparatus and camera, noting dimensions of the open field as 50 × 50 cm. Panel B shows trace diagrams of a representative control animal (blue lines) as being more dense compared to those of the LPS-injected animal (orange lines), suggesting that LPS decreases locomotor activity. Panels C through F show combined data represented as bar graphs for different measures related to locomotor activity, including time spent moving (panel C), time spent frozen (not moving, panel D; an inverse measure where higher values suggest less locomotion), movement speed (panel E), and total distance traveled (panel F). Across all four measures, statistical significance at $p < 0.001$ was observed. Colored dots represent data from individual animals (blue = control, orange = LPS).

If the open field is used for measuring time spent in each zone (assessing anxiety-like behaviors), a visual guideline may be drawn to identify the dimensions of the center area relative to the surround area. As with the locomotor activity readings, a trail may show the animal's location over the course of the session. Greater density in the center zone indicates lessened anxiety-like behavior.

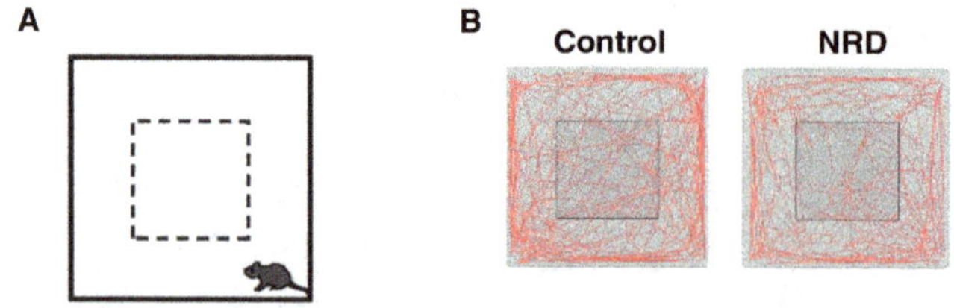

Figure 2.5 Center versus surround in an open field test. Source: Zhu Y, Ye Y, Zhou C, et al. Effect of sensory deprivation of nasal respiratory on behavior of C57BL/6 J Mice. *Brain Sci.* 2021; 11(12):1626. https://creativecommons.org/licenses/by/4.0/. Figure has been cropped.

The same representative data may be shown on a **heat map**. Heat maps use colors to represent the amount of time that the animal spends in that specific area over the course of testing. A standard heat map spectrum uses cool colors (blues, greens) to indicate less time spent in that area, while warm colors (oranges, reds) indicate more time spent there.

In Figure 2.5, the overhead schematic (panel A) shows the boundary used to differentiate the center from the surround. The trace diagram (panel B) shows that animals experiencing sensory deprivation of nasal respiratory breath (NRD; right) enter the center area less frequently compared to control animals (left).

In summary graphs, the *x*-axis shows groups.

If horizontal activity is measured using an infrared beam system, the *y*-axis may plot the number of beam breaks, and more beam breaks indicate more activity. If zones are being reported, the number of entries into a zone or percentage of beam breaks in a certain zone can be plotted on the *y*-axis. A greater percentage of beam breaks in the surround zone suggests heightened anxiety. Because counts of infrared beam breaks do not give information about time, reporting duration would be misleading.

If using an overhead camera system to track locomotion, several different measures might be plotted on the *y*-axis, among them total distance traveled, average velocity, number of rotations, or rearing as a percentage of total time. Overhead camera systems can present anxiety-like data on the *y*-axis in different ways, commonly plotting time spent in the center zone as a fraction of total time.

Interpreting the Data

Many lab animals have a natural desire to explore, which often manifests as increased locomotor activity. In OFT data, activity is usually highest over the first 10–20 minutes and then plateaus over the following minutes. Alternatively, exposing the animal to the OFT chamber prior to testing may help eliminate the influence of the desire to explore or curiosity on locomotor activity.

In a paradigm called **locomotor sensitization**, horizontal and vertical movement counts are increased following repeat exposure to drugs – for example psychomotor stimulants such as amphetamine – over the course of several days. In graphs reporting this

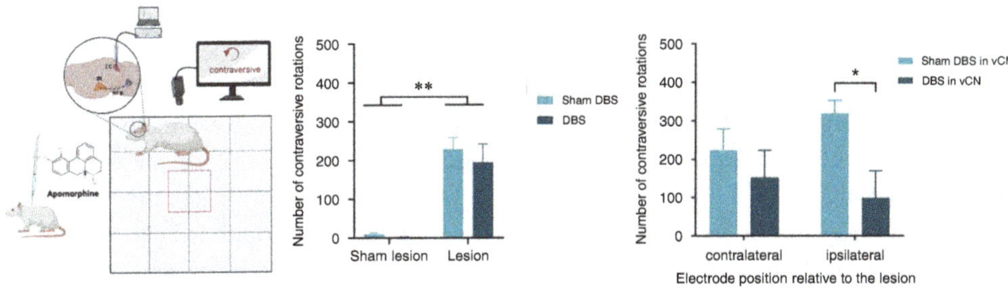

Figure 2.6 Apomorphine-induced rotation behavior. Source: Melo-Thomas L, Tacken L, Richter N, et al. Lateralization in hemi-Parkinsonian rats is affected by deep brain stimulation or glutamatergic neurotransmission in the inferior colliculus. *eNeuro*. 2022 Jul 11; 9(4):ENEURO.0076–22.2022. http://creativecommons.org/licenses/by/4.0/. Figures have been rearranged.

phenomenon, the *x*-axis usually plots session number (time) while the *y*-axis shows movement.

Atypical rotational movement may be induced by exposing the animal to apomorphine, a dopaminergic agonist. Exposure to apomorphine causes more turning (or **circling**) toward the side of the lesion. This is the **apomorphine-induced rotation test**, and is often used to assess the severity of dopaminergic lesion, which is an experimental model of Parkinson's disease.

Figure 2.6 shows results from a deep brain stimulation (DBS) experiment in a 6-OHDA lesion model of Parkinson's disease. In this model, animals are injected in one side of the brain with the neurotoxin 6-OHDA, which destroys dopamine cells in that half of the animal's brain (referred to as a lesion). The control group receives only a vehicle: an injection that carries no neurotoxin (sham lesion). On the left is an experimental protocol figure showing the systemic injection of apomorphine, the location of the deep brain stimulator in the inferior colliculus (IC), the open field apparatus, and the overhead camera for observation of which turning direction is contraversive (away from the lesioned hemisphere). In the middle of the figure is a bar graph showing group data. Sham-lesioned animals (left two bars) do not exhibit any contraversive turning, while 6-OHDA-lesioned animals (right two bars) do. DBS does not affect the number of turns. The bar graph on the right shows group data from a further experiment, in which a DBS electrode was either placed in the opposite hemisphere (contralateral) or the same hemisphere (ipsilateral) as the lesion. Turning was decreased only in the ipsilateral condition. A different control experiment here is the sham DBS, where an electrode is placed but no current is turned on.

Additional Resources

Võikar V, Stanford SC. The open field test. *Neuromethods*. 2023; 190:9–29.

2.2.2 Accelerating Rotarod

Background Information

The **accelerating rotarod** test assays fine motor coordination, motor learning, balance, and attention. In this test, an animal is placed on a rotarod: a cylinder (3 cm in diameter for mice, 6 cm for rats) that rotates, much like a treadmill. Over the course of the testing period, the rotarod gradually speeds up. If the animal does not walk quickly enough to keep up with the spinning rod, or if their balance is disrupted, they will fall off the rod and onto a soft platform below. The time until the animal falls is measured.

Many rotarods have large discs perpendicular to the rod that subdivide it into lanes. This allows multiple animals to be tested at the same time while minimizing interference between animals during testing. The rotarod is typically used for rodents.

The rotarod apparatus on the left in Figure 2.7 has separate lanes for each animal and a plate at the bottom to detect when an animal has fallen. On the right, data from a rotarod experiment is plotted over the course of 28 days for four different experimental groups. The researchers were curious as to whether the gene KLF11 is involved in motor performance deficits after traumatic brain injury (TBI). Prior to surgery, at day −1, animals were able to stay on the rotarod for around 130 seconds. The two control groups who received the sham surgery (dark- and light-gray circles) performed equally well during the month after the surgery, suggesting no influence of anesthesia or craniotomy on rotarod performance. The animals receiving a TBI on day 0 (TBI, red circles) performed significantly worse than the control group at a level of $p < 0.001$ (lower latency means they fell off sooner). Genetically modified "knockout mice" lacking the KLF11 gene (blue circles) that had received TBI performed significantly worse than the WT mice with TBI. The researchers concluded that the KLF11 gene codes for some factor that is neuroprotective in the event of TBI.

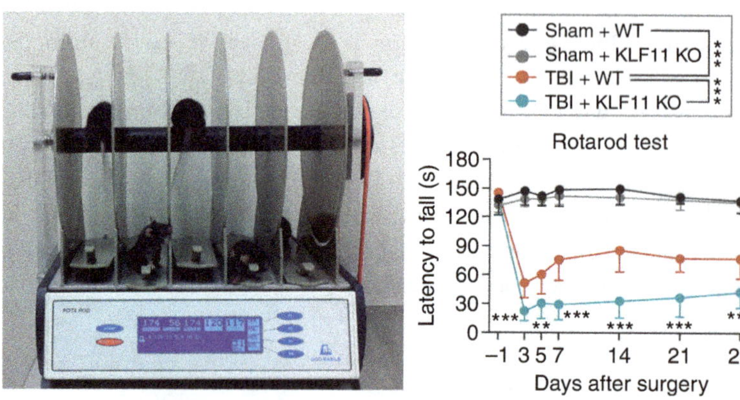

Figure 2.7 The rotarod test. Source: Left: Bmouzon, CC BY-SA 4.0 <https://creativecommons.org/licenses/by-sa/4.0>, via Wikimedia Commons. Right: Zhou C, Sun P, Hamblin MH, et al. Genetic deletion of Krüppel-like factor 11 aggravates traumatic brain injury. *J Neuroinflammation*. 2022; 19:281. http://creativecommons.org/licenses/by/4.0/.

Reading the Graphs

Summary graphs typically plot days of training (or training sessions) on the x-axis. Latency to fall (length of time until the animal falls off the rotarod, which carries the same information as time spent on the rotarod) is plotted on the y-axis, usually measured in hundreds of seconds. Data from multiple groups may be plotted on the same graph. Latency normally increases over trials (positive slope), but this is a training artifact as the animal is given more opportunities to practice on the apparatus. Longer latency to fall (higher y-axis values) suggests better performance on the rotarod.

Alternatively, graphs may plot distance traveled on the rotarod with values up to thousands of centimeters. Longer distances traveled suggests better performance.

Interpreting the Data

Performance on the rotarod is dependent on several neural circuits that are critical for motor control and balance, including cerebellum and basal ganglia. Diseases that model disruptions of these circuits, such as spinocerebellar ataxia or dopaminergic lesions of the midbrain, impair performance on the rotarod. Additionally, diseases resulting in poor motor control (such as dystonia), demyelination like that seen in multiple sclerosis, and traumatic brain injury are all known to impair performance on the rotarod task.

Psychoactive drugs can modify rotarod performance. Benzodiazepines and opioids decrease latency to fall, probably due to the sedative effects of these drugs. Haloperidol, a drug that blocks dopamine signaling, worsens performance, possibly through interacting with dopamine circuits of the basal ganglia.

Additional Resources

Shiotsuki H, Yoshimi K, Shimo Y, et al. A rotarod test for evaluation of motor skill learning. *J Neurosci Methods*. 2010; 189(2):180–185.

2.3 Pain

Pain is the sensation that alerts the organism that a part of the body is being injured. Pain can exist at the surface of the skin or deeper in our organs. Detecting pain can lead to reflexive withdrawal from a stimulus and can serve as a learning signal to inform the organism to avoid exposure to this injurious stimulus in the future. This type of healthy pain is called **nociceptive pain** and is probably evolutionarily protective.

Pain can be experienced in several different ways, and different behavioral tests are used to assess different forms of pain.

- **Mechanical pain** refers to the sensation of physical stimuli. Mechanical pain may have many different types of sensations, including pressure, crushing, pinching, stretching, rubbing, cutting, and more. In the lab, mechanical pain is usually elicited by a poking stimulus.

- **Thermal pain** refers to pain sensation from excessively hot or cold temperatures, both of which can be injurious. For humans, the typical heat threshold for the skin surface is around 43°C (109°F), and the cold threshold is around 15°C (59°F).
- **Chemical pain** is pain in response to the release of chemical factors by the body such as acetylcholine, adenosine, histamine, and serotonin, as well as inflammatory signaling molecules such as prostaglandins and cytokines. These chemical factors produce an inflammatory response among nociceptive neurons.

The reasons for studying pain are often related to disease.

- **Neuropathic pain** results from some injury to the nervous system that produces the sensation of pain despite the lack of injurious stimulus, and may lead to symptoms such as **hyperalgesia** (increased perception of the severity of a painful stimulus; lowered pain threshold), **allodynia** (pain perception from innocuous stimuli), or **spontaneous pain** (pain occurring in the absence of stimuli). Neuropathic pain may arise from a nerve injury, cancer or cancer treatment, diabetes, stroke, multiple sclerosis, or many other potential causes.
- **Inflammatory pain** is mechanistically distinct from neuropathic pain, and causes pain perception due to the influence of cell signaling factors such as cytokines. Some forms of inflammatory pain are protective, such as when inflammation leads to increased sensitivity at the site of injury; this may cause a person to avoid using the inflamed body part when doing so could damage it more. However, some forms of inflammatory pain may be brought on by nerve damage, spinal cord or vertebral injury, or rheumatoid arthritis, for example.
- **Phantom limb pain (PLP)** is the sensation of pain following the loss of a body part, and is a frequent side effect following amputation. Amputations are not often performed on nonhumans to study phantom limb pain; almost all studies of phantom limb pain recruit human participants.
- **Congenital insensitivity to pain** is a rare disease where the patient does not perceive pain at all. Because of their propensity to being injured frequently, they often have shortened lifespans.
- **Acute pain** can be induced experimentally as a way to screen for novel analgesic drugs.

Common nonhuman models of pain include:

- **Nerve ligation** (or **cuffing**, or **chronic constriction injury**, or **CCI**) is a surgical procedure performed on rodents by tying a restrictive band around a nerve, resulting in a model of neuropathic pain. Specific nerves can be targeted, such as the sciatic nerve or the L5 and L6 spinal nerve, both of which affect the ipsilateral hindpaw. This manipulation, when performed unilaterally, allows for comparison with an internal control, as pain measurements can be tested on the unaffected, contralateral hindpaw. Still, control animals experiencing **sham surgery** (a surgery that mimics every aspect of the nerve ligation without the intentional nerve injury) may be needed to control for the effect of anesthesia and the inflammatory effects of surgery.

- Injection of chemical compounds can cause temporary inflammatory pain. Different chemicals are used to induce inflammation at different parts of the body: carrageenan, **formalin**, **cisplatin**, and **complete Freunds adjuvant** or **CFA** are used to induce inflammation of the muscle and soft tissue, while carrageenan, collagenase, kaolin, or iodoacetate can mimic joint inflammation. These chemical methods often induce **edema** (swelling due to water accumulation) of the target body part.

Additional Resources

National Research Council (US) Committee on Recognition and Alleviation of Pain in Laboratory Animals. Models of pain. *Recognition and Alleviation of Pain in Laboratory Animals*. Washington, DC: National Academies Press (US); 2009. Section A. www.ncbi.nlm.nih.gov/books/NBK32654/.

2.3.1 Von Frey Fiber Assay

Background Information

The von Frey (pronounced "fry") fiber assay is used to measure the perception of poking mechanical pain or tactile sensation on the skin. The tools for performing this test are called **von Frey fibers** (also called **von Frey hairs**), a series of thin nylon filamentous rods of differing diameters. A fiber is pushed at a right angle into the surface of the skin, such as the palm of the hindpaw, until the fiber bends or the animal experiences pain (self-report in humans, or withdrawal response in nonhumans). Larger-diameter fibers are more stiff, and therefore require a greater amount of force applied until the fiber bends. Any further application of force is deflected sideways and is not felt on the skin. There are also electronic tools that can measure the withdrawal threshold, needing multiple trials with different stimulus intensities.

The von Frey fiber test can be performed on primates and rodents. It has also been used on Drosophila larvae, which have a mechanosensitive avoidance response.

Reading the Graphs

One von Frey assay may measure differences between groups or treatments at a single time point. Here, mechanical force is plotted on the *x*-axis in increasing values from left to right. Measures are reported in hundredths of grams up to grams (g) when measuring weight of the mechanical stimulus, or tenths of millinewtons to millinewtons (mN) when measuring force. The % pain responses may be plotted on the *y*-axis from 0 to 100. This plot creates curves, each curve depicting the group's responses under a range of von Frey fiber sizes. If the curve for the experimental group is leftward shifted compared to the control group's curve, the experimental group exhibits more sensitivity to mechanical pain, since the same amount of pressure produces a higher pain response than in the control group.

A different assay measures the development or treatment of allodynia over the course of several days after a manipulation. These graphs plot time on the *x*-axis in hours or days. The data at negative time points represents the baseline response before the manipulation. The *y*-axis may plot the paw withdrawal threshold (PWT) in grams or newtons. The threshold represents the thinnest fiber that causes the pain response. Another way to quantify this pain response is the 50% withdrawal, which may also be plotted on the *y*-axis. This is similar to the PWT, except multiple trials are performed, and the von Frey fiber stiffness that causes the pain response 50% of the time is recorded instead of the threshold. If these plots show a decrease in PWT or 50% withdrawal after the manipulation, this indicates heightened mechanical pain sensitivity. These values can also be determined using an electronic von Frey tester.

A researcher may also perform a measure of multiple trials observing responses after pressing the same thickness of fiber against the skin. Here, time would be plotted on the *x*-axis, and percentage of trials resulting in paw withdrawal or pain response would be plotted on the *y*-axis. In these experiments, elevations over baseline suggest increased mechanical pain sensitivity.

Figure 2.8 shows that the group treated with acetic acid (AA, red) has a lower withdrawal threshold compared to the control group (blue), indicative of heightened pain sensitivity. Exposing the animal to both AA and either nalbuphine (green) or PDTC (purple) increases the withdrawal threshold, suggesting decreased sensitivity even above the level of baseline.

A summary graph may simply show the behavioral response after the application of one selected size of von Frey fiber. For example, it may show different groups across the *x*-axis and pain threshold as a percentage of baseline on the *y*-axis. Here, a decrease in the withdrawal threshold indicates higher pain sensitivity. The control group should not show a change in *y*-axis scores.

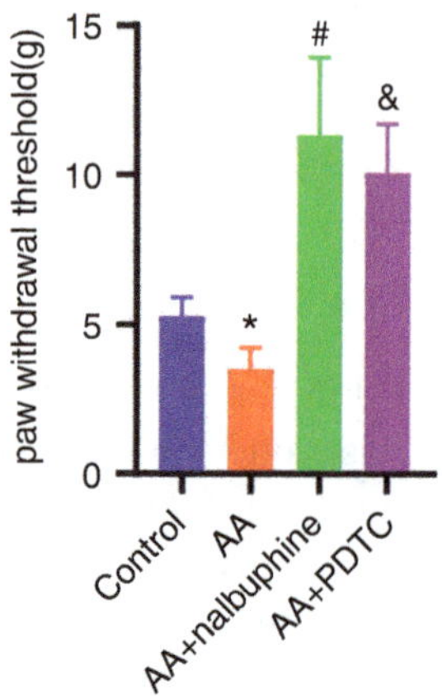

Figure 2.8 The paw withdrawal test. Source: Ruan D, Wang Y, Li S, et al. Nalbuphine alleviates inflammation by down-regulating NF-κB in an acute inflammatory visceral pain rat model. *BMC Pharmacol Toxicol.* 2022; 23(1):34. DOI: 10.1186/s40360-022-00573-7. Figure has been cropped and text label removed.

Interpreting the Data

A result showing increased sensitivity to pain indicates that the subjects experience more mechanical allodynia, since the animals now withdraw their paws in response to a less painful stimulus. Neuropathic and inflammatory pain causes increased sensitivity on the von Frey fiber test.

On the other hand, opioid drugs increase the paw withdrawal threshold, indicating that this test has strong predictive validity.

Additional Resources

Christensen SL, Hansen RB, Storm MA, et al. Von Frey testing revisited: Provision of an online algorithm for improved accuracy of 50% thresholds. *Eur J Pain*. 2020 Apr; 24 (4):783–790.

2.3.2 Hot Plate Assay, Cold Plate Assay, and Radiant Heat Test (or Hargreaves Method)

Background Information

Thermal pain is processed by the nervous system differently from mechanical pain. Therefore, modified behavioral tests have been developed to measure responses to thermal pain.

The animal is placed into a clear (commonly acrylic or plexiglass), narrow-diameter tube to minimize movement. Then, a body part, usually the hind paw, is placed onto a temperature controlled plate. Temperatures between 47° and 55°C are considered noxious heat (used in the **hot plate test**), while 4°C is noxious cold (used in the **cold plate test**). Alternatively, a device that emits progressively more intense heat may be pointed directly at the paw (**radiant heat test**, or the **Hargreaves method**). A maximum time of exposure (up to 1 minute) may be enforced, since prolonged exposure to the thermal stimuli may cause tissue damage. Rodents respond to these stimuli by biting, licking, or lifting the paw. Sometimes, they may jump to avoid the stimulus. They may also vocalize. Any of these behaviors suggest that the animal is experiencing pain, which ends the trial.

Similar hot plate assays for measuring pain have been adopted for Drosophila, and a radiant heat system can produce a thermal avoidance response in *C. elegans*. Thermal pain tests in humans are often done by immersing a part of the body in cold water until the participant voluntarily withdraws.

Reading the Graphs

Summary graphs may plot groups on the *x*-axis. The *y*-axis may plot:

- Number of responses during testing, where more responding is interpreted as heightened pain sensitivity.

- Latency to withdraw, a measure of the time it takes for the animal to exhibit one of many different pain responses. The higher the latency, the less sensitivity to thermal pain. Latency is typically in seconds or tens of seconds.
- **Maximum potential effect** (**MPE**). This value is calculated with this formula: (latency after treatment − baseline) ÷ (cut off time − baseline latency) × 100. The MPE value normalizes for an animal's intrinsic differences in sensitivity to pain. A higher MPE suggests less sensitivity.

In data from the hot plate test represented in Figure 2.9, morphine treatment (dark-blue squares) causes an analgesic effect, lasting around 80 minutes, compared to the control animals (gray circles). Treatment of morphine with high-dose cannabidivarin (CBDV; yellow triangles) potentiates the analgesic effect, but treatment with CBDV alone (light-blue diamonds) does not change heat pain responding.

Responding by the contralateral paw is a within-subject control, and these data are often plotted alongside the data from the ipsilateral paw.

Some experiments may assess the time course of the analgesic effect. These graphs show time on the *x*-axis, and measurements are taken periodically over the course of the experiment. A measure of sensitivity (such as latency to withdrawal) is plotted on the *y*-axis. In these plots, the rising phase (the left portion of the graph) suggests how quickly the drug takes effect, which may be a consequence of route of administration. The decay phase (falling phase; the right portion of the graph) informs us how quickly the drug effect fades, which may be a consequence of metabolism. The plateau of the graph suggests the degree of analgesia at its most effective.

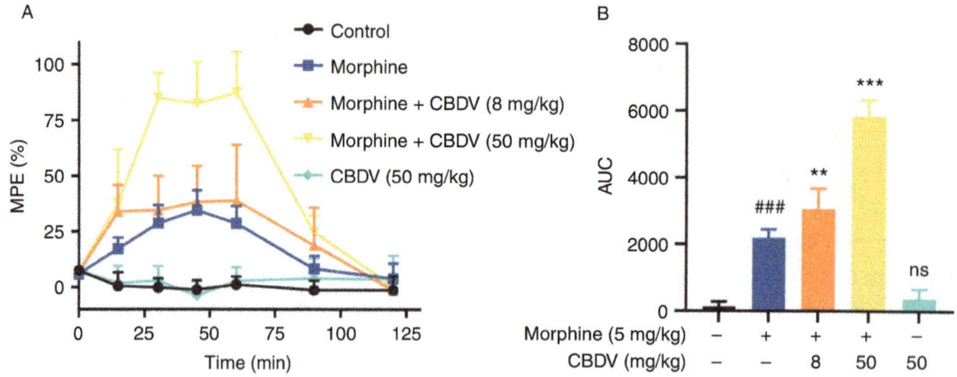

Figure 2.9 Morphine's effect on a hot plate test. Source: Wang X, Lin C, Wu S, et al. Cannabidivarin alleviates neuroinflammation by targeting TLR4 co-receptor MD2 and improves morphine-mediated analgesia. *Front Immunol.* 2022; 13:929222. https://creativecommons.org/licenses/by/4.0/.

Interpreting the Data

Analgesics may be delivered systemically, possibly by injection. Common methods are intraperitoneal (often abbreviated i.p.), or into the space around the gut; intravenous (i.v.), directly into the bloodstream; and subcutaneous (s.c.), underneath the skin. Because the drugs will be absorbed and distributed throughout the body, there is no way to restrict where the treatment ends up – although a local application of a topical anesthetic can also be tested.

When analgesic treatments are being studied, a reversal effect may be seen. For example, a surgically induced nerve injury may decrease latency compared to the contralateral (uninjured) paw, suggesting hypersensitivity to pain. Then, if a drug administration produces analgesia, the latency of pain responding may increase back to the values seen in the control condition.

Opioids are effective at inducing analgesia, and treatment with opioids increases the latency to pain response, which suggests good predictive validity.

The tests themselves are largely unnatural, since they require that the animal is kept in a small tube to restrict their movement. This is probably stress-inducing. Additionally, sources of radiant noxious heat used in a Hargreaves test are rare in nature, suggesting low ethological validity.

Additional Resources

Homberg JR. Measuring behaviour in rodents: Towards translational neuropsychiatric research. *Behav Brain Res*. 2013 Jan 1; 236(1):295–306.

2.4 Learning and Memory

Learning refers to the process of acquiring new pieces of information or skills that may influence future behavior. Behavioral tests can assess different types of learning: for example, how well a monkey can learn to push buttons in a certain order to receive a fruit drink reward (self-administration), or how quickly a rat can learn to find a platform hidden underwater (Morris water maze). Learning and memory are evolutionarily valuable cognitive functions, since being able to remember the location and nutritional value of foods is critical for survival.

There are several different forms of memory.

- **Declarative** (or **explicit**) **memories** have a concrete piece of explainable knowledge associated with the memory. Recalling these memories is typically a conscious and active process. In humans, examples of declarative memories include facts learned in elementary school, definitions of vocabulary words, or recalling the events of your day yesterday.
- **Procedural** (or **implicit**) **memories** are those based on knowledge that is acquired unconsciously. For example, people often perform a series of complex actions without

thinking about each individual step, such as while brushing teeth, getting dressed, or taking a shower. These memories may be informally called "muscle memory".

These divisions have been based primarily on human neuropsychology research, and parallels found in nonhuman memory processes are not perfectly analogous.

Many structures of the brain are important for learning and memory, but the most strongly implicated is the **hippocampus**. Much of the early work examining the hippocampus arose from the study of **Henry Molaison** (also known as **Patient HM**), a man with intractable epilepsy who was treated by surgical removal of his left and right hippocampus. Molaison was unable to learn new facts or create new memories about day-to-day activities, suggesting that declarative memory requires the hippocampus.

Besides the hippocampus, many other structures are involved in different forms of memory, including the amygdala, the prefrontal cortex, and the cerebellum just to name a few. Most likely, memories as we think of them exist as a network of cells distributed widely across the brain.

There are several complex processes involved in learning and memory.

- **Encoding**, the process of building the neural circuitry involved in the specific memory. In nonhuman neurological research, encoding largely happens during acquisition trials as the animal learns the behavioral task.
- **Storage**, the ability to actively maintain these networks over a period of time. To quantify storage capacity, delays of varying lengths may be introduced between the acquisition (learning) and testing phases.
- **Retrieval**, the ability to access the network when the moment arises. Retrieval is assessed during a testing trial.

Encoding, storage, and retrieval are believed to be the minimum processes required for learning. If the animal performs poorly on a behavioral test, it may be difficult to determine which of the three processes is impaired. Other memory-related processes include:

- **Relearning**, the adjusting of the circuit to different circumstances.
- **Forgetting**, the act of disassembling (or failing to maintain) circuits involved in certain memories.

Learning and memory processes are correlated with cellular and molecular level changes, which can be assessed by complementary methods.

At the cellular level, learning may be accompanied by **plasticity**: physical changes in cells or in the ways the cells communicate. Some types of plasticity, such as an increase in the dendritic spines, can be observed using microscopy techniques such as a Golgi stain.

At a molecular level, learning is likely to be a consequence of **long-term potentiation (LTP)**, the strengthening of a synapse over a time course of hours or longer; its opposite, **long-term depression (LTD)**, is the weakening of a synapse. LTP at glutamatergic synapses requires coincident activation of different receptor classes, notably the **NMDA receptor**. These receptors are permeable to Ca^{2+}, the ion that can activate several intracellular signaling pathways (the enzyme CaMKII, for example), which leads to increased synaptic strength. Some of these molecular-level changes can be observed using immunochemistry and electrophysiology.

A potential confound is that many behavioral paradigms that we discuss outside of this section involve the measurement of learning and memory to some degree. For example, the accelerating rotarod (Section 3.1.2) is used for studying motor activity and coordination, but it also requires the animal to learn how to respond on the apparatus as it speeds up, which is a procedural memory task. Animals that perform poorly on this test may have impaired motor learning capability.

Additional Resources

Frankland PW, Josselyn SA, Köhler S. The neurobiological foundation of memory retrieval. *Nat Neurosci.* 2019 Oct; 22(10):1576–1585.

2.4.1 Morris Water Maze (MWM)

Background Information

The **Morris water maze** (MWM) is a rodent behavioral paradigm that is used to measure **spatial navigation**, the skill of learning the positions of important areas in the environment. Good spatial navigational memory is probably selected for by evolutionary pressures, since rodents in the wild will need to search for food and water and remember these surroundings for future foraging trips.

The MWM apparatus is a circular pool of water (~1–2 meter diameter). Powdered milk or nontoxic paint has been added to make the water opaque, making it difficult to see through. Within the pool is a transparent platform (~5 cm diameter) beneath the surface of the water, placed in one quadrant of the pool, equidistant from the center and the wall. The platform is the maze exit: the animal is removed by the experimenter when they find the platform. Visual cues, such as pictures of shapes or textures, are placed along the outside of the pool and are visible from the inside. These cues serve to help the animal orient itself to the surroundings. Overhead, a camera is used to record the position of the animal.

On each trial, which may last a minute, the rodent is placed in the pool against the wall. The time it takes for the animal to reach the exit platform is recorded. Over time, if the animal learns that the platform is close to a certain visual cue, the time to reach the exit decreases. Trials are usually repeated over the course of several days.

Instead of learning the association between the visual cues and the exit, an animal may memorize a swim pattern to reach the exit. To eliminate this variable, the animal is placed in a different location on each trial.

A **probe** trial may be conducted, in which the researcher removes the platform and measures the time spent in the quadrant of the pool where the platform is expected.

Reading the Graphs

Representative images typically show a circle, which is an overhead representation of the pool, along with the exit platform. The pool may be visibly divided into four sections with each quadrant denoted by perpendicular lines or shaded with different colors, although the maze itself doesn't have borders or colors in the water.

Lines overlaid on each circle show the animal's position over the course of the post-training trial (like a trace diagram in the open field test). Animals that learn the behavior better will have a shorter line to the exit or more time in the exit quadrant. Animals that do not learn well will have a longer, more circuitous line, or may not preferably spend time in the quadrant of interest. Each trace diagram shows a representative animal from each of the different experimental conditions.

A similar way to present these data is with a heat map. Blue shades indicate less time spent in that area, while redder shades indicate more time spent. Animals who learn better will have more red color shades in the quadrant of the exit.

To demonstrate progressive learning of the MWM, summary graphs may plot day of training (or training session) on the x-axis across several sessions.

Different variables may be plotted on the y-axis.

- Latency to escape is a measurement of the time that has lapsed between when the animal is first put in the MWM and when they reach the exit, usually measured in tens of seconds. A steeper negative slope (or lower latency on the final test day) means better learning.
- Path length measures how far the animal traveled after being placed in the MWM before reaching the platform, usually reported in meters. Steeper negative slopes (shorter path length) indicate better learning, since the animal remembers where the exit is and goes straight to the target.
- Time spent in the quadrant of interest may be plotted as a fraction (or percentage) of total time; in these cases steeper positive slopes with values higher than 0.25 (or 25%) indicate better learning. Animals that do not learn will spend an equal amount of time in all quadrants, and will show no slope over time.

It is also common to present these same data, but only at a single time point post-training. In these summary graphs, different experimental manipulations are on the x-axis, while the variable of interest such as latency or path length is plotted on the y-axis.

Figure 2.10 shows results from a Morris water maze experiment. Panel c shows trace diagrams of mouse movement. Animals were exposed to either DMSO (a vehicle) or Aβ (experimental model of Alzheimer's pathology) via an intracerebroventricular injection. The Aβ-treated animals performed worse on the MWM (as shown in the third diagram): they travelled a farther total distance and took longer to reach the platform (the small circle) compared to the control group (shown in the first diagram). Oxytocin was delivered by intranasal spray. Oxytocin did not significantly change MWM performance for the DMSO-treated rats. However, oxytocin treatment improved the performance of the Aβ group (diagram 4), showing a reversal of effect. Panels d and e show bar graphs with individual data points summarizing group data.

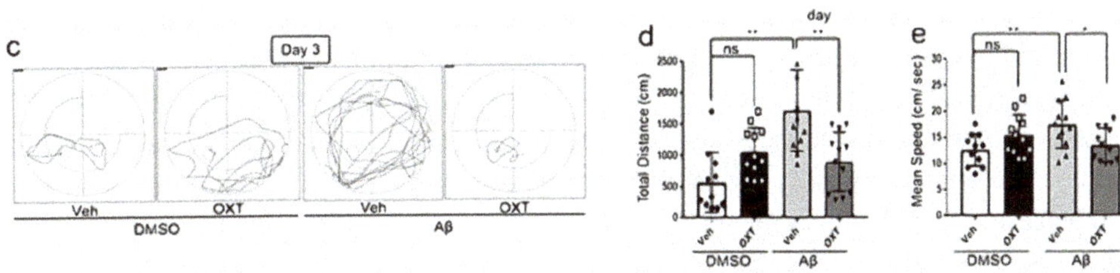

Figure 2.10 The Morris water maze. Source: Takahashi J, Ueta Y, Yamada D, et al. Intracerebroventricular administration of oxytocin and intranasal administration of the oxytocin derivative improve β-amyloid peptide (25–35)-induced memory impairment in mice. *Neuropsychopharmacol Rep.* 2022; 00(42): 492–501. DOI: 10.1002/npr2.12292. Epub 2022 Sep 19. PMID: 36117475; PMCID: PMC9773650. https://creativecommons.org/licenses/by/4.0/. Image cropped.

Interpreting the Data

Learning on the Morris water maze is dependent on structures including the hippocampus and the basal ganglia. For example, damage to the hippocampus from physical lesions or neurodegeneration causes worse performance (longer latency to exit, longer path length, or less time spent in the correct quadrant) on the MWM.

Chemicals also impair spatial learning. For example, the glutamate NMDA receptor is essential for long-term plasticity at synapses. Drugs that block this receptor also impair spatial learning. Drugs with amnesic effects, such as anesthetics or ethanol, decrease performance on the MWM, which suggests strong predictive validity since these drugs also impair memory in people.

Additional Resources

Morris RGM. Spatial localization does not require the presence of local cues. *Learn Motiv.* 1981; **12**:239–260.

2.4.2 Novel Object Recognition Task (NOR, or NORT)

Background Information

The **novel object recognition task** (NORT) is used as an assay of recognition memory. The NORT is based on the observation that animals, rodents especially, have a natural interest in exploring and interacting with objects they have not previously seen. An animal that does not form a memory of an object will consider it to be new and will spend more time interacting with it.

The chamber used in a NORT is equipped with video cameras to record the animal's behavior. The animal is considered to be exploring the object if their nose is within a few centimeters of it. The size of the testing chamber must be scaled appropriately for the age and size of the animal. If the testing chamber is too small, the animal may be scored as engaging with the object when they are just turning around. If the chamber is too large, they may spend too much time exploring the chamber instead of the objects.

Many different objects have been used in the NORT, including plastic eggs, glass vials, Lego blocks, candlesticks, coffee mugs, dog chew toys, and tennis balls. An object that is ideal for this task is one that is easily cleaned and resistant to damage by chewing. Objects should not be climbable and should be heavy enough so that the animals do not move them around too much. Also, objects should not resemble other stimuli in nature, since animals might, for example, avoid snake-like objects out of fear, or engage with food-like objects hungrily.

The test consists of four **phases**:

1. **Habituation phase** (also called the **acclimation phase**, **preconditioning phase**, or **pre-test phase**), when the animal is removed from the home cage and placed into the testing cage. No objects are introduced during this phase.
2. **Training** (or **sample**), when two of the same objects are placed on opposite sides of the chamber, with some space between the object and the wall.
3. **Delay** (or **retention**), when the animal is returned to the testing chamber with no objects introduced until a specified time.
4. **Testing**, when the object from training (also called a **familiar object**, abbreviated **F**) will be placed on one side of the chamber, while a new object (**novel object**, abbreviated **N**) will be placed on the opposite side. The novel object should be different from the familiar, possibly in shape, texture, or size, but it may share some traits in common such as color. During testing, the position of the objects (whether on the left or right side of the chamber) may be alternated, which eliminates the influence of any intrinsic or learned place preference. Only the first few minutes of the testing phase are analyzed, since this is when the novelty response is at its peak. If the animal stores recognition memory of the object from the training phase, then it will prefer to explore the novel object.

NORT is mostly performed in rats and mice but has been modified for pigs and monkeys as well.

Reading the graphs

In summary graphs, different groups may be plotted on the x-axis. Different measures may be on the y-axis:

- Number of exploration bouts of the novel object. More exploration of novel objects (or fewer exploration counts of the familiar object) suggest better familiarity recall. This value may be misleading, since a single exploration event that lasts for tens of seconds will only count as one event.
- Time spent exploring the novel object, typically in seconds. A longer time exploring the novel object suggests better recall.
- Percentage or fraction of time exploring the novel object. Generally, higher values indicate increased recognition memory. This value may be expressed in comparison to total time in the testing phase, or total time spent exploring the two objects. If only exploration time (not total test time) is in the denominator, then 50% (or 0.5) indicates that no memory of the familiar object was recalled during the testing phase.

- A **novelty discrimination index (NDI)** or **preference index**, which is a replot of the percentage time data and is calculated by:

  (time with novel object) − (time with familiar object) ÷ (total time exploring both novel + familiar objects).

  Values range from 1 to −1, with 1 indicating the animal spent the entire time engaging with the novel object, and −1 suggesting they spent the entire time with the familiar object. Higher scores suggest better familiarity memory recall. A 0 on this index means no discrimination between familiar and novel objects was observed, suggesting an impairment of memory.

Figure 2.11 shows data collected from a NORT. During training (panel A, left diagram), two objects (black squares) are introduced into the testing chamber. After a delay, one of the two objects is replaced by another (hatched circle; panel A, right diagram). Panel B shows that, with a short delay (15 minutes), both animals performed equally well. At longer delays (24 hours), the mice overexpressing a mutant tau protein (rTg4510) lost memory of the objects and could not discriminate which was old and which was new.

Interpreting the Data

Longer delay phases worsen performance on the NORT, akin to forgetting. At longer delays (greater than 10 minutes), the NORT is hippocampal-memory-dependent, since lesions disrupt performance on this task. But it is controversial how much the hippocampus is responsible for shorter delays, since these memories may be maintained by different brain structures.

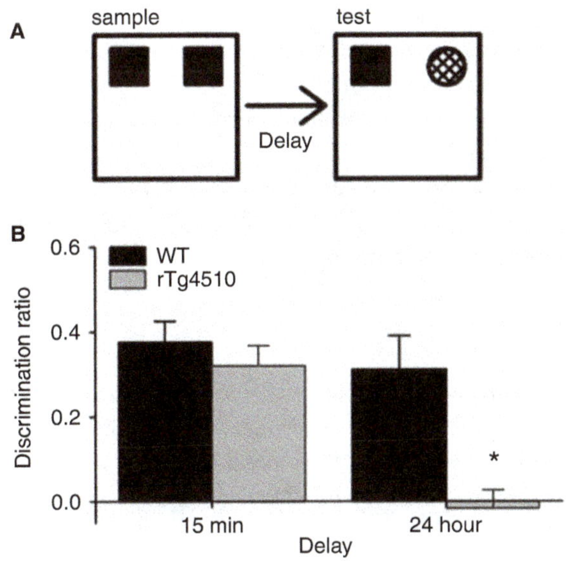

Figure 2.11 The novel object recognition test. Source: Scullion SE, Barker GRI, Warburton EC, et al. Muscarinic receptor-dependent long term depression in the perirhinal cortex and recognition memory are impaired in the rTg4510 mouse model of tauopathy. *Neurochem Res.* 2019; 44:617–626. http://creativecommons.org/licenses/by/4.0/.

Additional Resources

Ennaceur A, Delacour J. A new one-trial test for neurobiological studies of memory in rats. 1: Behavioral data. *Behav Brain Res*. 1988 Nov 1; 31(1):47–59. DOI: 10.1016/0166-4328(88)90157-x. PMID: 3228475.

Antunes M, Biala G. The novel object recognition memory: Neurobiology, test procedure, and its modifications. *Cogn Process*. 2012; 13:93–110.

2.4.3 Match-to-Sample (MTS) and Delayed-Nonmatch-to-Sample (DNMS)

Background Information

The match-to-sample (MTS) test is a paradigm for assessing working memory. In the standard MTS experiment on nonhuman primates, the animal is presented with an object placed above a small well containing a pellet of food (this is called the **baited** well). When the animal interacts with that stimulus, they receive the food. The animal is then presented with that stimulus again alongside a novel stimulus. Interacting again with the first stimulus provides the reward. Several trials (even into the hundreds) may be necessary before this memory is acquired. The memory is acquired when performance reaches a **success criterion**, which may be defined as receiving the reward in 90% of recent trials.

In a variant called the **delayed match-to-sample** test, a time window (called a **retention interval**) is allowed to pass between the training and testing. Animals tend to perform worse at longer time intervals. Delay intervals may range from tens of seconds to minutes. In the **nonmatch-to-sample test**, the animal is rewarded only when they engage with the new stimulus on testing. A **delayed nonmatch-to-sample (DNMS)** task combines both features, rewarding the animal for engaging with the novel stimulus after a delay. This is typically the most difficult variant of this task.

Different types of stimuli can be presented to form this type of memory, including visual, olfactory, and auditory stimuli.

These tests are normally done in nonhuman primates, but they have been modified for rodents, dogs, honeybees, and chickens. Many variations of these tests have been modified for humans; the test is similar to matching pairs of face-down playing cards.

Reading the Graphs

Researchers may be curious about how long it takes to learn these behaviors. These graphs plot trial number (or testing day) on the x-axis and success rate on the y-axis. Since there are only two options presented during testing, 50% is considered guessing, indicating there was no success at performing the behavior. A steeper slope suggests those animals learned the behavior faster.

Some experiments examine how long the memory persists within a single testing session. These data are plotted with increasing intervals of delay on the x-axis, while accuracy, represented as number of rewards or a percentage of successes, is plotted on the y-axis.

Sometimes the y-axis may show **trials-to-criterion**, which is the number of stimuli presentations until the animal receives the reward 90% of the time. Fewer trials-to-criterion suggests faster learning.

Figure 2.12 is a schematic of the delayed nonmatch-to-sample test. A monkey is rewarded for selecting the blue pyramid after the delay in the first trial, since it does not match the red cube sample (panel A, first test). Panel B shows data from trials with both young and aged monkeys. Aged animals (blue circles) take several more trials before they reach 90% correct nonmatches. The longer the delay, the worse the animals perform, with the deficit being more pronounced among aged animals (panel C).

Interpreting the Data

These behaviors are guided by the medial temporal lobe, the prefrontal cortex, and other cortical areas. This task is often considered similar to human declarative memory.

Using the delayed test paradigm may be a way to separate learning from recall. At shorter delays, performance on the task more meaningfully measures acquisition of the memory, while longer delays are more of an assay of retrieval of the memory. However, this interpretation may be confounded by working memory processes instead of declarative memory.

Additional Resources

Cooper CP, Shafer AT, Armstrong NM, et al. Recognition memory is associated with distinct patterns of regional gray matter volumes in young and aged monkeys. *Cereb Cortex*. 2022 Feb 19; 32(5):933–948.

2.4.4 Conditional Fear Learning

Background Information

Conditional fear learning is a paradigm used to quantify how strongly an animal gains knowledge about environmental stimuli associated with fear. In rodents, the test chamber contains a light that turns on and a speaker that plays sounds, typically pure sine-wave tones in the 3 to 12.5 kHz range. These cues are typically only present for a duration of seconds. The chamber also has a metal grid or bars on the floor that the animal grips onto with their whole paw. A painful electrical current can be delivered across the floor; this current is usually just a few milliAmps (mA) or less.

Performing the experiment consists of three phases:

1. Acclimation (or habituation). The animal is placed into the chamber and allowed to roam and explore their surroundings. During this phase, the light may turn on and at least two different tones may play. This is to eliminate the influence of novelty, since animals may change their behavior when first exposed to new environments or stimuli.
2. **Acquisition** (or training, or learning). The light cue and tone may be activated while a foot shock is delivered. A control condition presents a different stimulus without the

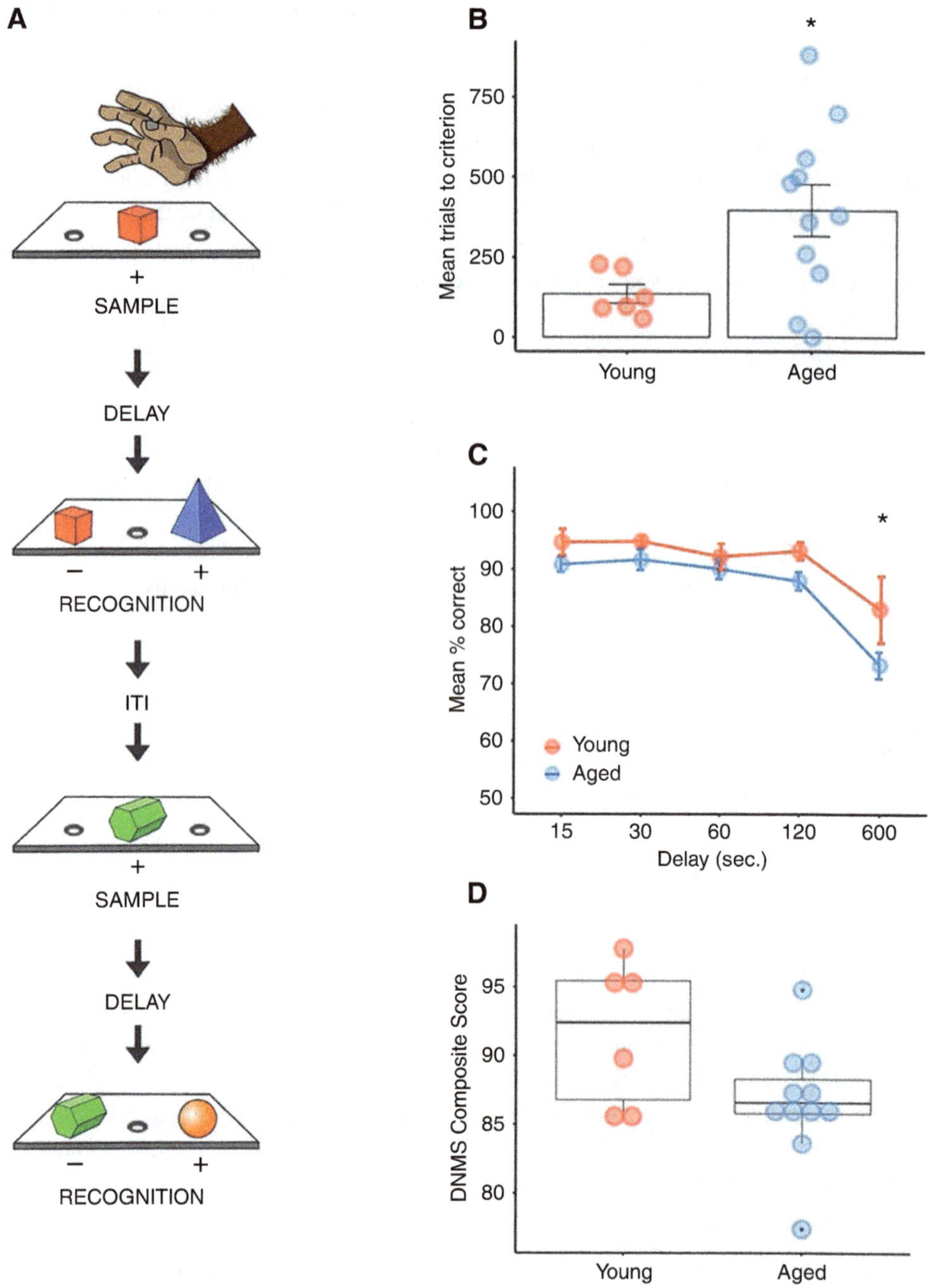

Figure 2.12 The delayed nonmatch-to-sample test. Source: Cooper CP, Shafer AT, Armstrong NM, et al. Recognition memory is associated with distinct patterns of regional gray matter volumes in young and aged monkeys. *Cereb Cortex.* 2022 Feb 19; 32(5):933–948.

foot shock. With repeat pairings of the environmental cues and the foot shock, the animal learns to associate the cues with the inevitable painful experience. This acquisition phase may take a few sessions.

3. **Testing** (or **recall**). The light and tone are presented without the foot shock. When the animal anticipates an incoming painful stimulus, they stop moving, a behavior called **freezing**. An animal with stronger fear memory will freeze longer.

A fourth step can also be performed following the testing phase called **extinction** (or relearning). Here, the light and tone are presented in the absence of foot shocks as in testing, but over several sessions, the previously learned associations weaken as the animal relearns that the stimuli no longer warn about an incoming foot shock. Usually, extinction takes more sessions than acquisition.

A control group may be a nonconditioned group, which is presented only with the tone and light but no foot shock. These are expected not to freeze during testing.

Figure 2.13 represents a foot shock test. During the habituation phase (left), the animal is given free access to the test chamber. In the training phase (middle), the sound is paired with the shock. During testing (right), the sound is played but there is no shock. Freezing is recorded.

Reading the Graphs

Summary graphs may show two different measures:

1. Behavior during testing phase with different group data plotted on the x-axis and freezing on the y-axis. Usually, freezing is expressed as a fraction or percentage of the duration of stimulus presentation. Freezing may last for up to 50%, and more freezing indicates more fear learning.
2. Behavior over multiple training sessions, with testing sessions (usually separated by days) plotted on the x-axis and time freezing on the y-axis. These graphs are helpful for showing how quickly a group learns extinction. Each curve represents data from a single group, and multiple groups are usually plotted on the same graph.

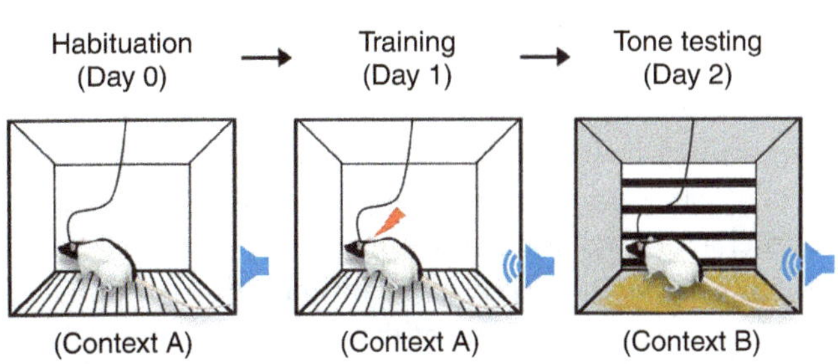

Figure 2.13 The foot shock test. Source: Zambetti PR, Schuessler BP, Lecamp BE, et al. Ecological analysis of Pavlovian fear conditioning in rats. *Commun Biol.* 2022; 5:830. http://creativecommons.org/licenses/by/4.0/. Image cropped.

Interpreting the Data

Generally, longer freezing times indicate better learning of the fear-associated stimulus.

This paradigm relies heavily on the principles of **Pavlovian** (or **classical**) conditioning. The light and sound cues are the positive conditioned stimulus (CS+) while the foot shock is the unconditioned stimulus (US). A control condition – light and tone not paired with the foot shock – is the negative conditioned stimulus (CS–). Freezing during the testing phase is the conditioned response (CR). Pavlovian learning is more implicit than declarative.

Learning on this paradigm is dependent on amygdala function, particularly of the basolateral amygdala. Lesions of amygdala, for example, block learning on the task, and animals do not freeze during the testing phase. In comparison, hippocampal or cortical lesions do not block this fear learning. Other brain circuits, such as in the prefrontal cortex and cerebellum, are also implicated in fear learning. The thalamus and sensory cortices are involved in pain processing, so these connections are also implicated in these studies.

This behavioral paradigm is used as a rodent model for post-traumatic stress disorder (PTSD). Drugs that improve PTSD in humans decrease freezing time in rodents, suggesting good predictive validity.

Pure sine-wave tones and electric foot shocks are rarely found in nature, so this test suffers from poor ethological validity.

Additional Resources

Curzon P, Rustay NR, Browman KE. Cued and contextual fear conditioning for rodents. In Buccafusco JJ, editor. *Methods of Behavior Analysis in Neuroscience*. 2nd edition. Boca Raton, FL: CRC Press/Taylor & Francis; 2009. Chapter 2. www.ncbi.nlm.nih.gov/books/NBK5223/

2.5 Mental Disorders

Mental disorders are strongly correlated with poor health outcomes and premature death. Most of them are probably influenced by both genetics and environment.

Some of the more well-known mental disorders include anxiety, depression, and substance use disorder. Anxiety affects about 7% of people worldwide with variance across cultures. Depression also has a worldwide prevalence of around 7%, with numbers reaching as high as 17% depending on age group, young adults being at the highest risk. Substance use disorder, formerly described as "drug abuse," refers to compulsive use of drugs, illicit or not. Around 15% of Americans meet the criteria for substance use disorder.

In humans, the criteria for diagnosing these conditions are outlined in the ***Diagnostic and Statistical Manual of Mental Disorders*, fifth edition** (**DSM-V** or **DSM-5**). However, in nonhumans, it is difficult to measure some of the criteria (e.g. suicidal ideation in depression) or is just not applicable (e.g. failure to fulfill obligations at work in substance use disorder). Researchers therefore developed a variety of behavioral tests to model some of the DSM-V criteria.

Because of the burden that these diseases place on individuals and society, researchers have developed nonhuman behavioral tests that can help aid in drug development. Novel antidepressants and **anxiolytics** (drugs that decrease anxiety) are often tested in nonhumans before moving to human clinical trials. On the other hand, the effect of **anxiogenics** (drugs that produce an anxiety-like state), such as caffeine or high dose THC, can also be measured using these tests.

As a major caveat to this discussion, behavioral tests only serve as a tool that models certain aspects of complex mental diseases, and do not replicate the full extent of the human condition. For example, we don't have nonhuman behavioral tests that can measure guilt, which is involved in anxiety, depression, and substance use disorder.

Additional Resources

Castagné V, Moser P, Porsolt RD. Behavioral assessment of antidepressant activity in rodents. In Buccafusco JJ, editor. *Methods of Behavior Analysis in Neuroscience*. 2nd edition. Boca Raton, FL: CRC Press/Taylor & Francis; 2009. Chapter 6. www.ncbi.nlm.nih.gov/books/NBK5222/

2.5.1 Light/Dark Box (LDB) and Elevated Plus Maze (EPM)

Background Information

These behavioral tests are used as proxy measures of anxiety-like behaviors. Generally, rodents have an innate aversion to areas they perceive as risky and will avoid these spaces. In both types of test, animal position is tracked with an overhead camera.

The **light/dark box** (LDB) is made up of two separate chambers, usually of equal size. One chamber is brightly lit, while the other is darkened. There is a small hole between the two chambers which allows the animals free movement between the chambers. On testing, the animal is usually placed in the light side of the box and given the opportunity to move back and forth. Prey animals such as rodents often avoid the brightly lit area because they are more exposed to predation.

The **elevated plus maze** (EPM) is a test apparatus placed some distance above the ground. The maze has a square platform in the center and four narrow platforms extending from the center, each of which is called an **arm**. Two opposite arms have no walls, called the **open arms**, which allows the animal to look over the edge. The other two opposite arms are surrounded by walls, and these are called the **closed arms**. During testing, the animal is placed on the center platform and allowed to move freely between any of the arms. Animals may tend to prefer the closed arms because they perceive less risk of falling.

The LDB has been adopted for other animals, including goldfish, tilapias, and zebrafish, where they show a similar avoidance of light called **scototaxis**. However, the EPM is designed for rodents, and has been adapted for mice, rats, guinea pigs, and gerbils.

Figure 2.14 shows cartoon representations of two different behavioral tests often used to measure anxiety. In both cases, more time spent in the "riskier" parts of the apparatus

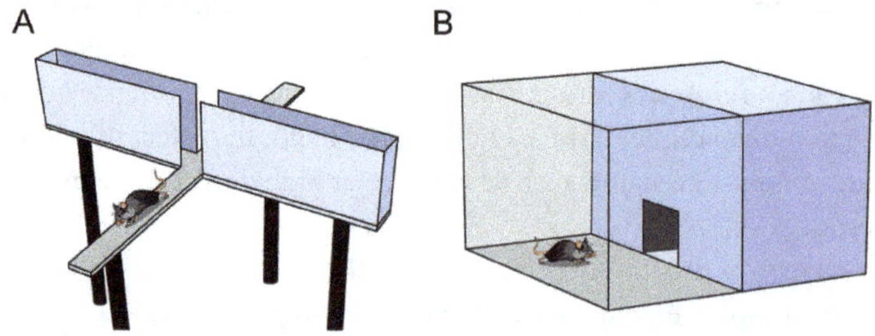

Figure 2.14 Two anxiety-testing paradigms: the elevated plus maze and the light/dark box. Source: La-Vu M, Tobias BC, Schuette PJ, Adhikari A. To approach or avoid: An introductory overview of the study of anxiety using rodent assays. *Front Behav Neurosci.* 2020; 14:145. http://creativecommons.org/licenses/by/4.0/.

indicates less anxiety. A: an elevated plus maze has two arms that are open (riskier) and two arms that are closed off. B: a light/dark box has a brightly lit chamber (riskier) and a darkened chamber, with the chambers connected by a passage.

Reading the Graphs

Representative data may show a representation of the chamber overlaid with animal movement over the duration of testing (a trace diagram). In the EPM, the closed versus open arms would be denoted in some way since the walls may not be visible in the overhead view.

Combined data may show averages from different groups on the *x*-axis. The *y*-axis may plot:

- Number (or %) of entries. Fewer entries into the light box or the open arms of the maze suggest more anxiety-like behavior. However, this number may be misleading, since an animal that spends the entire time in the risky condition (low anxiety-like behavior) may still have a small number of entries. This value does not always consider changes in locomotor activity, which is a possible confounding variable since a sluggish animal may have low entries altogether.
- Time (or % of time) spent. Groups that spend less time in the risky condition (light box or open arms) show more anxiety-like behavior.
- Mean duration per entry. This variable is a measurement of the mean number of seconds the animal remains in either the light box or the open arms.
- Number of transitions between boxes or arms. This measure controls for activity or exploratory behavior, and is ideally unaffected by changes in anxiety state.

Figure 2.15 represents data from an experiment in which the circadian rhythms of mice were disrupted before they were placed in the EPM. They entered the open arm less frequently (left graph) and spent less time there (right graph) than the control group, indicating increased anxiety-like behaviors.

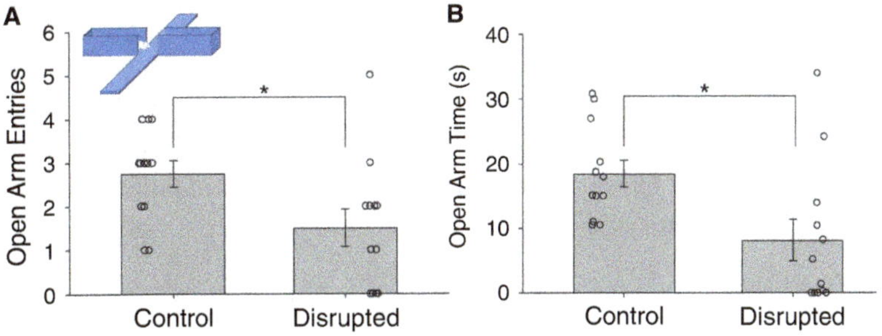

Figure 2.15 The elevated plus maze and circadian rhythm disruption. Source: Ameen RW, Warshawski A, Fu L, et al. Early life circadian rhythm disruption in mice alters brain and behavior in adulthood. *Sci Rep.* 2022; 12:7366. http://creativecommons.org/licenses/by/4.0/.

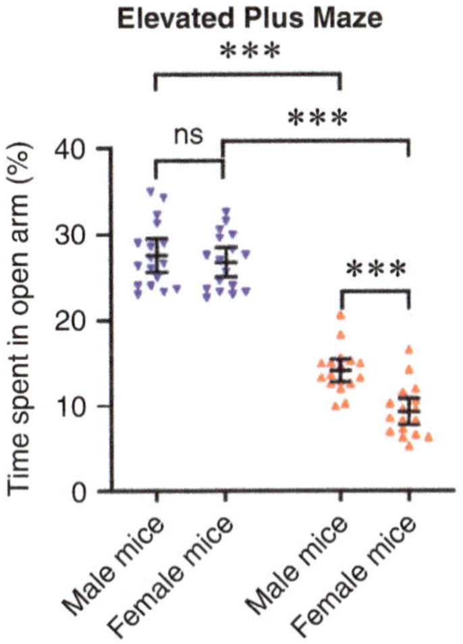

Figure 2.16 The elevated plus maze, physical stress, and gender. Source: Ghosh S, Mohammed, Z, Singh I. Bruton's tyrosine kinase drives neuroinflammation and anxiogenic behavior in mouse models of stress. *J Neuroinflammation.* 2021; 18:289. http://creativecommons.org/licenses/by/4.0/. Image cropped.

Figure 2.16 shows a comparison between the behavior of male and female mice that have been physically stressed before being placed in the EPM. The percentage of time spent in open arms was the same in the control group of mice, both male and female (blue triangles), and was around 30% of the testing time. The physically stressed animals (red triangles) showed a decrease in open arm time, suggesting heightened anxiety (right two groups compared to left two groups). This effect was stronger in female mice compared to male mice (right-most group compared to second-to-right-most group).

Interpreting the Data

The classic experiments using these paradigms on rodents demonstrated that benzodiazepines increase the time spent in the light chamber or on the open arms. These drugs, which include diazepam, are commonly prescribed in humans as anxiolytics, which suggests strong predictive validity. On the other hand, there is an anxiogenic effect of physical, psychosocial, or prenatal stress, which decreases time spent in the light chamber or on the open arms.

Additional Resources

Bourin M, Hascoët M. The mouse light/dark box test. *Anim Models Anxiety Disord.* 2003; 463(1):55–65.

Kraeuter AK, Guest PC, Sarnyai Z. The elevated plus maze test for measuring anxiety-like behavior in rodents. *Methods Mol Biol.* 2019; 1916:69–74.

2.5.2 Tail Suspension Test (TST) and Forced Swim Test (FST; also called Porsolt Test)

Background Information

One of the clinical symptoms of depression in humans is despair, a feeling of hopelessness about one's circumstances. The tail suspension test and forced swim test are two different rodent models of despair or resignation.

In the **tail suspension test (TST)**, a rodent is suspended upside down by the tail (maybe by a piece of adhesive tape) above a safe surface. Since this position is uncomfortable, the animal struggles to right itself. The animal remains here on the order of minutes. When the animal stops its movement for longer than 2 seconds, this is considered a sign of despair, and the time spent immobile is measured.

In the **forced swim test (FST**; also called the **Porsolt test**), the animal is placed into a narrow (between 10 and 30 cm in diameter) cylinder that has been partially filled with water. Animals are tested for minutes in each trial. Typically, animals will at first kick their legs to stay afloat, while longer time spent immobile suggests despair.

The FST has been adapted for Drosophila.

Reading the Graphs

Data from the TST and FST are typically presented as summary graphs with group data plotted on the *x*-axis.

The *y*-axis usually plots time spent (or % time) immobile. Longer immobility time suggests they are experiencing depressive-like behavior. Treatments that decrease immobility time are suspected to have antidepressant effects.

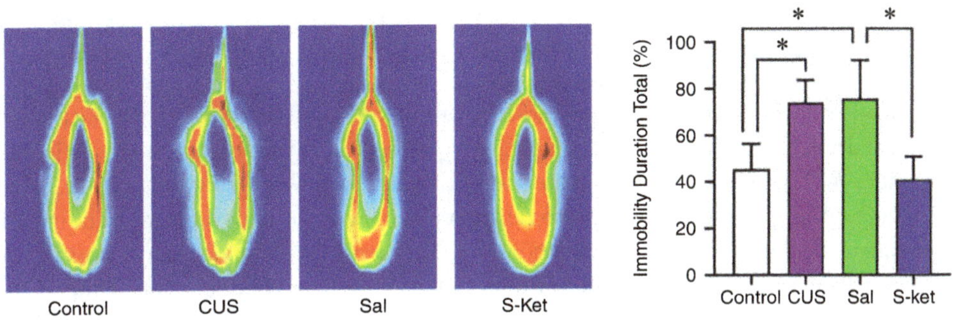

Figure 2.17 The tail suspension test. Source: Hou L, Miao J, Meng H, et al. Sirtuin type 1 mediates the antidepressant effect of S-ketamine in a chronic unpredictable stress model. *Front Psychiatry.* 2022; 13:855810. https://creativecommons.org/licenses/by/4.0/. Image cropped.

A heat map may also be used to represent the TST, as shown in Figure 2.17 (left four images). The heat map shows the movement of a mouse in the tail suspension test, where red indicates more movement. Mice that have been exposed to chronic unpredictable stress (CUS) or injected with saline (Sal) spend more time immobile, while exposure to ketamine (S-Ket) reverses the immobility caused by the CUS. The bar graph on the right plots these data.

Interpreting the Data

These tests of despair are also used to measure the depressive aspect of models for **bipolar disorder**, a human disease characterized by alternating periods of depression and mania (elevated mood state and hyperactivity).

As a potential confounding variable, both the TST and the FST induce a stress response.

The correlation between freezing behavior, the main observable variable on these assays, and depression is controversial. Freezing response may be a coping mechanism to conserve energy rather than an expression of despair.

In people with depression, treatment with antidepressant drugs usually goes on for weeks before a clinical improvement is noticed. By contrast, acute exposure to antidepressants in the rodent quickly improves their performance on either of these tests. Therefore, these tests may have limited predictive validity.

Additional Resources

Steru L, Chermat R, Thierry B, et al. The tail suspension test: A new method for screening antidepressants in mice. *Psychopharmacol.* 1985; 85:367–370.

Molendijk ML, de Kloet ER. Coping with the forced swim stressor: Current state-of-the-art. *Behav Brain Res.* 2019; 364:1–10. DOI: 10.1016/j.bbr.2019.02.005.

2.5.3 Two-Bottle Free Choice (2BC, TBC) Test and Sucrose Preference Test

Background Information

The **two-bottle free choice test** is used to evaluate animal preference for, or dislike of, two different drinks. Their test cage is equipped with two bottles. Animals are placed singly into the test cage and given time to habituate to drinking standard water from the two bottles. In a testing session, the contents of one bottle are replaced with the experimental solution. On subsequent testing sessions, the positions of the experimental and control bottles are switched back and forth to prevent an effect of conditioning. The amount of liquid the animal drinks from each bottle is then quantified. The experiment may be performed for several days (up to 20).

This paradigm is mainly used in research to answer questions about substance use; the most common is ethanol, the psychoactive ingredient of alcohol, since it is consumed as a liquid. Other drugs, including nicotine and morphine, can also be studied in this paradigm. As a drug administration paradigm, the two-bottle free choice test can also be used to study different elements of substance use, including decision making, motivation, withdrawal, the effect of other substances that increase or decrease drug taking, and the influence of genetics or early experiences on drug seeking.

The paradigm can also be used to study the process of chemoreception and taste, such as in experiments to see how deleting certain genes changes preference scores toward specific flavor profiles.

Modifications to the test include:

- Limited access by including the experimental solution only once every other day, or only during the animal's light (or dark) phase.
- Access to more than two bottles, perhaps to evaluate a preference for specific concentrations of substance.
- A **sucrose preference test**, where one bottle is filled with a solution of up to 5% sucrose. A decrease in preference toward sucrose may be indicative of **anhedonia**, a lack of pleasure, which is one of the symptoms for diagnosing depression in people.

Percentages of solutions may be written as **v/v**, which refers to volume per 100 ml (volume) of water; this is common when mixing liquid with liquid, such as in ethanol administration. Doses vary between experiments and may be ramped up over the course of testing days.

Figure 2.18 presents group data from a two-bottle free choice test in which the SorCS2 knockout mice (red traces and bar) drank less ethanol (EtOH, measured in grams per hour per gram of body weight) than the wild type control mice (black traces and bar). The SorCS2 protein forms complexes with receptors such as TrkB that are involved in plasticity, suggesting that learning may be involved in EtOH preference.

Experimenters may choose to add **adulterants** to the water, which are chemicals that change the flavor of the liquid. This is common to promote the consumption of bitter-tasting compounds, such as morphine water. Frequently used adulterants include sucrose or saccharin, which make a drink more palatable and therefore more preferred. On the other hand, adulterants

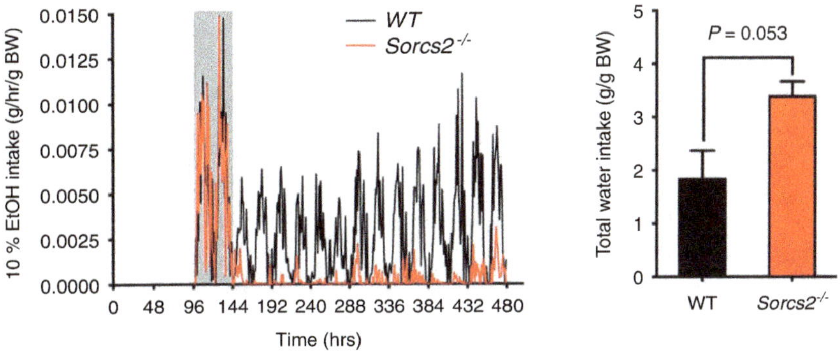

Figure 2.18 The two-bottle free choice test. Source: Olsen D, Kaas M, Lundhede J, et al. Reduced alcohol seeking and withdrawal symptoms in mice lacking the BDNF Receptor SorCS2. *Front Pharmacol.* 2019; 10:499. https://creativecommons.org/licenses/by/4.0/. Image cropped, text labels replaced, panels reorganized.

may be used to discourage drinking; commonly **quinine**, the bitter ingredient found in tonic water, is used. As a caveat, adulterants can inherently change preference toward the drink (sucrose is intrinsically rewarding, for example), so they are usually added into the control bottle as well.

These tests are easily modified for nonhuman primates. In Drosophila, a similar test is called the **capillary feeding assay (CAFE)**.

Reading the Graphs

In summary graphs showing long-term changes in preference, the *x*-axis plots time over multiple days of testing, where each data point represents the average daily consumption of the experimental solution. If the concentration of the substance is changed over the course of the experiment, the dosages may be indicated as overlaying text.

There are a few different variables that can be measured to represent the amount of substance consumed on the *y*-axis.

- Lick total, a measurement collected by liquid containers called **lickometers**. The data may report absolute number of licks or the ratio between licks of experimental solution versus control solution.
- Liquid intake or consumption, determined through daily measurements of the remaining solution. This variable is typically measured in units of milliliters per kilogram of animal body weight each day (ml/kg/day). The mass of the liquid consumed can also be reported (measured in grams instead of milliliters).
- Relative preference, represented as a percentage (or fraction), where 100% (or 1) indicates that the animal drank only from the experimental solution. 50% (or 0.5) indicates no preference for experimental solution versus control. This measure normalizes for overall liquid consumption but does not show absolute values of how much liquid was drunk.

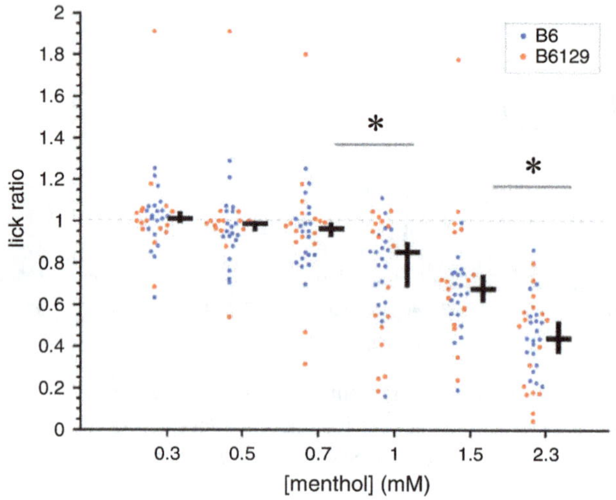

Figure 2.19 Aversive response in a two-bottle choice test. Source: Lemon CH, Norris JE, Heldmann BA. The TRPA1 ion channel contributes to sensory-guided avoidance of menthol in mice. *eNeuro.* 2019 17 Oct; 6(6). ENEURO.0304-19.2019. https://creativecommons.org/licenses/by/4.0/.

In the data shown in Figure 2.19, the adulterant menthol is aversive, as indicated by a lick ratio less than 1 (below the dashed line) in both the B6 and the B6129 strains of mice (blue and red dots). This aversion is dose-dependent, as higher concentrations (right on the *x*-axis) result in lower lick ratios.

Total fluid intake, the sum of experimental and control liquids consumed, is an important control variable, especially when a treatment causes thirst or has a **diuretic** (increasing urine output) effect.

Another important control is to prepare a cage containing two bottles filled with experimental and control liquids, but no animal. Sipper tubes may leak liquids over time due to gravity or lose volume to evaporation, which represents a decrease of liquid not consumed by the animal. These control data may be subtracted from the measured amount to provide a more accurate measurement of consumption.

Interpreting the Data

Generally, more consumption of a solution indicates preference, while decreased consumption indicates dislike.

Because almost all ethanol use in people is through oral administration, this assay suggests good ethological validity. However, other drugs tested using this behavioral paradigm such as nicotine or morphine are not commonly taken orally by humans. The **route of administration** (how the drug enters the body) has a huge effect on how the drug influences the body, with oral administration being one of the slower routes. In these cases, low ethological validity may be a weakness of this paradigm.

Additional Resources

Frie JA, Khokhar JY. An open source automated two-bottle choice test apparatus for rats. *HardwareX*. 2019 Apr; 5:e00061.

2.5.4 Self-Administration and Intracranial Self-Stimulation (ICSS)

Background Information

Self-administration is an **operant conditioning** (also called **instrumental conditioning**, or **Skinnerian conditioning**) learning paradigm that is used to assess how much an animal is willing to work for a rewarding stimulus. The animal is trained to interact with some **operant**, such as pressing a lever or poking their nose into an opening called a **port**. Following this behavioral response, the animal receives the rewarding stimulus. Commonly, a set of cues are associated with the operant, such as presentation of a light or a sound. After a reinforcer is delivered, a post-reinforcement pause (or **lockout**) is enforced where further responding does not provide reward. The testing session may last up to an hour.

Primary rewards are biologically rewarding stimuli that do not require much training. These include food, drink, social interaction, sex, and certain commonly misused drugs. For food rewards, interacting with the operant may cause a food pellet to fall into a trough (or a receptacle, or **magazine**) or otherwise easily accessible chamber. For liquid rewards, the animal may be equipped with a direct cheek tube that delivers a small amount of the liquid directly into the mouth. In studying substance use, an operant response might deliver the drug to the animal intravenously via an indwelling catheter driven by a pump. Alternatively, the drug dissolved in liquid may be infused directly into a specific area, such as into the ventricles (**intraventricular**) or into brain areas (**intracranial**).

A closely related paradigm, **intracranial self-stimulation** (**ICSS**), involves the installation of a stimulating probe into the brain. Interacting with the operant causes direct electrical stimulation of that brain area. Optogenetics can also be used in ICSS: light-sensitive proteins can be expressed selectively in brain populations, and an intracranial indwelling fiberoptic cable can deliver light in response to operant engagement.

A primary reward or the stimulation of a rewarding brain circuit can also be called a **reinforcer**.

An **inactive** operant or delivery of a control substance should also be available to the animal to eliminate the effects of boredom leading to increased activity, curiosity regarding the engagement with the operant, the novelty of the sounds associated with reward delivery such as activation of the infusion pump in IV drug self-administration, or the sensation of increased blood volume in IV self-administration.

Figure 2.20 shows an operant conditioning box, with nose-poke holes and lights on the wall and the food trough in the center (panel C). The tether at the top (panel B) allows the animal the freedom to move around the chamber.

Table 2.1 Types of reward delivery schedules

	Interval (delivery based on responding after a specified time interval)	Ratio (delivery based on a specified number of operant responses)
Fixed (predictable delivery of reinforcer)	Fixed interval (FIX)	Fixed ratio (FRX)
Variable (less predictable delivery of reinforcer)	Variable interval (VIX)	Variable ratio (VRX)

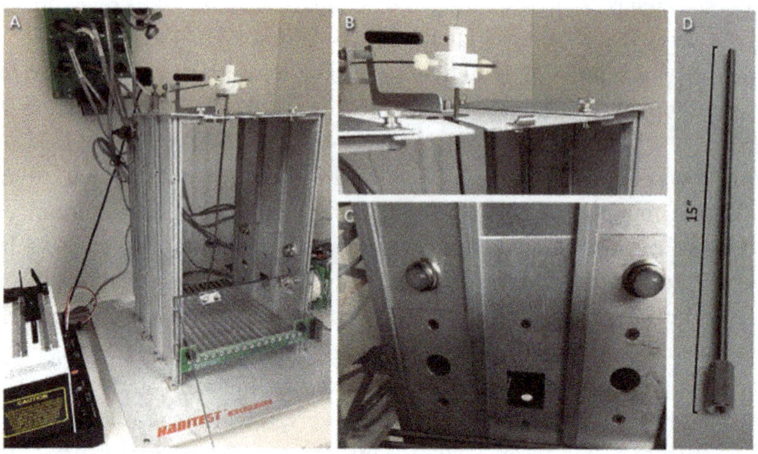

Figure 2.20 A self-administration chamber with food as reward. Source: Valles G, Huebschman JL, Chow E, et al. Jugular vein catheter design and cocaine self-administration using mice: A comprehensive method. *Front Behav Neurosci.* 2022 Jun 15; 16:880845. https://creativecommons.org/licenses/by/4.0/.

Rewards are delivered on different schedules, as shown in Table 2.1. Some schedules depend on the number of operant responses (ratio), while others depend on the passing of time (interval). Some schedules have no randomness built into the delivery of reward (fixed), while others introduce some aspect of probability (variable). X indicates a number (time interval or number of responses) after which the delivery of reward takes place.

Interval schedules are usually in minutes, so an FI5 would mean that the first operant response after 5 minutes have passed will result in delivery of a reward. A VI5 means that an operant response will lead to reinforcer delivery on average once every 5 minutes.

For ratio schedules, X is the number of operant responses. An FR5 would mean that the reinforcer would be delivered every 5 responses. A VR5 means that an operant response will lead to reinforcer delivery on average once every 5 operant responses.

A **progressive ratio (PR)** schedule may also be used. Progressive ratio schedules use a geometric growth formula to calculate how many operant responses are necessary before the delivery of reward. An example PR formula may be as follows:

Number of operant responses needed for next delivery (rounded up) = $[5e^{(R\times0.2)}] - 5$ where R is the number of past reinforcers delivered plus 1. Under this progressive ratio, the reinforcers are delivered after the first, second, third, fourth, ninth, etc., response on the operant.

Each of these delivery schedules produces slightly different patterns of responding. Generally, VR schedules produce the most robust responding on the operant.

Extinction can also be measured using this self-administration paradigm. In extinction, the animal can interact with the operants and is exposed to all associated cues, but no reward is delivered. Extinction may last for several days, during which time responding on the drug-paired operant decreases gradually. After extinction, the operant may become active again, and the reward may then be delivered; this session is called **reinstatement**. Animals often respond highly during reinstatement.

These studies are done in both humans and nonhumans. In nonmammalian studies, self-administration is usually done via a choice assay, where the animal simply selects one stimulus over another, but these paradigms are not considered operant conditioning.

Reading the Graphs

Since experiments are often repeated over the course of several days, the *x*-axis plots consecutive days or testing sessions.

The *y*-axis plots the number of reinforcers delivered or operant responses. In progressive ratio schedules, these values may also be called the **break point**, which represents the number of responses when the animal is no longer willing to work for a single infusion. Because of the progressive ratio formula, break point responses correspond to exponentially increasing operant responses, so it takes many more responses to receive the reinforcer at high break points.

Responding on both the active and inactive operants may be plotted on the same graph. Inactive operant responses are generally lower than the active operant. During extinction testing, responding on the (formerly) active lever decreases to the level of inactive responding.

The data represented in Figure 2.21 show that, during extinction, animals that had been trained to lever-press for methamphetamine (filled circles) pressed less when they no longer received the reward.

Interpreting the Data

If the number of reinforcers delivered under a certain circumstance are higher, this indicates the animal wants the reinforcer more; smaller numbers indicate the animal is less willing to "work" for the reinforcer.

Interventions that decrease the willingness to work for a substance result in less operant responding. Alternatively, different genetic populations may have differences in rates of use.

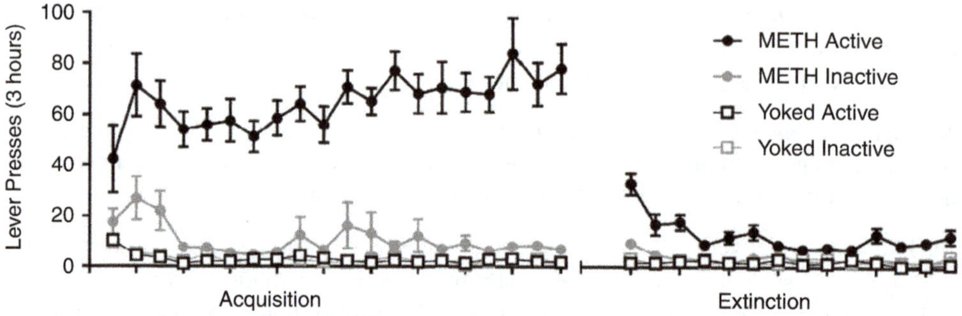

Figure 2.21 A self-administration chamber delivering methamphetamine. Source: Robinson KJ, Everett NA, Baracz SJ, et al. The effect of self-administered methamphetamine on GABAergic interneuron populations and functional connectivity of the nucleus accumbens and prefrontal cortex. *Psychopharmacol.* 2022; 239:2903–2919. http://creativecommons.org/licenses/by/4.0/. Image cropped and text labels removed.

Extinction and reinstatement can be considered learning processes, as both forgetting (the operant no longer provides reward) and relearning (the operant gives reward again) are components of memory. Extinction may be analogous to the human condition of drug-seeking or drug-wanting during withdrawal or abstinence.

Additional Resources

Banks ML, Czoty PW, Negus SS. Utility of nonhuman primates in substance use disorders research. *ILAR J.* 2017 Dec 1; 58(2):202–215.

2.5.5 Conditioned Place Preference and Conditioned Place Aversion

Background Information

Conditioned place preference (CPP) and **conditioned place aversion** (CPA) are tests used to quantify how much an animal likes (CPP) or dislikes (CPA) a condition or substance. This paradigm is based on the principles of Pavlovian (or classical) conditioning: an animal that likes a particular feeling forms an association with the specific environmental cues, and will voluntarily choose to spend more time in those surroundings if given the chance. On the other hand, CPA is observed when an animal that dislikes the feeling avoids those cues.

The test apparatus has two different chambers. Each chamber has unique environmental cues, such as different-colored walls (light, dark, specific colors, stripes) or flooring material (bedding, a cross-grid, a series of bars). Some CPP devices have a neutral middle chamber that contains no significant environmental cues, which serves as a hallway to connect the two chambers. There is also a door that can be dropped in from the top, which is to restrict movement of animals between the chambers. CPP chambers are equipped with

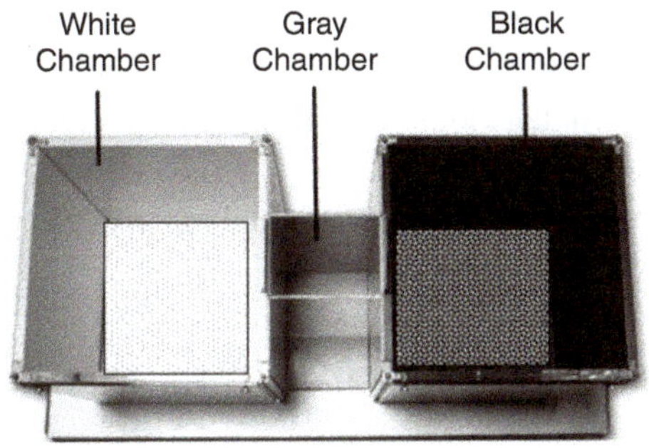

Figure 2.22 The conditioned place preference chamber. Source: Webber-Waugh A, Thaxter Nesbeth K, Anderson-Johnson P, et al. Drug seeking behavior of amphetamine addicted Sprague-Dawley rats is eliminated after nutritional supplementation. *J Behav Brain Sci.* 2017; 7:585–597. http://creativecommons.org/licenses/by/4.0/. Text labels have been replaced.

the capacity to measure either movement or animal location, possibly using an overhead video recording of animal movement or counts of infrared beam breaks.

Figure 2.22 shows a three-chambered conditioned place preference box containing a light side (left), a neutral chamber (middle), and a dark chamber (right). The test is performed in three different phases or sessions.

1. The first is the acclimation phase (also called habituation phase), where the animal is removed from their home cage and given time to explore all chambers of the CPP apparatus. In this phase, even without conditioning, some animals may have an intrinsic aversion to the light side and will be likely to avoid it (as in a light/dark box setting: see Section 2.5.1).
2. In the **conditioning phase** (sometimes also called a **training** or **learning phase**), the animal is treated with the experimental manipulation and then is placed into their least preferred room as determined by the acclimation period. The doors are lowered, and they are restricted to this room and cannot move between the chambers. In a following training session, the animal is treated with the control manipulation and is then restricted to the other chamber. These learning sessions may be repeated, generally with fewer than 5 pairings of each condition. In a three-room apparatus, the middle chamber is unpaired with any treatment. It is common to pair the light chamber with a preferred treatment, which would require the animal to overcome their dislike of the light chamber.
3. In the **preference testing phase**, the animal is not treated with any manipulation. They are placed in one of the chambers (or the middle neutral chamber) and are free to move between the chambers. The location or movement of the animal is measured during the course of the test. Trials typically last on the order of minutes to tens of minutes.

Common manipulations include injection of a drug the animal finds rewarding, such as psychostimulants (e.g. cocaine). An injection of saline is the most common control for this manipulation. Optogenetic manipulations can also be performed, where some light-sensitive ion channels have been introduced into specific neural circuits using a viral vector and a fiberoptic cable is permanently implanted into the brain. The circuits can then be activated during the conditioning phase when paired with one chamber. Injection of a vector that carries only a fluorescent tag along with the indwelling fiberoptic cable is an appropriate control for these experiments.

Many subjects exhibit CPP in the laboratory, including *C. elegans*, fish, rodents, nonhuman primates, and people.

Reading the Graphs

Sample traces may be shown, depicting an overhead view of the chamber and the animal's location as a trail during the testing session (akin to a trace diagram, as described in Section 2.2.1). These graphs show a summary of animal movement over the duration of the session. A higher density of lines in one chamber than the other indicates a stronger preference for that chamber (or an aversion to the other chamber), while equal density of lines indicate no change in preference.

An alternative to showing the trace diagram is a heat map of animal location. Usually, cooler colors (blues) indicate less time spent in that specific area, while warmer colors (reds) indicate more time spent in that area and suggest preference.

CPP/CPA data can be summarized in different ways. Nearly all of them will plot treatment groups on the *x*-axis. Some may plot the effect as a "before-and-after," showing data from the acclimation phase followed by data from the preference testing phase. In a plot showing before-and-after, data points from the same animal will be connected by a left-to-right line. A completely horizontal line indicates no change in preference for that animal.

Time spent in the manipulation-paired chamber (also called dwell time) during the testing phase may be plotted on the *y*-axis. The values depend on the duration of the trials but will often be on the order of hundreds of seconds to minutes. More time spent suggests stronger preference.

Some graphs convert time spent into percent time spent in the conditioned chamber, calculated by this formula: time spent in conditioned chamber ÷ total time × 100. This data can also be represented as a fraction, with values ranging from 0 to 1. When plotted over multiple sessions, a dashed line may be drawn horizontally at the 50% or 0.5 mark, which indicates no preference or aversion. Scores higher than 50% (or 0.5 if a fraction is plotted) represent preference, while scores less than 50% indicate aversion.

In Figure 2.23, the representative heat map shows animal location in warmer colors (here, light blue in comparison to dark blue) in a three-chamber CPP testing apparatus. Experimenters tested whether infusion of an active monoclonal antibody (mAb) or a control antibody (IgG) produced a CPP in a model of neuropathic pain, the partial transection of the infraorbital nerve (p-IONx). In the sham-operated mice, neither mAb nor IgG treatment produced a preference. However, a preference was observed for the mAb-paired chamber (upper chamber) in the p-IONX mice (right), suggesting that the active mAb relieved the pain.

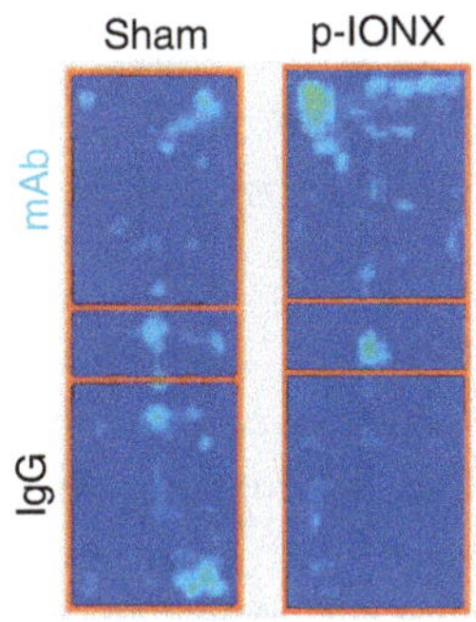

Figure 2.23 Heat map of conditioned place preference. Source: Du Y, Xu CL, Yu J, et al. HMGB1 in the mPFC governs comorbid anxiety in neuropathic pain. *J Headache Pain*. 2022; 23:102. http://creativecommons.org/licenses/by/4.0/. Image cropped.

Other graphs plot a conditioned place preference score (or preference index) which is commonly calculated by this formula: time spent in the conditioned chamber minus time spent in the neutral chamber. These units will be in seconds, and may be labeled **delta time spent**. Positive values represent a preference, while negative values represent an aversion. A score of zero indicates no preference or aversion, and zero is expected for the negative control conditions.

Data are presented differently when *C. elegans* are used as the model. In these experiments, the word **chemotaxis** may be used, which refers to how the animal's movement is influenced by the presence of chemicals. Groups are usually on the *x*-axis. The number of animals that prefer one side of the lawn is plotted along the *y*-axis. Alternatively, the fraction or percentage of animals on one side of the lawn, which might be labeled as a chemotaxis index, may be plotted on the *y*-axis. A higher chemotaxis index (closer to 1) suggests a preference toward the experimental section of the lawn, while 0 represents no preference.

Interpreting the Data

In Pavlovian terms, the paired chamber is the **conditioned stimulus** (**CS+**), the unpaired chamber is the CS−, and spending more time in the paired chamber during testing is a **conditioned response** (**CR**).

These behavioral tests also have a memory component, since the animal must recall the environment in which the drug effect was felt. Pavlovian memories are more implicit than they are declarative.

Additional Resources

McKendrick G, Graziane NM. Drug-induced conditioned place preference and its practical use in substance use disorder research. *Front Behav Neurosci*. 2020 Sep 29; 14:582147.

2.6 Social Behaviors

Most experimental animals, rodents and primates especially, are social animals that engage in complex behaviors toward other members of their species. Social interaction has various functions:

- It conveys valuable survival information. Honeybees (*Apis mellifera*) perform a waggle dance after returning from an expeditionary trip to inform hive-mates about where a food source is located and how much food it contains. Ants release different chemical signals (pheromones), some of which warn nearby ants about predator location.
- It promotes animal hygiene. Monkeys inspect the fur of fellow monkeys to help them remove harmful parasites such as ticks and fleas. Self-cleaning of fur can help maintain body temperature and decrease stress.
- It encourages physical and psychological growth. **Rough and tumble play** is a set of behaviors such as tickling, pouncing, and wrestling, and is most often observed in juvenile males across several species of mammals from humans to rodents. From an evolutionary perspective, rough and tumble play might promote success in finding mates during adolescence.

Many social behaviors are innate and can be learned through normal exposure to others of the species. Expression of social behaviors is sensitive to many variables, including the animal's mental and physical state as well as their development.

Additional Resources

Kim SW, Kim M, Shin HS. Affective empathy and prosocial behavior in rodents. *Curr Opin Neurobiol*. 2021 Jun; 68:181–189.

Panadeiro V, Rodriguez A, Henry J, et al. A review of 28 free animal-tracking software applications: Current features and limitations. *Lab Anim*. 2021; 50:246–254.

2.6.1 Ultrasonic Vocalizations

Background Information

Ultrasonic vocalizations (USVs) are communicative calls used by rodents. These specific calls are vocal sounds in the range of 30,000 to 110,000 Hz (more commonly written as 30–110 kilohertz, kHz). These pitches are above the hearing range of humans and other predators, suggesting that USVs have been selected for by evolutionary pressures to remain undetectable in the face of danger.

USVs serve a variety of social communicative functions.

- Pups emit USVs when they are socially isolated or cold, perhaps as a call to attract attention from the mother.
- Adults emit USVs when they encounter strangers of their own species, perhaps as a show of aggression, to enforce territoriality, or to establish a social hierarchy.
- Adults also emit USVs as part of courtship and during mating.

Outside of communicative USVs, changes in USVs are also observed in nonhuman models of autism, which may parallel deficits in communication in autism. USVs are also studied in the context of sensorimotor processes and are affected in neurodegeneration and aging.

Most studies examining USVs are done in rats and mice, but many other rodents also emit USVs, including hamsters, gerbils, and voles.

A standard audio recording system includes a microphone placed above the lid of the cage combined with a camera system to accurately attribute sounds from multiple animals in the same cage.

Reading the Graphs

Occasionally, sample audio **waveforms** are shown. The *x*-axis shows time, and the *y*-axis shows the amplitude of the sound. These graphs can show information about amplitude (volume), vocalization duration, and intervals between vocalizations, but they cannot meaningfully show information about specific frequencies unless the data have been filtered to show those frequencies.

A more common way to display sample recordings is with a **spectrogram** (also called **sonogram**). Spectrograms display time on the *x*-axis, usually on the scale of tens to hundreds of milliseconds. The *y*-axis plots frequency, with a range that might run from 0 at the bottom to 110 kHz at the top. The third component shown on a spectrogram is signal intensity, or USV loudness, which might range from −60 to −30 decibels (dB). Spectrograms can be in grayscale or in color. In grayscale, the background is white and higher signal intensity is represented by darker shades. In color spectrograms, the background is black or blue and the signal intensity is represented on a color spectrum, where redder shades indicate higher intensity.

The spectrogram in Figure 2.24 shows the passage of time (left to right, top to bottom, in seconds), and the frequency of each vocalization is plotted on the *y*-axis. Darker signals

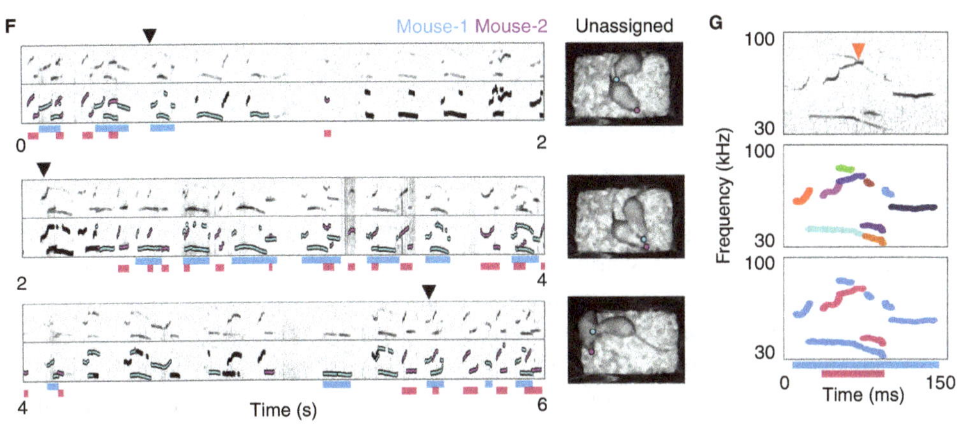

Figure 2.24 Spectrogram of ultrasonic vocalization. Source: Matsumoto J, Kanno K, Kato M, et al. Acoustic camera system for measuring ultrasound communication in mice. *iScience*. 2022; 25(8). http://creativecommons.org/licenses/by/4.0/.

indicate louder vocalization. The recording device is able to differentiate the sounds coming from two different mice in the same cage, one mouse's sounds shown in blue and the other's in purple.

Several features may be extracted from the spectrograms and shown in a summary graph:

- Number of USVs per unit time. Total USVs may be further subdivided by ethologically relevant frequencies, such as 22 kHz or 50 kHz calls.
- Syllables and cadence. A USV longer than 2 ms with more than 10 ms between USVs count as a syllable. The number of syllables per bout may also be reported.
- Signal maxima. Some maximum values that may be reported include amplitude (or intensity, or volume) and frequency.
- Patterns of vocalizations. Many groups name the USVs based on the shape that appears on the spectrogram, with names such as ramp, trill, inverted-U, or chevron, among others.

Interpreting the Data

Adult rats emit two clearly discernible categories of USVs. The **22 kHz call** indicates an aversive state, emitted by a rat experiencing social defeat or anxiety, being exposed to predators or unknown threats, and during drug withdrawal. On the other hand, the **50 kHz call** is indicative of a rewarding state, emitted during positive experiences such as play and sexual contact.

Additional Resources

Brudzynski SM. Biological functions of rat ultrasonic vocalizations, arousal mechanisms, and call initiation. *Brain Sci.* 2021; 11(5):605. https://doi.org/10.3390/brainsci11050605 20–125kHz

2.6.2 Partner Preference Paradigm

Background Information

Unlike most mammals, **prairie voles** (*Microtus ochrogaster*) in the wild exhibit **social monogamy**, the behavior of sharing living space and parental duties after mating. This complex behavioral trait, also called **pair bonding**, can be measured and observed in the laboratory using a **partner preference paradigm**.

The behavioral apparatus consists of three chambers. Prior to behavioral testing, opposite-sex prairie voles are paired for 24 hours, enough time for mating to take place. (In a related paradigm involving voles of the same sex, the partners are called **peers**.) During testing, one of the **partner** (or **mated**) **voles** is tethered via a leash or harness to one of the end chambers. A third vole, who has never met either of the pair, is tethered to the other end chamber. This unpaired vole serves as a control for social interaction. The leash is short enough that neither vole can leave their chambers. The chamber in the middle is a neutral room; this is where the other paired vole is placed. The movement and location of this vole is then observed and tracked via an overhead camera. The testing period typically lasts on the order of a few hours.

This behavioral test has been modified for other rodents, including mice and gerbils. Since social monogamy is not the norm among mammals, most other animals do not show a strong preference for their partners.

Reading the Graphs

Summary graphs usually only show data collected from a single testing period, with different groups plotted across the x-axis. The y-axis may plot:

- Time the untethered vole spends in each chamber. Data from all three chambers (neutral, paired, and unpaired) may be plotted here. If a partner preference is formed, the untethered vole will spend more time with the previously mated vole compared to the neutral room or the unmated vole.
- **Partner preference index**. These data summarize the time spent in each chamber normalized to time. The index is calculated by this formula: time spent with partner vole − time spent with stranger vole ÷ total time spent interacting. Values range from 1 to −1, with numbers closer to 1 suggesting partner preference. A 0 suggests no preference between voles. This index controls for social interaction and ignores time spent in the third chamber.
- Time spent **huddling** (or **huddling counts**) with other voles. Huddling is side-by-side contact that partner voles are more likely to display compared to strangers. Higher huddling times (or counts) are expected if a preference has been formed.

Figure 2.25 is a side view of a partner preference testing chamber. This design allows for interaction with either the partner or the stranger vole, but no huddling. The box and whiskers plot quantification shows a statistically significant increase in time spent with the partner compared to the stranger vole.

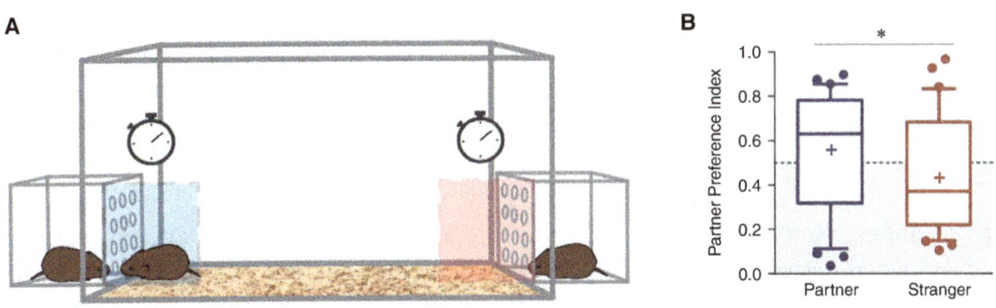

Figure 2.25 The partner preference paradigm. Source: Fernanda López-Gutiérrez M, Gracia-Tabuenca Z, Ortiz JJ, et al. Brain functional networks associated with social bonding in monogamous voles. *eLife*. 2021; 10:e55081. http://creativecommons.org/licenses/by/4.0/.

Interpreting the Data

This test has been used to determine which neurohormone signals are implicated in vole social monogamy. Using chemicals that either block or mimic neurohormones, it was discovered that both vasopressin and oxytocin are involved in the formation of partner preference. The test has also shown that commonly misused drugs such as alcohol and amphetamine modify partner preference.

Additional Resources

Beery AK. Familiarity and mate preference assessment with the partner preference test. *Curr Protoc*. 2021 Jun; 1(6):e173. DOI:10.1002/cpz1.173.PMID:34152696;PMCID: PMC8221176

2.7 Survival Analysis: Kaplan–Meier Curve and Cumulative Risk Curve

Background Information

The **Kaplan–Meier curve** is a graphical representation of a **survival analysis**. While "survival" might seem to imply time until death, many curves are used to show time until some event of interest occurs. These curves are often used in the cancer biology and medical literature, but they have applications in neuroscience as well, plotting such data as time to stroke, relapse of drug use, or risk of dementia. In all cases, they are still considered measures of "survival".

Kaplan–Meier curves can be used to plot both clinical human and nonhuman data. It has become rare to see Kaplan–Meier curves plotting death events in mammalian animal models, since modern experimental endpoints generally suggest euthanasia before natural death. These curves can also be used to measure survival of an *in vitro* preparation, such as when quantifying deaths of neurons in cell cultures after exposure to high doses of toxic substances.

Reading the Graphs

The *x*-axis plots time. The units will usually depend on the outcome of interest. In human clinical studies, time is often measured in months or years. In nonhuman mammalian studies, the scale is usually on days to months. In studies using nonmammals or cells *in vitro*, the scale may be as short as hours.

While often called a "curve," the data are more accurately described as a "series of steps." Information about survival may be collected at irregular intervals, especially in human studies where it is difficult to collect patient results on a daily basis. Time points are not measured continuously; although the data are shown with connected lines, the vertical parts of the graph do not technically carry any meaning and are only included to improve the readability of the graph.

The more common curve has a y-axis plotting cumulative survival (or survival probability, or just probability). These values may be represented as a fraction (0 to 1) or as a percentage (0% to 100%). The curve starts at the top left of the graph, since none of the subjects or patients has experienced the event at the beginning of the experiment. Whenever an event is reported during the course of the study (moving to the right on the x-axis), a new "step down" is added that represents the fraction of subjects or patients who experienced the event at that given time point. These curves have a negative slope, since events occur as time increases. Once a subject or patient reports the event, they are excluded from future data points.

On some Kaplan–Meier survival curves, the y-axis plots cumulative risk. Cumulative risk plots may express the data as a fraction or percentage of a population. If the population is the limited sample, these numbers will range from 0 to 1 (fraction) or 0% to 100% (percentage). If the population is the general population at large, the fraction or percentage may be very low, since the denominator includes the total population outside of the study. These plots start at the bottom left of the graph, since none of the subjects or patients has experienced the event at the beginning of the experiment. They show positive slopes, and each step up indicates another event.

Usually, two or more curves appear on the same graph. This allows for a comparison between, for example, treatments or interventions, differential effects of gene expression on survival, or survival differences between demographically distinct groups.

Figure 2.26 represents survival analysis of mice in a model of brain cancer. The main experimental question is whether exposure to radiation worsens survival

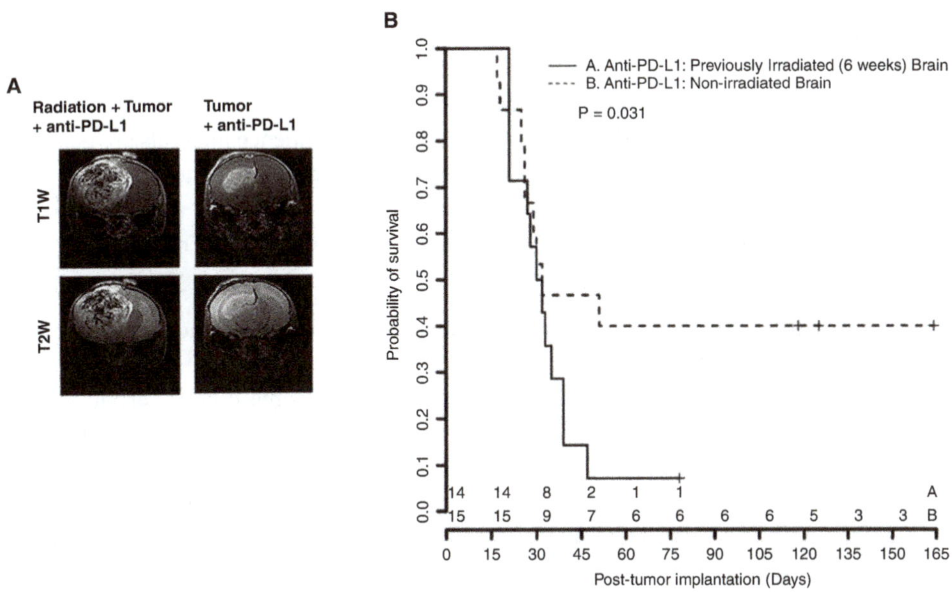

Figure 2.26 Kaplan–Meier curves. Source: Garbow JR, Johanns TM, Ge X, et al. Irradiation-modulated murine brain microenvironment enhances GL261-tumor growth and inhibits anti-PD-L1 immunotherapy. *Front Oncol.* 2021; 11:693146. http://creativecommons.org/licenses/by/4.0/.

outcome, even when cancer treatment (anti-PD-L1) is delivered. The panel on the left shows magnetic resonance under T1- or T2-weighted images taken in the coronal plane of mouse brains that have been implanted with glioblastoma tumor cells. Animals exposed to radiation show larger and more invasive lesions. On the right is a Kaplan–Meier analysis of the two conditions. Mice with irradiated brains (solid line) have worse survival outcomes at a statistical significance level of $p = 0.031$. Less than 10% of the irradiated mice were still alive by 50 days after tumor implantation. Mice not exposed to radiation (dotted line) had better survival outcomes. Numbers at the bottom of the graph above the x-axis correspond to animals still alive at each time point for the two groups.

Interpreting the Data

The data plotted in a Kaplan–Meier curve are nonparametric and are usually analyzed with a log rank test, which is the sum of chi-squared tests performed at each time point. The p-values for the log rank test are reported. When the p-value is less than 0.05, we conclude there is a statistical difference between the two groups. If the curves plot survival, the higher curve indicates survival is increased in that condition, while a lower curve suggests that survival is decreased. If plotting risk, higher curves indicate increased risk, while lower curves indicate decreased risk.

Some Kaplan–Meier curves show **median survival points**. These represent the time at which 50% of the subjects or patients experience the event. They can be graphically represented with a horizontal line drawn from 0.5 (or 50%) on the y-axis that extends until it intersects with the curves. A vertical line may be drawn downwards from this intersection to the x-axis. If the curve plots survival, a median survival point further to the right indicates longer survival times and better outcomes.

These graphs may also plot 95% confidence intervals. Confidence intervals are generally represented as a large block of color above and below each "step" of the curve. A large confidence interval is often a sign of a small sample size.

Sometimes, data points representing individuals will get **censored**. Censored data points indicate two things:

1. A censored data point along the curve indicates that a patient had dropped out of the study or was otherwise unable to be followed up with. These patients may be denoted along each curve with an X, a vertical line, or some other overlaid symbol to indicate the time point when they left the study. In these cases, all future data points have a denominator that is smaller by the number of censored data points thus far. In other words, the occurrence of each future event makes up a larger percentage of remaining patients (the steps will look taller, especially if the sample size is small).
2. Other censored data points include patients who never experienced the event after the conclusion of the study. In these cases, the assumption is that their survival is at least as long as the duration of the study.

Additional Resources

Rich JT, Neely JG, Paniello RC, et al. A practical guide to understanding Kaplan–Meier curves. *Otolaryngol Head Neck Surg*. 2010 Sep; 143(3):331–336. PMID: 20723767; PMCID: PMC3932959.

Summary

Nonhumans interact with their surroundings in different ways. Animals will naturally approach food when hungry and move away from sources of painful heat. They play with one another, seek out mating partners, and understand when neutral stimuli predict something good. Through careful observation that is the foundation of modern science, laboratory tests can be developed to understand these behaviors – and many more.

This chapter describes some of the techniques used to study and present nonhuman behavioral data. Some behaviors are more straightforward to observe, such as movement in an open space or sensitivity to pain. Others are much more subtle and complex, such as feelings of hopelessness or verbal communication. Regardless, neuroscientists have made great strides in understanding how animals behave.

Key Terms

- accelerating rotarod
- acquisition
- *ad libitum*
- adulterants
- *Aplysia californica*
- apomorphine-induced rotation test
- birdsong
- brain–computer interface
- break point
- C57 Black 6 (C57BL/6)
- *C. elegans*
- chemical pain
- conditional fear learning
- conditioned place preference/aversion
- conditioned response
- conditioned stimulus (CS+)
- conditioning phase
- declarative memory
- delayed match-to-sample
- delayed nonmatch-to-sample
- *Diagnostic and Statistical Manual of Mental Disorders*, fifth edition (DSM-V/DSM-5)
- *Drosophila melanogaster*

- elevated plus maze
- encoding
- environmental enrichment
- ethological validity
- extinction
- face validity
- fine motor skills
- fixed interval/ratio
- forced swim test
- freezing
- gait analysis
- gill withdrawal reflex
- habituation phase
- heat map
- hippocampus
- home cage
- hot plate assay
- huddling
- Institutional Animal Care and Use Committee (IACUC)
- inbred
- inflammatory pain
- instrumental conditioning
- intracranial self-stimulation (ICSS)
- Kaplan–Meier curve
- lawn
- learning phase
- lickometer
- light/dark box
- locomotion
- locomotor sensitization
- long-term potentiation
- long-term depression
- macaque monkey
- match-to-sample task
- maximum potential effect (MPE)
- Molaison, Henry
- Montoya staircase test
- Morris water maze
- nerve ligation
- neuropathic pain
- NMDA receptor
- nociceptive pain

- nonhuman primate
- nonmatch-to-sample task
- novel object recognition test
- novelty discrimination index (NDI)
- open field test
- operant conditioning
- outbred
- pair bonding
- partner preference paradigm
- Pavlovian conditioning
- prairie vole
- preconditioning phase
- predictive validity
- preference index
- primary reward
- procedural memory
- progressive ratio
- radiant heat test
- reflex
- reinforcer
- reinstatement
- relearning
- retrieval
- rough and tumble play
- route of administration
- self-administration
- sham surgery
- Skinnerian conditioning
- spatial navigation
- spectrogram
- Sprague-Dawley rats
- stereotypies
- stock
- storage
- strain
- sucrose preference test
- survival analysis
- tail suspension test
- trace diagram
- two-bottle choice test
- ultrasonic vocalizations
- validity

- variable interval/ratio
- vole
- von Frey fibers
- von Frey test
- weaning
- zebra finch
- zebrafish

CHAPTER THREE

Gross Anatomy and Imaging

3.1 Introduction to Gross Anatomy and Imaging

One of the earliest methods of scientifically understanding the correlation between brain and behavior was **post-mortem dissection** (or **autopsy**) of the patient. This provided important evidence early in the history of neuroscience, such as Paul Broca's 1861 examination of patients with aphasia and their corresponding localized brain damage. Although post-mortem analyses can provide a great deal of information at the cellular and molecular level, they are limited in their usefulness because they cannot diagnose a patient in a meaningful time frame for treatment.

However, live imaging methods have been developed since Broca's time, which offer the advantage of being minimally invasive. These imaging strategies are often used in human research and to help verify a clinical diagnosis, but most of the technology has also been adapted for studying larger nonhumans.

In this chapter, you will become familiar with some of the tools used to image the nervous system on a gross anatomical scale. The information collected by these strategies allows the researcher to ask questions about anatomical differences ("Is the severity of frontotemporal dementia associated with smaller brain volume?") or functional differences ("Can changes in cortical neurons firing activity predict how severe a seizure will be?").

Learning Objectives

By the end of this chapter, you will be able to:

- Apply the concepts of resolution to imaging techniques
- Use and understand the anatomical language of imaging techniques
- Describe the theory and application of structural and functional imaging techniques
- Understand the figures used to present anatomical and functional imaging data

3.1.1 Resolution

Imaging methods are often concerned with **resolution**, the capacity to accurately identify two distinct items or events. Informally, techniques are described as having either "high" or "low" resolution. High-resolution techniques provide more accurate information, often at the tradeoff of greater cost, more intensive memory usage, increased risks to the participant, or more time needed to collect that information.

Resolution has two different components, spatial and temporal resolution.

Spatial resolution refers to the ability to differentiate events across physical distances. For imaging the human brain, low-spatial-resolution strategies such as the electroencephalogram (EEG, discussed in Section 3.7) can only approximate areas of activity on the order of centimeters, thereby subdividing the cortical lobes into a few rough areas. High-spatial-resolution strategies such as magnetic resonance imaging (MRI, Section 3.5) can identify differences in volumes as small as a tenth of a millimeter cubed.

Temporal resolution is the capacity to differentiate two events across time. In functional imaging, it is typically estimated in units of minutes to milliseconds. Some imaging methods are not concerned with changes over short windows of time, as when computed axial tomography (CAT scan, Section 3.3) is used for diagnosing the presence of brain tumors and planning their surgical removal. A low-temporal-resolution method such as fMRI provides information on the order of seconds to tens of seconds; a high-temporal-resolution strategy such as EEG can provide information on the millisecond scale.

Figure 3.1 illustrates spatial and temporal resolution. On the left, an image with low spatial resolution is not able to distinguish between two signals close to one another, so signals may be averaged together over the limit of resolution. Pixels are a way to think about spatial resolution; fewer pixels means lower resolution, producing a grainier and lower-fidelity image. On the right of Figure 3.1, a low-temporal-resolution strategy may not be able to detect the precise moment that a change in signal occurs, instead averaging that signal across time.

3.1.2 Anatomical Language

Some anatomical terms are often used to describe nervous system structures in both the human and nonhuman literature.

1. **Anterior** to **posterior**. In the brain, the anterior to posterior axis runs from the "front" toward the "back" of the brain. Sometimes, **frontal** may be used to describe anterior structures. In the spinal cord, anterior is the part that is closer to the "front" of the body, while the posterior spinal cord is closer to the "back" of the body. The words **rostral**

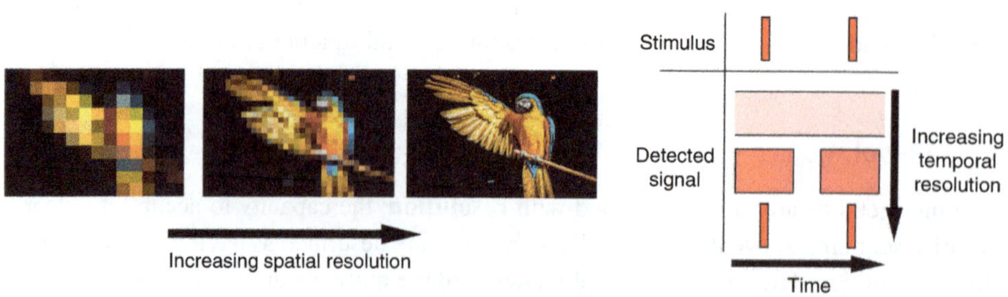

Figure 3.1 Spatial and temporal resolution. Source: https://pixabay.com/photos/parrot-yellow-macaw-bird-perched-3601194/.

(front) and **caudal** (back) may also be used; these are more common in the nonhuman literature.

2. **Dorsal** to **ventral**. Dorsal refers to the "top" surface of the brain, such as those structures closer toward the top of the skull, while ventral refers to structures closer to the "bottom" side of the brain. Sometimes, **superior** (or the prefix **supra-**) is used to refer to dorsal structures, as in the term "suprachiasmatic nucleus," a part of the hypothalamus immediately dorsal to the optic chiasm. Alternatively, **inferior** (or the prefix **-infero**) may be used to refer to ventral structures. However, the ventral spinal cord corresponds to the anterior spinal cord, and the dorsal spinal cord is the posterior spinal cord.
3. **Medial** to **lateral**. The nervous system is anatomically symmetrical. In the brain, medial structures are those closer toward the longitudinal fissure that divides the brain into two hemispheres. In the spinal cord, "medial" refers to structures closer to the midline, the line of symmetry. Lateral refers to structures farther from the midline.

These terms are only anatomical descriptions and are rarely useful in providing any functional information. They can be used in combination with one another, such as when describing subnuclei of the thalamus (ventral posterior medial nucleus, for example) or broad regions of the cortex (such as the posterior inferior frontal gyrus).

Structures may also be described in relation to anatomical landmarks:

1. The **midline** is the line of symmetry that runs down the middle of the brain, or down the center of the spinal cord. In the brain, it corresponds to the longitudinal fissure, the major sulcus (groove) from the anterior to the posterior where the two hemispheres appear to be separated.
2. **Bregma** is a point on the skull at the intersection of the midline and the point where the frontal bone and the two parietal bones fuse as the infant skull develops.
3. The **interaural midpoint** refers to the intersection between the midline and an imaginary line drawn from one ear canal across the dorsal surface of the skull to the other ear canal.
4. **Lambda** is the intersection of the midline and the extrapolation of the lateral sutures between the parietal bones and the occipital bone. Lambda is just a little bit anterior to the interaural point.

Figure 3.2 shows anatomical landmarks on the skull that can be used to identify brain structures, both in cartoon drawing (left) and in a photo (right). In these images, the anterior direction is to the left.

3.1.3 Planes of Imaging

Many figures showing anatomical or functional images concern themselves with **planes of imaging** (also called **projections** or **slices**). Since the nervous system is a three-dimensional structure, there are at least three ways the brain and spinal cord may be viewed.

1. **Axial** (sometimes **transaxial**, or **transverse**) images of the human brain are those showing slices of the brain parallel to the ground if the person is standing upright. In the nonhuman literature, these slices are more often called **horizontal** sections.

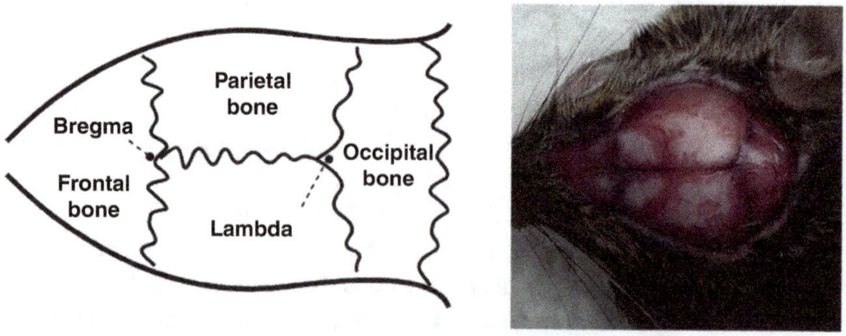

Figure 3.2 Anatomical landmarks on the surface of the rodent skull. Source: Zhou P, Liu Z, Wu H, et al. Automatically detecting bregma and lambda points in rodent skull anatomy images. *PLOS ONE*. 2020; 15(12):e0244378. https://creativecommons.org/licenses/by/4.0/. Image cropped.

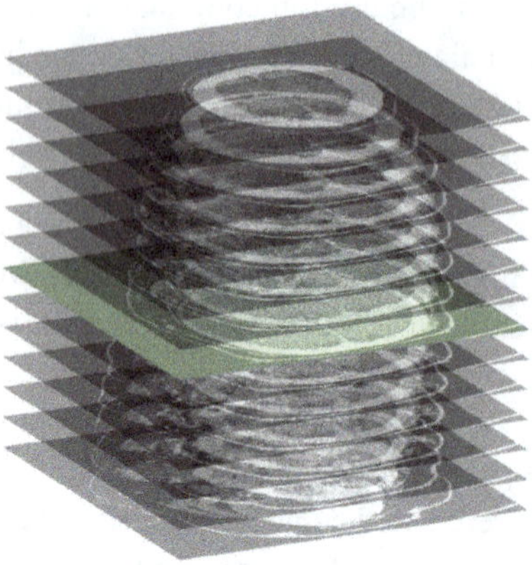

Figure 3.3 Computed tomography. Source: De-Giorgio F, Ciasca G, Fecondo G, et al. Post mortem computed tomography meets radiomics: A case series on fractal analysis of post mortem changes in the brain. *Int J Legal Med*. 2022; 136: 719–727. http://creativecommons.org/licenses/by/4.0/. Image cropped and text removed.

2. **Frontal** (or **vertical**) projections of the human brain are those taken as if parallel to the front of the person's face. In nonhumans, this projection is also called a **coronal** section.
3. **Lateral** (or **longitudinal**) views are planes of brain images that are parallel to the midline (central sulcus), as if cutting from anterior to posterior in the brain. Cutting directly along the midline produces a view called the **midsagittal** plane, and slices made parallel to that may be called **parasagittal** slices.

Figure 3.3 shows how using computed tomography to capture a series of images in one plane (axial) allows for reconstruction in any other plane.

In the spinal cord, typically transverse slices (also called **cross sections**) are shown, which are those that are parallel to the ground if the person is standing upright. Sometimes, sagittal views of the spinal cord (oriented up and down, as if imaging the person as they stand) may be shown, but these are typically done with a focus on the bony structures of the spinal column, since multiple vertebrae can be seen in the same image.

Some imaging strategies rely on **tomography** (derived from Greek *tomos*, meaning to cut) to produce a three-dimensional reconstruction of the nervous system with help from computer systems. Even though the scanner collects images in only one plane at a time (usually the axial plane as the person lies on their back and moves through the scanner headfirst), a tomography system allows the experimenter to visualize the system in any plane.

Anatomical images may also contain two intersecting lines at right angles ("**crosshairs**") that span the length of each image, drawn on top of each orientation. These lines inform the reader of the location that each image is taken from. For example, the coronal image will have a vertical line that shows us where along the medial–lateral axis the parasagittal image is taken from; the horizontal line shows us where the horizontal image is taken along the dorsal–ventral axis. Alternatively, this same information can also be presented by showing a number next to each projection; these will correspond to the measurements along each axis that the section is taken from.

In Figure 3.4, three planes of images of the same human brain show an axial view (on the left), a frontal view (middle), and a lateral view (right). Letters are used to indicate orientation: A for anterior, R for right hemisphere, S for superior, and P for posterior. The horizontal crosshair on the axial slice shows the location of the frontal image, while the vertical crosshair shows the location of the lateral image.

3.2 Dissection

Background Information

Post-mortem dissection is one of the oldest methods to examine the morphology of the nervous system. Before dissection, the tissue is treated with a **fixative**, which preserves biological tissue through chemicals such as paraformaldehyde (PFA) or formalin. Fixation creates cross-linkages

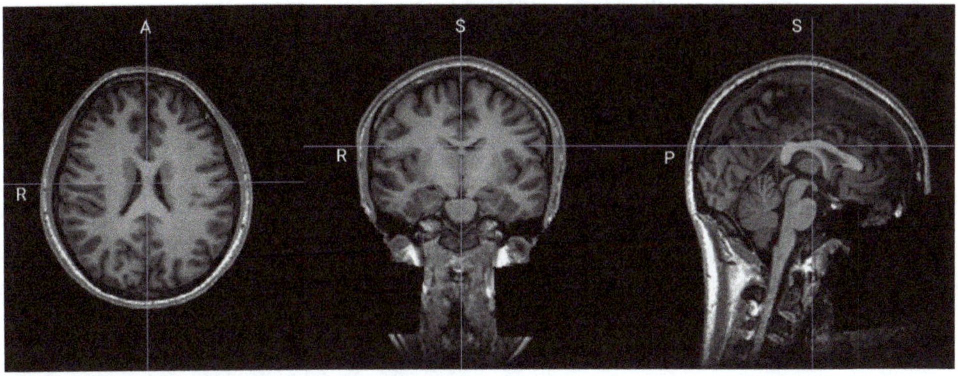

Figure 3.4 Three planes of imaging a human brain. Source: Nugent AC, Thomas AG, Mahoney M, et al. The NIMH intramural healthy volunteer dataset: A comprehensive MEG, MRI, and behavioral resource. *Scientific Data*. 2022; 9: Article 518.

of proteins and inactivates many enzymes, resulting in tissue that is resistant to degradation. Then the tissue is **sliced** (or **sectioned**) thinly with a tool such as a **cryostat** or a **microtome**. It is common to fix and section brains for use in microscopic analyses.

Another purpose of dissection is to acutely isolate tissue, such as slices of brain or spinal cord, from the living animal. This is one way to collect samples for some forms of electrophysiology experiment.

Many times, illustrations of representative tissue with outlines will be shown instead of actual photographs. These images may be shown to illustrate:

- The location of injection sites in viral-mediated transfection or toxin injection experiments.
- The location of electrode placement or cells recorded in an electrophysiology experiment.
- The location of fiberoptic placement in *in vivo* optogenetic experiments.
- Sites of **lesions**, areas of observable cell loss. These might be shown in human case studies to correlate the site of a lesion with a behavioral deficit (as in the work of Paul Broca, who examined the brain of Patient Tan post-mortem and discovered that a specific part of Tan's brain was injured which correlated with his aphasia). In nonhuman experimental studies, the brain can be intentionally lesioned (usually by high electrical stimulation) to verify the placement of stimulating or recording electrodes. This approach is commonly performed in *in vivo* electrophysiology studies.
- Summary schematics proposing novel neuronal circuitry (connectivity, or projection) paradigms.
- The presence or absence of major anatomical abnormalities, verifiable in photographs of sections.

Reading and Interpreting the Images

Change in tissue volume is one variable that can be measured using dissection. Photographs of the tissue may be shown. Scale bars are commonly presented, usually on the order of millimeters for mice and centimeters for monkeys. Regions of interest may be pointed to with arrows or otherwise outlined or highlighted. These data are usually quantified in group summary graphs, which may plot different groups or manipulations on the *x*-axis and report area in square meters on the *y*-axis.

Outlines of representative brains are commonly shown. In the rodent literature, usually consecutive sections of coronal slices are shown. Each slice is identified by its position along the anterior–posterior axis by a number, which indicates the distance from bregma. Positive values indicate distance anterior to bregma, while negative values indicate distance posterior to bregma. For example, a mouse slice may be notated as +2.2 mm AP (which stands for anterior–posterior axis) or bregma +2.2, meaning that the slice is taken 2.2 mm anterior to bregma.

While bregma is the most widely used landmark for identifying coronal slices, the interaural axis or lambda may also be used. As with bregma, positive values are anterior to the marker while negative values are posterior to the marker.

If parasagittal slices are shown, they are identified by their position on the medial–lateral (ML) axis; for mouse brains, this is typically reported in millimeters lateral from the midline. Since the brain is symmetrical across the midline, distances on the left hemisphere are mirrored by distances on the right. Sometimes, negative values refer to the left hemisphere while positive values refer to the right hemisphere.

Figure 3.5 shows a parasagittal slice of an opossum brain. The tissue has been treated with a chemical process (a Nissl stain, described in Section 4.6 of this book) that allows distinction between white and gray matter. Here, the rostral-most part of the brain (olfactory bulb) is to the left while the caudal-most parts (cerebellum, brain stem) are to the right. The dorsal aspect is at the top of the image, and the ventral aspect is at the bottom. The brain section is placed on a grid, as you might see in a brain atlas. The numbers correspond to millimeters relative to the anatomical landmark on the skull called lambda, where the solid black lines intersect.

If horizontal slices are shown, these may be reported in meters ventral from the dorsal-most surface of the brain at the level of the dura (but dorsal–ventral measurements may also be taken from the skull surface). These may be reported as 3 mm DV (dorsal–ventral). Negative or positive is irrelevant; only the absolute value matters.

It is also possible to make **oblique** sections at any intermediate degree. This may be done to preserve neuronal structures such as white matter tracts, which may be useful in electrophysiology. Usually, oblique slices are not shown.

In the spinal cord, slices are usually shown with the dorsal surface toward the top. This can be verified by the shape of the gray matter, the "inner" portion of the spinal cord that loosely resembles butterfly wings. The gray matter is more likely to extend all the way to the surface on the dorsal side of the spinal cord, but not the ventral side.

The conventions regarding the three-dimensional coordinates of brain structures are also used in **stereotaxic** (or **stereotactic**) **surgery**. Figure 3.6 shows a stereotaxic frame placed around the patient's head to allow for accurate targeting of brain structures during surgery.

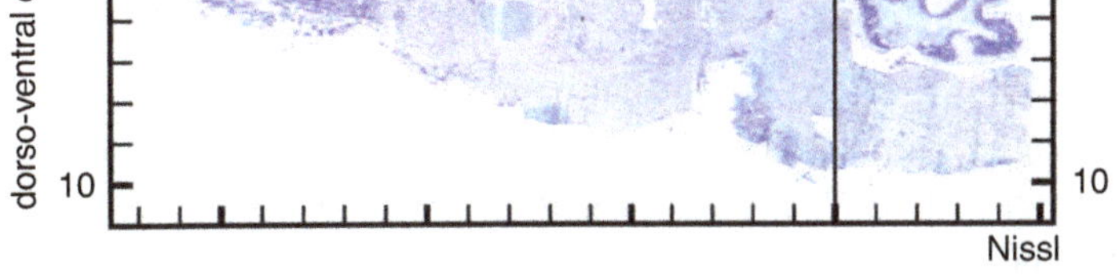

Figure 3.5 A parasagittal slice of an opossum brain. Source: Majka P, Chlodzinska N, Turlejski K, et al. A three-dimensional stereotaxic atlas of the gray short-tailed opossum (*Monodelphis domestica*) brain. *Brain Struct Funct.* 2018; 223:1779–1795. http://creativecommons.org/licenses/by/4.0/. Image cropped.

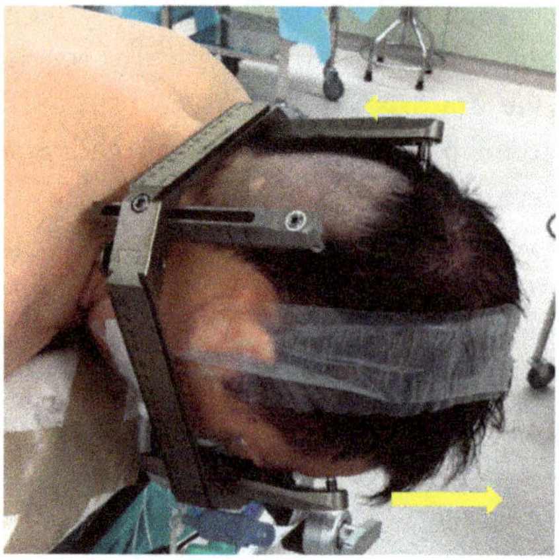

Figure 3.6 A stereotaxic frame. Source: Hirano Y, Shinya Y, Aono T, et al. The role of stereotactic frame-based biopsy for brainstem tumors in the era of molecular-based diagnosis and treatment decisions. *Curr Oncol.* 2022; 29(7):4558–4565. https://creativecommons.org/licenses/by/4.0/. Image cropped.

Dissection illustrations often use bold solid lines to indicate the boundaries of physical tissue: the outline of the brain and the ventricular system will be solid. Solid lines may also be used to separate clear anatomical boundaries, such as those between white and gray matter as in the spinal cord or the corpus callosum in the brain. Sometimes, in images of primate brains, major **sulci** (grooves in the brain) such as the central sulcus or lateral fissure may also be highlighted in solid lines (the brains of rodents and smaller animals do not have sulci).

There may also be dashed lines that are used to outline generally accepted structural or anatomical divisions, such as the border between primary motor cortex and supplemental motor area, or borders between layers of cortex, for example.

An identifying marker may be added to indicate the location of recordings, the placement of electrodes, an injection site, or other accurate sites of interest. These are often shown as a small shape, maybe a filled circle or square. The identified cells or target sites for injections should fall in the boundary that is generally accepted according to a standardized atlas. Data points outside these areas are outliers and not typically shown since they are excluded from analysis.

Additional Resources

Allen Reference Atlas – Mouse Brain. atlas.brain-map.org.

Bakker R, Tiesinga P, Kötter R. The scalable brain atlas: instant web-based access to public brain atlases and related content. *Neuroinform*. 2015; 13:353–366. http://link.springer.com/content/pdf/10.1007/s12021-014-9258-x.

Paxinos G, Franklin KBJ. *Paxinos and Franklin's The Mouse Brain in Stereotaxic Coordinates*. London: Academic Press; 2019.

3.3 Computed Axial Tomography (CT/CAT Scan)

Background Information

The computed (or computerized) axial tomography scan (**CAT scan**, or **CT scan**) is a medical imaging tool that relies on capturing information using x-rays. During the scan, an x-ray device revolves around a person as they move through the scanner, and a computer collects the x-rays and creates a three-dimensional reconstruction of the structures. Because of the ease of capturing information and the speed of the test, the CAT scan is the gold standard for diagnosing intracranial medical conditions, such as a stroke or hemorrhage. To improve the strength of the signal, a contrast agent may be injected intravenously before scanning. The most common contrast agent for nervous system imaging is an iodine injection.

The CAT scan is used much more frequently for clinical diagnoses than in neuroscience research. When CAT scan images do appear in publications, they are usually presented in case studies describing injuries, rare **congenital** (meaning "since birth") conditions, or diseases such as multiple sclerosis. The scan is a strictly anatomical analysis. Sometimes, a functional imaging method such as a **PET scan** (described in Section 3.4) may be performed alongside the CAT scan to overcome this limitation.

CAT scans are not generally performed in nonhumans, since dissection would provide more information at a higher spatial resolution. It is also difficult for nonhumans to remain still in the scanner without anesthesia.

Reading the Images

CAT scan images are shown only in black, white, and shades of gray (a color scheme called **grayscale**). Materials of high density (such as bone) are shown in lighter shades, while substances of low density (such as the air surrounding the head) appear darker.

Information from all angles is captured by the scan, but typically only one angle is shown in the publication. Most commonly, the **axial** (also called **transverse** or **horizontal**) view is shown. Sometimes, the **frontal** (also called **coronal** or **vertical**) or the **lateral** (also called **parasagittal**) view may also be shown.

There are some unwritten conventions in the orientation of brain CAT scans.

- Axial view: upwards is **rostral** (or **frontal**, or **anterior**, as if the patient is lying down facing upwards). The right half of the image is the left hemisphere of the brain; left and right hemispheres may be indicated by the letters L and R.
- Frontal view: upwards is **dorsal** (or the **superior aspect**, as if the patient is facing you). The right half of the image is the left half of the brain, and vice versa.
- Lateral view: the left side of the image is usually the frontal aspect of the patient, as if the person were looking to the left. This can be verified by looking for the cerebellum and brain stem, which are at the posterior aspect of the brain.

As for scans of the spinal cord: in lateral projections, the left side of the scan is usually the frontal aspect of the patient. In axial projections, upwards is often ventral, while downwards is the dorsal aspect of the spinal cord (as if the patient is lying down on their back). This can be verified by the presence of the **processes** (protrusions of bone), which are only on the dorsal aspect of the vertebrae and will point downward.

Figure 3.7 shows a CAT scan taken of the spinal cord at chest level. The bright shape in the center at the bottom of the image, circled in red, is the vertebra, and three spiny processes are pointing downwards, one straight down and two at angles. This image is as if the person is lying on their back (dorsal is downwards in the image).

Although CAT scans can be used to quickly image the spinal cord and the vertebrae, the MRI offers higher spatial resolution, which might be needed because of the size of the spinal cord.

Interpreting the Scans

In the healthy brain, axial and frontal images should be grossly symmetrical across the midline in both tissue density (shading) and shape, while lateral images are always asymmetrical. In projections that should be symmetrical, a distortion of the midline between the hemispheres is called a **midline shift**. These midline shifts may happen if there is more substance than would be predicted (such as a tumor), which pushes out other tissue; this is called a **mass effect**.

One of the notable landmarks that appear in many images are the ventricles, large spaces in the center of the brain that are filled with **cerebrospinal fluid (CSF)**. Because CSF is mostly water, they will appear darker compared to the surrounding brain tissue. The lateral ventricles are expected to be roughly symmetrical as well.

Figure 3.8 shows a CAT scan (axial view) of a human brain with an intracerebral hematoma (ICH, bright white mass) producing a midline shift, which pushes both lateral

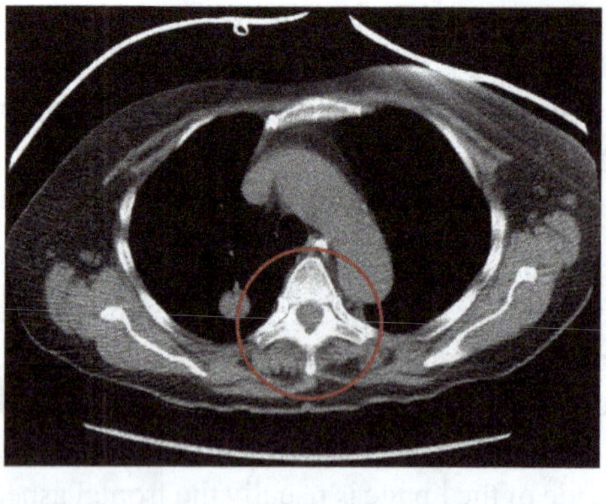

Figure 3.7 A CAT scan of the spinal cord. Source: Albertina B, Watson M, Holback C, et al. Radiology data from The Cancer Genome Atlas Lung Adenocarcinoma [TCGA-LUAD] collection. The Cancer Imaging Archive. 2016. https://creativecommons.org/licenses/by/3.0/.

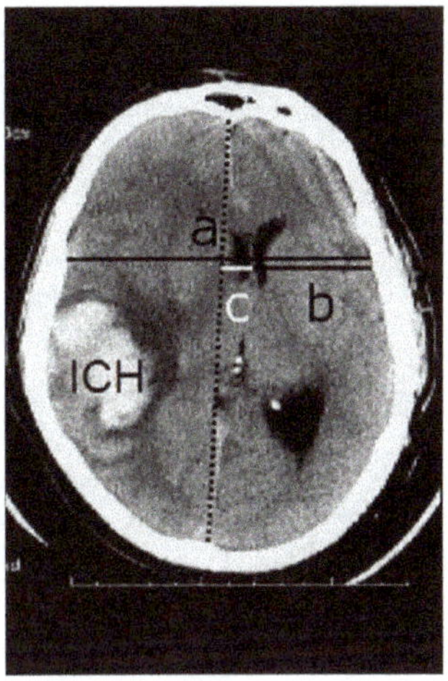

Figure 3.8 A CAT scan showing a midline shift. Source: Liao CC, Chen YF, Xiao F. Brain midline shift measurement and its automation: A review of techniques and algorithms. *International Journal of Biomedical Imaging.* 2018; article ID 4303161, 13 pages. https://creativecommons.org/licenses/by/4.0/.

ventricles to one side of the midline (vertical dotted line). The severity of the midline shift, c, is calculated by the formula $c = a \div 2 - b$. In the healthy brain, c is expected to be 0, but here we see the ICH has displaced the midline so that c (represented by the horizontal white line in the image) is greater than 0.

Scale bars are not usually presented, and statistical tests are not typically performed. Usually, diagnosis of CAT scans is subjective and performed by experts. Some of the more common reasons an atypical CAT scan is shown in a publication include:

- Intracranial bleeding (hemorrhage; or **intracranial hemorrhage**). Acute blood will appear as **hyperdense** and will appear lighter than brain tissue on a CAT scan. Chronic blood appears as **hypodense**, which appears darker than the surrounding tissue. The shape of the blood region will provide diagnostic information as to the location of the bleeding (extradural, subdural, etc.).
- Tumors. Tumors are unexpected growths of tissue, and they appear hyperdense in the CAT scan. Sometimes, the surrounding brain tissue appears as hypodense due to edema, the movement of water into that space.
- Hydrocephalus. This results from the expansion of the ventricles, possibly due to improper clearance of the cerebrospinal fluid. This condition is characterized by larger than expected ventricles and a decrease in brain tissue. Hydrocephalus is usually symmetrical.
- Brain atrophy seen in dementias. A CAT scan may detect decreased tissue size by a pronounced dark outline between the brain and the skull and a widening of the sulci (grooves) of the cortex.

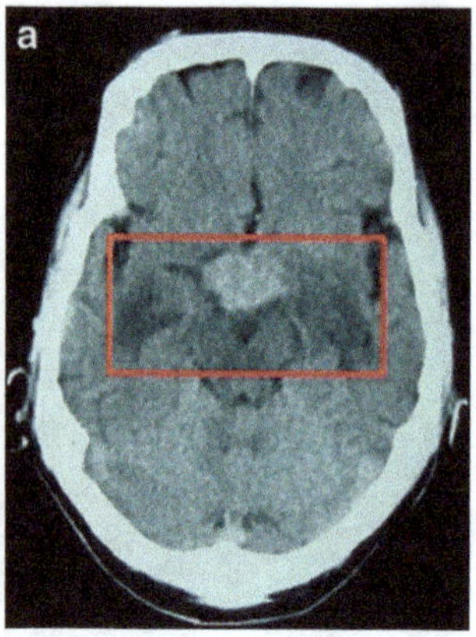

Figure 3.9 A CAT scan showing tissues of different densities. Source: Bataduwaarachchi VR, Tissera N. Paraneoplastic limbic encephalitis with associated hypothalamitis mimicking a hyperdense hypothalamic tumor: A case report. *BMC Med Imaging*. 2016; 16:8. https://creativecommons.org/licenses/by/4.0/. Image cropped.

- Other abnormalities in the tissue, such as cysts, calcification, or granulomas. These may appear as asymmetrical differences in density.
- Unusual cases of extreme anatomical anomalies: for example, people who have had a surgical intervention such as a hemispherectomy, people born without parts of their brain, or people who have survived various skull injuries.

Figure 3.9 shows an axial view of the brain of a 64-year-old man. A hyperdensity (a mass) is shown in the hypothalamus with surrounding hypodensity (edema, or swelling due to excess water). Note that the anterior part of the brain is at the top of the image.

Additional Resources

Broder JS. Head computed tomography interpretation in trauma: A primer. *Psychiatr Clin North Am*. 2010 Dec; 33(4):821–854.

3.4 Positron Emission Tomography (PET Scan)

Background Information

A positron emission tomography is a functional imaging scan. It requires the injection of a radioactive chemical called a **radiotracer** (or just **tracer**). Radiotracers are identified by their chemical name and the radioactive component by atomic symbol and radioisotope. In choline C-11, for example, one of the carbon atoms of the molecule choline has been replaced by radioactive C-11. The radioactive compound decays over the course of minutes, and when it does, it emits a positively charged electron, a particle called a **positron**. Because of the ability to produce positrons, radiotracers may also be called **positron emitting radiotracers**, or **PERs**. This positron interacts with nearby electrons, thus destroying itself and the electron in an **annihilation event**. During this event, two **gamma radiation** particles are emitted in opposite directions. The PET scanner uses gamma radiation detectors which revolve around the person as they move through the tunnel-shaped scanner. Then, the computer creates a three-dimensional reconstruction to identify areas where the radiation signal is found.

The PET imaging technique can be used to collect different categories of information, such as:

- Patterns of brain activity as measured by increased metabolic activity. This was the original design of the earliest PET experiments. When energy usage of a region of brain tissue increases, so does the demand for glucose, a source of cellular energy. Then, a radiotracer such as **fluorodeoxyglucose** (F18-FDG, or just **FDG**), which is an analog of glucose, will accumulate in areas with high energy demand. This causes the radiotracer to remain in this area longer, leading to a stronger radioactive signal.
- Detection of tumors. Tumors take more FDG into their cells since they are patches of rapidly reproducing tissue that require high energy consumption.
- The expression patterns of certain proteins that form a complex with another substrate, such as receptors, transporters, or enzymes. This principle relies on injecting a **radioligand** (radiotracer compound that binds to the target of interest) into the blood, allowing the ligand to bind to its target, then using the scan to detect where the signal is located, indicating the presence and approximate quantity of the target. The radioligand used depends on the target. For example, **[11C]-raclopride** is a selective antagonist for the dopamine D2 receptor, so a strong PET signal indicates high levels of the D2 receptor in that given area. **[18F]-fluorodopa** is a substrate for the enzyme AADC, which is an enzyme that is part of the dopaminergic synthesis pathway, so a stronger PET signal indicates AADC presence and activity. **PIB** (Pittsburgh Compound B) binds to beta-amyloid plaques, which may be useful in early detection of Alzheimer's disease.
- **Receptor** or **enzyme occupancy studies**, which provide information about the percentage of receptors/enzymes that are bound by a compound and about the time course of action of that drug. This may be helpful in understanding the pharmacodynamic/pharmacokinetic and blood brain barrier permeability properties of drugs being developed.
- Blood flow. PET can be used to track changes in **regional cerebral blood flow** (rCBF), a measure of how much blood is going to a particular area of the brain. This may be used clinically to study blood vessel integrity. For research studies, temporary increases in rCBF serve as a proxy for brain area activation, although a similar measure is better detected with functional magnetic resonance imaging (described in Section 3.5.2). The most often-used radiotracer for measuring blood flow is intravenous **[O15]-water**, which dissolves in the blood plasma and can be tracked over time.

In Figure 3.10, cerebral blood flow (CBF) during resting state is measured with **arterial spin labeling** (**ASL**, discussed in Section 3.5.1) on the left, and with [O15]-water on the right, across different areas of the brain in three sections (axial, frontal, and lateral, top to bottom).

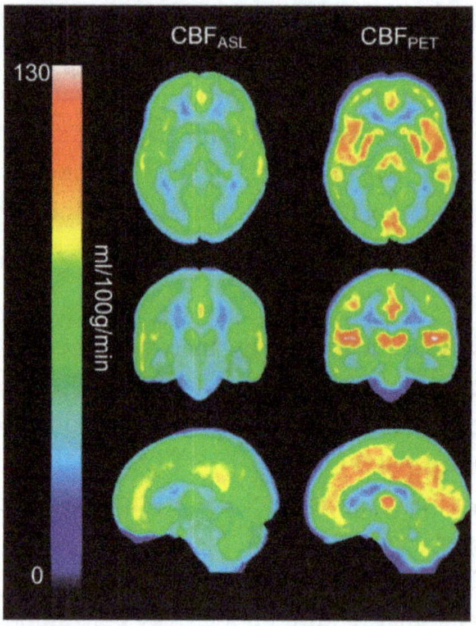

Figure 3.10 A PET scan showing cerebral blood flow. Source: Fahlström M, Appel L, Kumlien E, et al. Evaluation of arterial spin labeling MRI: Comparison with ^{15}O-water PET on an integrated PET/MR scanner. *Diagnostics.* 2021; 11(5):821. https://creativecommons.org/licenses/by/4.0/. Image cropped.

PET offers poor spatial resolution on the order of a few millimeters. To counteract this shortcoming, many PET scanners are combined with a higher-resolution structural imaging technique, such as a CAT or MRI scan. PET also offers low temporal resolution on the order of seconds since it depends on changes in blood flow, and blood vessel dilation happens on this time frame.

PET scans have uses in both clinical diagnostics and research into biomarkers or changes that precede the onset of severe symptoms of a disease. Most PET scan machines are built for human imaging, but there are also small-animal machines for imaging rodents. In these cases, the animal may need to be anesthetized, which introduces a confounding variable.

Reading and Interpreting the Images

Representative images from PET scans may show three planes of the brain in grayscale (shades of black, gray, and white). The grayscale images provide anatomical information about the location of the PET signal.

Overlaid on top of these images are areas of different colors showing where a significant PET signal was detected, with a spectrum usually included alongside the PET images. Different colors indicate different ***z*-scores**, which is a statistical calculation of how many standard deviations those data are above or below the mean in a normally distributed data set. A larger *z*-score indicates stronger change in PET signal; typical ranges are from 0 to 4. *Z*-scores may have a negative or positive value; negative values indicate decreases in signal, while positive values indicate increases in signal. A common example spectrum is black through red, orange, yellow, and white, with white being the highest z-value detected under the conditions of the experiment, and therefore the strongest difference in signal. Another spectrum may plot both negative and positive z-values, setting the middle of the spectrum at a z-value of 0.

In Figure 3.11, each row shows data from different patients, all three of whom have epilepsy. FDG-PET results (colors) overlaid on anatomical coronal MRI images (grayscale) show hypometabolism (blues) of tissue in some areas of the medial temporal lobe. Larger negative z-values indicate stronger decrease in signal.

In measures of regional blood flow, a representative color map may be presented indicating the amount of blood flow. The image is expected to be bilaterally symmetrical. Summary data often plot averages of blood flow, which is usually in the range of tens of milliliters of blood per 100 grams of brain tissue per minute.

In radioligand binding, pharmacodynamics, and occupancy studies, different values may be reported. Representative images may also show brain sections overlaid with color plots of the **standard uptake value ratio (SUVr)**, which is the intensity of PET signal in comparison to some reference control tissue, often the cerebellar cortex. The PET signal may range from 0 up, and units are reported in grams per milliliter (g/ml). Higher PET signal indicates stronger binding or greater presence of the target substrate (receptor, enzyme, protein).

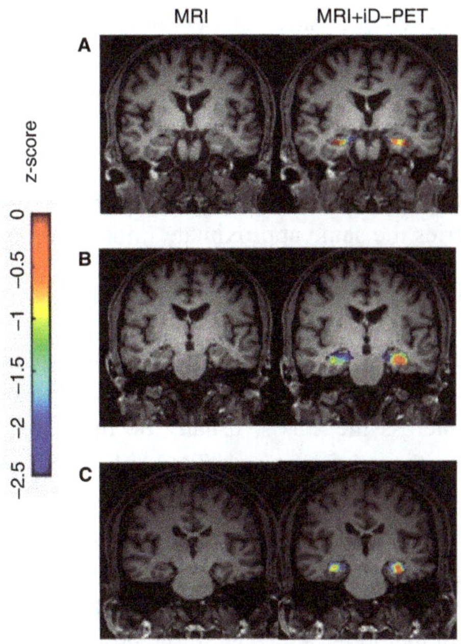

Figure 3.11 A PET scan overlaid with MRI images. Source: Quigg M, Kundu B. Dynamic FDG-PET demonstration of functional brain abnormalities. *Ann Clin Transl Neurol.* 2022; 9:1487–1497. https://creativecommons.org/licenses/by/4.0/.

As with SUVr, **total volume of distribution** (abbreviated as $\mathbf{V_T}$) may be shown as an overlay on brain slices, presented as colors across a spectrum. Higher V_T indicates more uptake of that radioligand. This volume, reported in milliliters per cubic millimeter, will vary depending on the substrate.

A color spectrum may also be used to illustrate a **nondisplaceable binding potential** ($\mathbf{BP_{ND}}$). These values are compared with a control area that shows minimal binding signal, which may be cerebellar gray matter.

Representative images might show the signal pattern in the control condition compared to the experimental condition.

Instead of presenting images, only data tables may be shown. Here, researchers may report changes in PET signal at different areas in the brain under different conditions. To describe precisely where the signal is observed, coordinates (X, Y, and Z) may be reported based on a **standardized brain volume** such as the Talairach space or the Montreal Neurological Institute (MNI) space (these are both systems that are used to map the locations of brain structures). Significant differences between the PET signal of the control and experimental groups may be reported as a *z*-score. *Z*-scores are calculated for each region of interest (ROI). A higher *z*-score means the PET signal is much stronger compared to the control condition.

Other items that may be reported in a table include:

- Region of the brain, identified by name according to a standardized brain atlas, such as hippocampus or anterior cingulate gyrus.
- Brodmann area (BA) or region, using numbers to identify parts of the cortex based on their microscopic properties and organization of neural structure.
- Number of voxels. A **voxel** is a **vo**lumized pi**xel**, which represents the smallest unit of 3D space in the brain that can be distinguished from its surroundings (higher spatial resolution methods produce smaller voxels). When reported, this value is the size of each locus of heightened PET signal. Voxel size is usually in cubic millimeters; therefore, number of voxels carries the same approximate information as the variable volume of PET signal.
- *P*-value, the result of a statistical test for significance.

A **time activity curve** (**TAC**) may also be presented in an occupancy study. These are group summaries shown to evaluate the speed of uptake and elimination of radioactivity signal. These plots show time across the *x*-axis, usually on the order of tens of minutes, and standard uptake values on the *y*-axis. A single TAC only shows one region of interest, but data from several brain areas or different experimental groups may be plotted on the same graph. These curves all have similar shapes, with a characteristic rapid rising phase after time zero when the drug is administered representing the uptake of drug into the brain, and then a slow decline over the course of the following tens of minutes representing the removal of the drug from the brain. Areas with low protein/enzyme expression will have a smaller SUV (shorter curve peak and plateau); areas of high expression will have a higher SUV (taller peak and plateau).

Additional Resources

Guedj E, Varrone A, Boellaard R, et al. EANM procedure guidelines for brain PET imaging using [18F]FDG, version 3. *Eur J Nucl Med Mol Imaging*. 2022 Jan; 49(2):632–651. DOI: 10.1007/s00259-021-05603-w. Epub 2021 Dec 9. Erratum in *Eur J Nucl Med Mol Imaging*. 2022 Mar 7; PMID: 34882261; PMCID: PMC8803744.

3.5 Magnetic Resonance Imaging (MRI)

Background Information

The **magnetic resonance imaging** machine is a tool that relies on using a combination of a powerful electromagnet and a radio wave emitter to collect information about protons. As a person goes through the scanner, the magnet causes protons to align with or directly against the magnetic field (the direction of the magnetic field is abbreviated **B0**). Then, emitted pulses of radio waves (radiofrequency, or **RF pulse**) knock the protons out of alignment into a higher-energy state. The delay between the magnetic field and the RF pulse is called the **echo time** (TE). As the protons return to alignment with B0, a process called **relaxation**, they emit energy, which can then be detected. The theory is that protons of different substances, such as water or hemoglobin, will respond to the magnetic field and RF pulse in different ways. The analysis of the data and the experimental paradigm can be changed to measure different features. For example, **functional MRI** (**fMRI**) is capable of measuring changes in oxygenated blood flow as a proxy for activity, and **diffusion tensor imaging** (**DTI**) can sense differences in water movement as a proxy for the anatomical distinction between white matter and gray matter.

The MRI provides only structural anatomical information, and produces similar information to a CAT scan, although at a higher spatial resolution and with better discriminative power. The stronger the electromagnet, the higher spatial resolution can be obtained (temporal resolution is not affected by magnet strength). Magnet strength is measured in **tesla (t)**, or rarely **gauss**: 10,000 gauss is 1 tesla. Standard MRI magnet strengths range from 1.5 t to 7 t. Medical MRIs are often 1.5 t, while research MRIs are 3 t. A 3 t magnet provides resolution up to 1 cubic millimeter, while the less common 7 t magnet provides spatial resolution up to 0.1 cubic millimeter, which allows for differentiation of cortical layers, a feat called **laminar imaging**. To provide some real-world context, a 1 t electromagnet is strong enough to pick up a car.

MRI is mostly performed for clinical purposes, such as in the diagnosis of meningitis, multiple sclerosis, brain tumors, or traumatic injury. In research publications, MRI images may be shown to provide high-resolution anatomical outlines of the brain or spinal cord. Most MRI machines are built for humans, but small-animal MRI machines can also be used for studying an anesthetized animal.

MRI is noninvasive, but there are still risks. People with implanted metallic medical devices, such as pacemakers or artificial joints, should not enter the scanner. Participants may be allergic to a contrast agent, which might be injected before scanning.

Reading the Scans

Multiple images collected from an MRI may be shown, and the conventions for how these images are displayed are similar to those of a CAT scan:

- Axial slices are commonly shown. Typically, the top part of the image is **rostral**, and the left side of the image is the right half of the brain, as if you were viewing the patient from the top of their head as they are lying down facing upwards.
- In frontal views, the dorsal surface is up and the left half of the image is the right hemisphere of the brain.
- In a lateral image, the front (anterior) aspect of the patient may be facing to the left with dorsal to the top. As other landmarks which may help identify the orientation, the anterior portion of the brain tends to taper more; the cerebellum and spinal cord may be seen in the posterior end.

There are three main ways to collect anatomical data with MRI. Interpreting the images differs depending on which is used. All MRIs present images in shades of black, white, and gray (grayscale).

- **T1-weighted images**. In these images, fat appears as white, while fluids appear as dark. In terms of nervous system structures, white matter will appear lighter and the ventricles will appear dark. Sometimes, a gadolinium-based contrast agent (GBCA) is given via an IV injection before MRI scanning, which enhances the T1 signal in blood vessels and other abnormalities.
- **T2-weighted images**. In T2-weighted images, water will appear in lighter shades and fat will appear dark. Therefore, you will expect to see white in the ventricles, while the white matter appears dark. Inflammation appears as light shades.
- **Fluid-attenuated inversion recovery (FLAIR)**. FLAIR images are T2-weighted images that are set to show water as dark. FLAIR is especially useful for helping in the diagnosis of meningitis and multiple sclerosis.

Figure 3.12 shows axial views of a human brain as imaged by MRI. A T1-weighted image is on the left, a T2-weighted one in the middle, and an image collected using FLAIR is on the right. Each of these image types is ideal for imaging different features of the brain. In all images, the anterior aspect is up. Note how the ventricles, CSF-filled spaces shaped like a pair of outward-facing parentheses close to the middle, appear dark in T1 and FLAIR, but light in T2. Also, the white matter such as the corpus callosum, which connects the two hemispheres, appears white in T1, but dark on T2 and FLAIR.

Quantitative information about anatomy can also be collected from MRI and reported in averages. Possible quantifiable measures include brain or ventricle volume, cortical or white matter thickness, and even approximation of specific clearly defined brain areas.

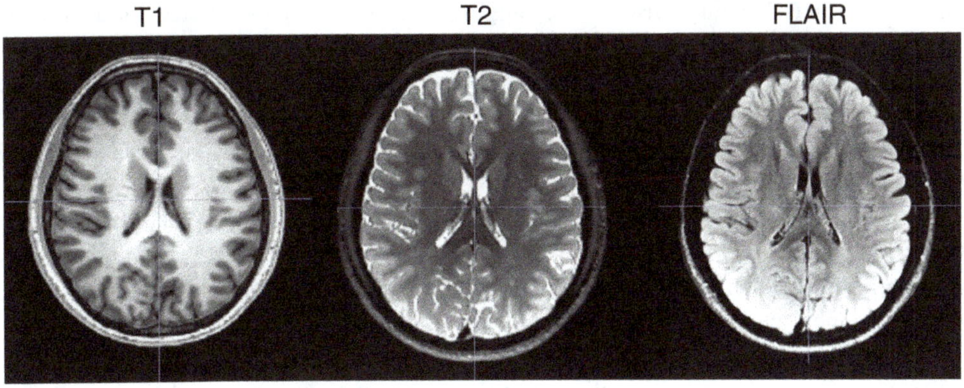

Figure 3.12 Three ways to collect MRI data. Source: Nugent AC, Thomas AG, Mahoney M, et al. The NIMH intramural healthy volunteer dataset: A comprehensive MEG, MRI, and behavioral resource. *Scientific Data*. 2022; 9, Article 518.

Interpreting the Data

Shrinkage in brain volume, increases in ventricle volume, and decreases in cortical thickness is correlated with severity of cognitive decline and aging, and more pronounced in Alzheimer's disease.

As for the interpretation of qualitative information, a diagnosis is often done by experts. As with CT scans, the brain should be roughly symmetrical around the midline on axial and frontal projections. The most relevant features of MRI images shown in case studies are typically asymmetries, such as the presence of a tumor that causes a midline shift. Tumors are generally light on T1, but may contain darker patches as well.

In multiple sclerosis, demyelination of axons causes lesions or plaques, which can appear as dark spots on T1 (light spots on T2). Lesions may or may not be bilateral. Multiple sclerosis lesions can also be quantified and tracked over time.

Additional Resources

Symms M, Jäger HR, Schmierer K, et al. A review of structural magnetic resonance neuroimaging. *Journal of Neurology, Neurosurgery & Psychiatry*. 2004; 75:1235–1244.

3.5.1 Arterial Spin Labeling (ASL)

Background Information

Arterial spin labeling is a method to measure **cerebral blood flow** (**CBF**, also called **blood perfusion**) using MRI. A radiofrequency pulse is delivered at the level of the neck, which causes the protons of the water in the blood to align in a specific manner (a process called

inverting), thus labeling (also called **tagging**) that blood. This labeled blood travels upwards through the vessels in the brain. The protons of this labeled blood decay back to the more stable energy configuration over the course of seconds, and this energy decay can be detected. These signals are then compared with a control or baseline scan taken several minutes after all the labeled protons have relaxed. The difference in signal between the tagged blood and the baseline is therefore a measure of blood flow, a measure abbreviated as **ΔM**.

Common applications of ASL are for studying disorders of brain vasculature, including blood brain barrier dysfunction or stroke. It may also be useful for studying central nervous system diseases, such as cancer, Alzheimer's or frontotemporal dementias, and epilepsy. Currently, most applications of ASL are for research purposes rather than clinical.

ASL offers the advantage that it is completely noninvasive. No contrast agents need to be injected before imaging, which eliminates the exposure to radiation and risk of allergic reaction to the agent. However, this means that ASL suffers from a poor signal-to-noise ratio, so detecting a genuine biological signal may be difficult.

Reading the Scans

Usually, ASL scans shown are in the axial (transverse, or horizontal) view, with anterior sections of the brain toward the top of the image (as if the person was lying down facing upwards). The left half of the image represents the right hemisphere of the brain.

Images of results may be either grayscale or **pseudocolor** images. Grayscale images are the output of the ASL. In these images, darker shades indicate less blood perfusion, while lighter shades indicate more perfusion. Pseudocolor images have colors added to better illustrate differences in results. Common pseudocolor palettes include a spectrum from cool to warm colors (dark blues to bright reds), with warmer colors (reds) indicating increased perfusion. Alternative palettes may also be used and indicated. These color palettes may be used to show changes from baseline, with one spectrum showing increases in perfusion and a different spectrum showing a decrease in perfusion. A scale indicating the numerical values of each color is often presented next to the spectrum of colors.

Figure 3.13 shows axial MRI images of ASL in a patient with epileptic seizures before medication (left image) and after (right image). Anterior is up. The cerebellum shows

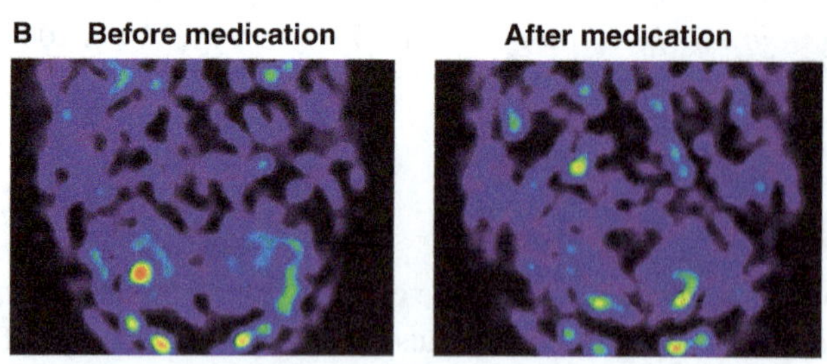

Figure 3.13 Arterial spin labelling in MRI. Source: Sato K, Nakahara K, Obata K, et al. Hyperperfusion in the cerebellum lobule VIIb in patients with epileptic seizures. *BMC Neurol.* 2022; 22:352. http://creativecommons.org/licenses/by/4.0/. Image cropped.

increased cerebral blood flow before medication (more greens and reds near the bottom portion of left image). After medication (right image), the cerebellar areas show less cerebral blood flow (fewer reds, yellows, and greens).

Interpreting the Data

Cerebral blood flow (CBF) may be reported as numbers in a table or graph rather than through scans. Units are reported in milliliters (ml) of blood per 100 grams of tissue each minute (sometimes written as ml g-1 min-1). Expected values in the human brain are on the order of tens to 100 in healthy brain tissue, decreasing with advanced age, but there are regional differences in this value.

In research applications, it may be more meaningful to analyze a specific region of interest (ROI) based on a hypothesis. In a passive scan (no active tasks), as with most imaging methods, significant asymmetries (in views that should be symmetrical, like axial or frontal views) may be indicative of clinically relevant disease. For example, neurodegeneration or a stroke produces hypoperfusion (less blood flow); tumors or inflammation produce hyperperfusion (more blood flow). Epilepsy, acute infection, and migraine may produce a mixed pattern of perfusion.

During real-time task performance, localized hyperperfusion (increases in blood flow) can be seen during task performance in brain areas related to the task. For example, when presented with visual stimuli, the visual cortex signals increase in intensity; cognitive tasks increase signals in the frontal lobes, and so on.

ASL is being tested as a potential biomarker which may predict complex central nervous system diseases ranging from dementia to depression, and the pattern of regional perfusion changes may be correlated with the disease state. However, ASL does not provide any causative explanations.

Additional Resources

Borogo A, Asllani I. Arterial spin labeling (ASL) fMRI: Advantages, theoretical constraints and experimental challenges in neurosciences. *Int J Biomed Imaging*. 2012; article ID 818456, 13 pages. https://doi.org/10.1155/2012/818456.

Bambach S, Smith M, Morris PP, Campeau NG, Ho ML. Arterial spin labeling applications in pediatric and adult neurologic disorders. *J Magn Reson Imaging*. 2022 Mar; 55(3):698–719. DOI: 10.1002/jmri.27438. Epub 2020 Dec 11. PMID: 33314349. http://creativecommons.org/licenses/by/3.0/.

3.5.2 Functional Magnetic Resonance Imaging (fMRI)

Background Information

Functional MRI (fMRI) is a technique used to visualize brain areas that experience changes in oxygenated blood flow over time. It is based on the observation that oxygenated hemoglobin has a different magnetic response from deoxygenated hemoglobin. Looking for changes allows the MRI to detect a **blood oxygenation level dependent (BOLD) signal** (also called a **hemodynamic response, HRF**). The fMRI can locate areas where this difference is observed. The dilation of blood vessels and subsequent increase in oxygenated blood flow is used as a proxy for brain activity based on the assumption that increased blood flow correlates with increased neuronal energy expenditure.

In research, fMRI experiments are divided into two types of study designs, each asking a different set of questions.

1. **Resting state fMRI (rs-fMRI)**. In these experiments, the participant is asked to lie in the scanner and instructed to think of nothing in particular, typically with eyes closed. Resting state fMRI can be used to answer questions about the connectivity of brain regions. Notably, the **default mode network** is a series of structures which decrease their BOLD signal when a person is engaged in a mental task. Questions related to network differences between populations of people are also answered with rs-fMRI. For example, scientists may ask if the total connectivity between the left insula and the left orbitofrontal cortex are less connected among people with major depressive disorder compared to those without depression.

   Figure 3.14 shows a series of axial images of a standardized brain volume. The study was an fMRI resting state comparison of connectivity between brain areas in two populations. *Z*-values represent where each brain slice is positioned along the ventral–dorsal axis, with negative values approaching the ventral surface (the dorsal-most image is at the bottom right). In these images, anterior is upwards. Colors are used to indicate the results of seed-to-voxel statistical analysis, here showing that the connection between left cerebellum and left habenula was stronger in healthy controls than in subjects with major depressive disorder.
2. **Task-based design**. Here, the person is engaged in a task while inside the scanner, allowing the researchers to observe differences in BOLD signal in real time. Example tasks may include **passive tasks**, such as viewing a series of faces, or **active tasks**, where the participant has to press a button whenever a high-calorie food appears in front of them. The stimuli (such as faces or foods in the previous examples) may be presented either by block or by events:

   a. **Block design**. Typically, the stimuli from the same condition are presented over the course of 15–60 seconds at a time. Block design experiments produce a larger BOLD signal since the stimulus is present for longer, allowing ample time for blood vessel dilation.
   b. **Event-related design**. The stimuli from conditions are interspersed in a randomized order, and only presented for a few seconds. Event-related design benefits from randomization and eliminates the effect of expectation.

For example, consider images of faces as the experimental stimuli, and images of inanimate objects as the control stimuli. A block design might show several faces sequentially over the course of a minute, followed by a minute of various scrambled colors, then a minute of

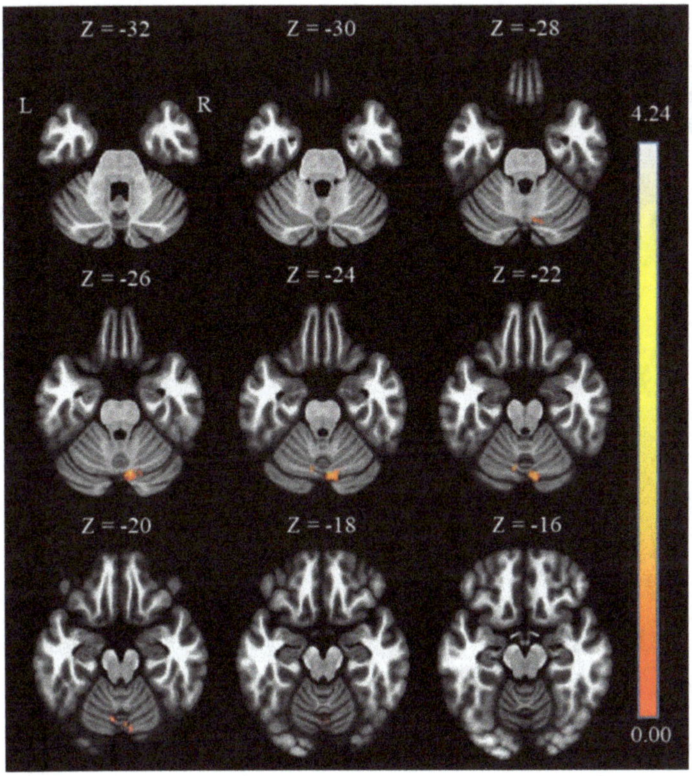

Figure 3.14 A resting state fMRI. Source: Jung J-Y, Cho S-E, Kim N, Kang C-K, Kang S-G. Decreased resting-state functional connectivity of the habenula-cerebellar in a major depressive disorder. *Front Psychiatry*. 2022; 13:925823. https://creativecommons.org/licenses/by/4.0/. Image cropped.

different inanimate objects. An event-related design might show, for two seconds each, a face, a face, an object, a face, an object, an object, and so on.

A commonly used task in task-based behavioral fMRI looks for correlations between circuits of the brain that increase in BOLD signal while a person is engaged in a passive or active task. For example, when viewing faces (a passive task), the BOLD signal in a part of the medial temporal lobe called the fusiform face area increases. FMRI has many applications in research but can also be used in clinical diagnostics.

Reading the Images

Images that represent fMRI data often include a grayscale anatomical representation of an "average" or representative brain as collected by the MRI. Overlaid on this image are a spectrum of colors which represent statistical differences in BOLD signal.

In fMRI studies, it is preferable to predefine a region of interest (ROI) for focused analysis. These ROIs are brain structures where a difference might be expected based on

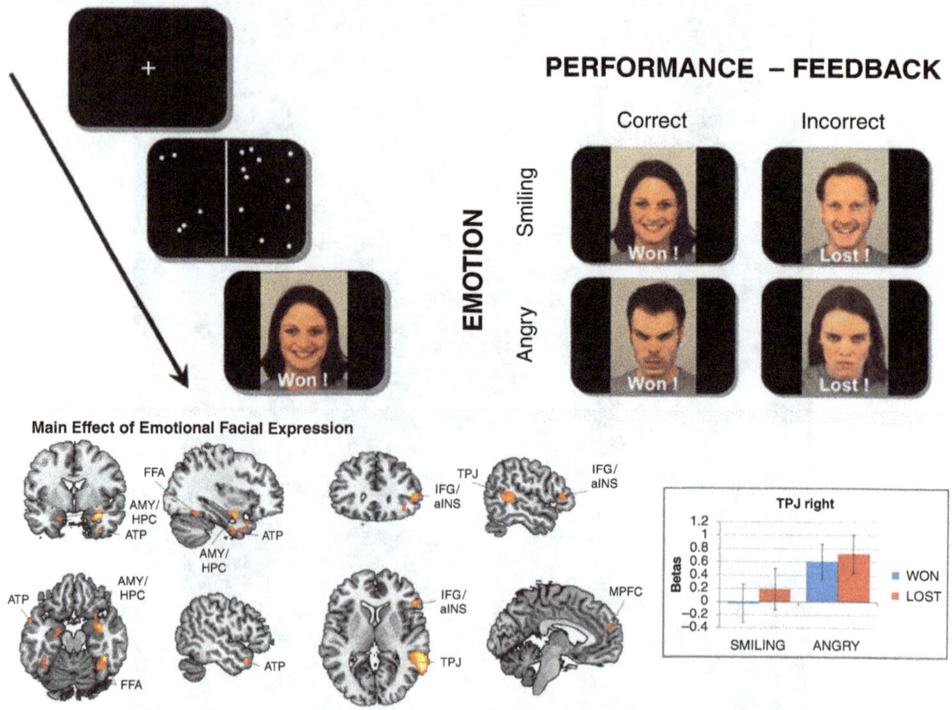

Figure 3.15 An fMRI experiment. Source: Miller JG, Shrestha S, Reiss AL, et al. Neural bases of social feedback processing and self–other distinction in late childhood: The role of attachment and age. *Cogn Affect Behav Neurosci.* 2020; 20:503–520. http://creativecommons.org/licenses/by/4.0/. Image cropped and text label removed.

the previous literature. This focused approach makes the study more hypothesis-based than some, although many fMRI studies function as a screen for finding future areas of interest.

Figure 3.15 represents a social feedback processing task conducted while the participant was in an fMRI. At the top is an experimental protocol figure outlining the task. A person fixates on the white plus symbol and then is shown two fields with white dots. They are asked to select the field which contains more dots. In this example, they selected the right-hand field. They are then given feedback showing whether they "Won" or "Lost." Happy or angry faces also appear along with the feedback. Some winning subjects would see a happy face, and some an angry face, as shown at the top right of the figure. At the bottom left, changes in BOLD signal are reported across several brain areas, including the bilateral amygdala (AMY), hippocampus (HPC), and fusiform face area (FFA). The bar graph at the bottom right shows raw activation values for the right temporoparietal junction (TPJ), which showed activation only upon seeing angry faces, regardless of whether the player won (blue bars) or lost (red bars).

Interpreting the Data

Because the degree to which brain blood vessels dilate is very small, false positives (or type I errors) are a major concern in fMRI data. The average fMRI scan will run more than a thousand comparisons, of which many may report statistical significance due to noise where none truly exists: an infamous study once discovered BOLD signal in the brain of a dead salmon using standard analysis methods. To help reduce the number of false positives, the threshold for statistical significance (p-value) is often much lower than 0.05, commonly using $p < 0.001$ as a standard threshold for determining significance.

Resting state fMRI studies may be difficult to interpret, since it is very difficult to obtain true resting brain conditions while in the bizarre conditions of a scanner. Participants often experience mind-wandering and sometimes even fall asleep.

Additional Resources

Soares JM, Magalhães R, Moreira PS, et al. A hitchhiker's guide to functional magnetic resonance imaging. *Front Neurosci.* 2016; 10:515. DOI: 10.3389/fnins.2016.00515.

3.5.3 Diffusion Tensor Imaging (DTI) and Tractography

Background Information

Diffusion tensor imaging is an imaging method to identify the direction and to quantify the amount of **white matter** (myelinated axons of neurons; sometimes abbreviated **WM**) in a brain. This is a useful tool for understanding the **connectome**, a map of which cells are connected to which other cells. It is a modification of the MRI, specifically looking at differences in the movement of protons found in water molecules.

DTI relies on understanding **Brownian motion**, the random movement of particles (water) suspended in a fluid (extracellular space, CSF). Imagine a cup full of water. Here, the molecules of water are distributed homogeneously, so a water molecule will be free to move in any direction. This process is called **isotropic diffusion**. However, in biological material, such as along a white matter tract, much of the tissue is oriented along one direction. In this heterogeneous distribution of matter, a water molecule in that space diffuses faster along the same direction as the axons ("with the grain") and slower perpendicularly across the tract ("against the grain"). This is **anisotropic diffusion**. The scanner observes where anisotropy is high, and creates images based on the differences in diffusion rate across tissue.

A white matter tract may also be called a **fasciculus**, a **lemniscus**, or more historically, a **band**. Many are named based on their relative location in the surrounding tissue (e.g. the medial lemniscus, which carries ascending proprioceptive information into the thalamus), or using a convention of "origin–end" (such as the corticospinal tract, which carries motor information from the cortex into the spinal cord). A few are named based on their appearance, such as the arcuate fasciculus, which is shaped like an arc (it connects language-related structures in the temporal lobe with the frontal lobe). Occasionally, they are named on their function (optic radiations carry visual information from the thalamus to the visual cortex). The same white matter tract may have multiple names (optic radiations are also called the geniculocalcarine tract).

As with most MRI-based technology, DTI is predominantly performed in humans. Case–control observational studies are commonly the design of a DTI study, but sometimes case studies or experimental studies are performed. White matter connectivity is decreased in demyelinating diseases such as multiple sclerosis, during healthy aging, and in stroke.

Reading the Images

Scanning with a DTI produces a **diffusion weighted image (DWI)**. These provide information about only white matter tracts, and do not often provide other structural information about brain anatomy. To overcome this limitation, the DWI may be presented overlaid on a grayscale image showing the gross anatomical features as captured by the MRI (or a representative typical brain template, such as the Montreal Neurological Institute brain or Talairach space).

In a color map of the DWI, different color hues may indicate the directionality of a particular white matter tract. A typical color scheme uses blue for dorsal/ventral (top/bottom), green for anterior/posterior (front/back), and red for lateral (side to side), but other color schemes may also be used.

Color maps may also be used to highlight specific, well-defined white matter tracts. Figure 3.16 shows a tractography map produced by DTI overlaid on a side view of the brain showing well-defined white matter tracts. In this example, four major white matter bundles have been labeled with colors (blue for superior longitudinal fasciculus, green for uncinate fasciculus, yellow for inferior fronto-occipital fasciculus, and orange for inferior longitudinal fasciculus).

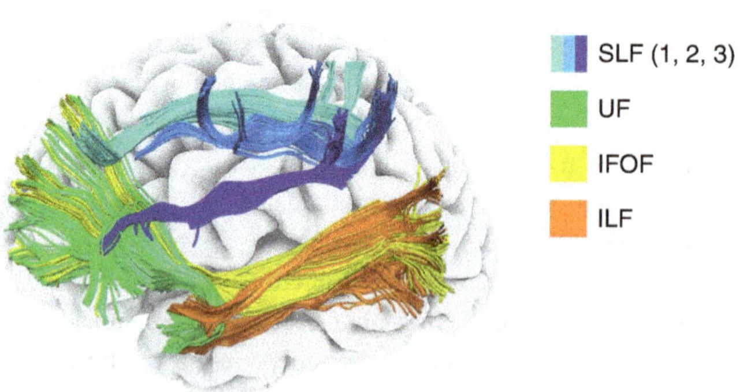

Figure 3.16 A DTI scan. Source: Saini F, Dell'Acqua F, Strydom A. Structural connectivity in Down syndrome and Alzheimer's disease. *Front Neurosci.* 2022; 16:908413. DOI: 10.3389/fnins.2022.908413. https://creativecommons.org/licenses/by/4.0/.

Because differences in white matter volume may not be visible from representative images, data will usually be quantified and presented in a table or summary graph. Some values that may be reported in the DTI analysis include:

- **Fractional anisotropy** (**FA**), which is the main dependent variable reported in a DTI experiment. FA is a measurement of molecular movement in three-dimensional space in a particular voxel. An FA value of 0 indicates complete isotropic diffusion, while a value of 1 is movement only along a single direction. FA values are usually reported for specific regions of interest, white matter tracts being the most common ROIs. Typical values are nearly 0 in CSF (ventricles), 0.1 in gray-matter-rich areas, 0.4 to 0.6 in smaller white matter tracts, and 0.7 to 0.9 in dense white matter tracts (corpus callosum). These values are unitless.
- **Apparent diffusion coefficient** (**ADC**, also **apparent dispersion coefficient**, sometimes also called **mean diffusivity** or **MD**) is a measurement of water diffusivity across the tissue, specifically the Brownian movement of protons found in water molecules. ADC is measured in units of mm^2/s, and typical measurements range from 0.5×10^{-3} in brain tissue up to 3×10^{-3} in CSF. For a specific ROI, the measurement of diffusivity may be divided into two independent measurements.
    - **Axial diffusivity** (**AD**) refers to the diffusion movement along the longest vector, which is the same direction as the white matter tract.
    - **Radial diffusivity** (**RD**) is an average of the diffusion vectors in the other two directions, against the white matter tract. These three vectors are called **eigenvectors**; the longest is the **primary eigenvector**, denoted by the lowercase Greek letter lambda (λ_1), while the shorter ones are λ_2 and λ_3.

Interpreting the Data

A major limitation of FA is that it does not tell us about the directionality of the tract, and we cannot conclude which direction the axons are projecting using DTI analysis methods.

FA values depend on the integrity of white matter. A smaller FA value may indicate that the participant has damage to their white matter, possibly due to demyelinating diseases such as multiple sclerosis. Smaller FA is associated with more severe disability. Increased RD in a white matter tract may also indicate demyelination.

The DTI in Figure 3.17 has traced the corticospinal tract of a patient who survived a left hemisphere stroke, showing a smaller number of white matter fibers (colors) in the left hemisphere (labeled L, shown on the right in both images). Axial (left-hand image) and frontal (right-hand image) views are shown.

Additional Resources

O'Donnell LJ, Westin CF. An introduction to diffusion tensor image analysis. *Neurosurg Clin N Am*. 2011 Apr; 22(2):185–96, viii. DOI: 10.1016/j.nec.2010.12.004. PMID: 21435570; PMCID: PMC3163395.

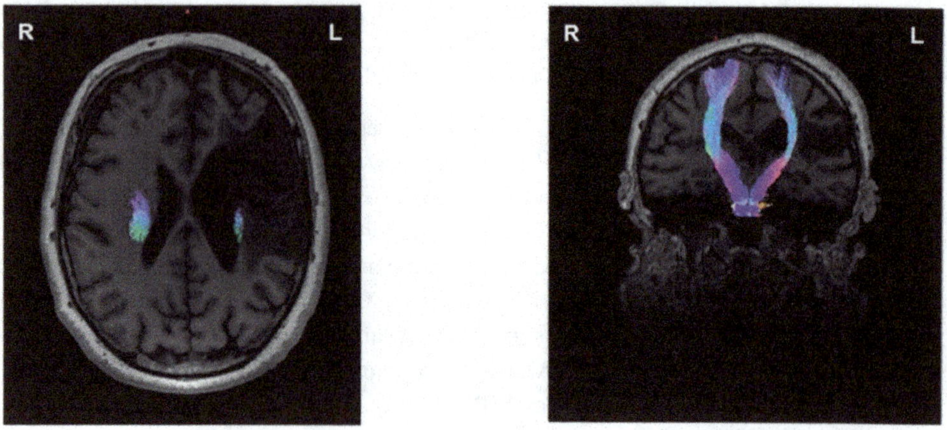

Figure 3.17 A DTI of a patient who has had a stroke. Source: Ciceron C, Sappey-Marinier D, Riffo P, et al. Case report: True motor recovery of upper limb beyond 5 years post-stroke. *Front Neurol.* 2022; 13:804528. DOI: 10.3389/fneur.2022.804528. https://creativecommons.org/licenses/by/4.0/. Image cropped.

3.6 Single Photon Emission Computed Tomography (SPECT)

Background Information

SPECT is a measurement of changes in blood perfusion under different circumstances. The patient is injected intravenously with a radioactive tracer compound, identified by a number followed by the atomic symbol, usually in brackets, such as [123I]. That chemical undergoes gamma radiation decay over time. The emission of this photon is then detected by the SPECT machine. Since the machine collects information as it rotates around the person's head and feeds that into a computer for reconstruction, SPECT is a three-dimensional imaging method. It is noninvasive, and typically performed in humans, but it can be done in monkeys and in smaller animals using microSPECT.

SPECT can be used to assess regional cerebral blood flow (rCBF). Other scans can be used to approximate receptor binding; in these experiments, a radioactive version of the ligand for the receptor of interest is used.

SPECT offers relatively poor spatial resolution, roughly on the order of 2 to 4 cubic millimeters. Because the gamma emission is low energy, the particles scatter when they interact with other particles in the body, so the machine that detects the location of the photon cannot do so accurately. Since only one photon is emitted, the scanner is less able to precisely locate where the photon came from than a PET scan. Additionally, the scan provides no structural information, so it may be presented along with structural imaging methods such as CT or MRI.

Another weakness is that SPECT has poor temporal resolution, typically on the order of seconds, since movement of the radiotracer throughout the brain depends on changes in blood flow.

Since SPECT can perform readings of overall brain activity, it can be used in studying dementia and cognitive decline.

Reading the Images

The axial view is the most common presentation of SPECT images, as if the person is lying down and looking upwards. The left side of the image corresponds to the right half of the brain.

SPECT scans are usually shown as **heat maps**. These heat maps often use a color spectrum where black indicates no signal, cool colors (blues and greens) indicate weak signal, warm colors (oranges and reds) indicate strong signal, and white is the strongest signal.

SPECT images in research studies are typically representative data. Often, data from a control participant will be compared with data from the atypical participant.

Figure 3.18 represents the results of three months of globus pallidus deep brain stimulation, a treatment sometimes prescribed for movement disorders such as dystonia or Parkinson's disease. On the left, the Toronto Western Spasmodic Torticollis Rating Scale (TWSTRS) is a measure taken by observation of the patient. A lower score suggests less severe dystonia. The black lines are the group average, while the gray lines are individual scores. Symptoms were less severe after one week and after three months of treatment. Right: SPECT scans of axial brain slices moving from ventral-most (upper left) to dorsal-most (bottom right). Z indicates the level along the dorsal–ventral axis, with smaller numbers indicating more ventral images. Here, SPECT is used to measure regional cerebral blood flow in specific brain areas, decreasing (blues and greens; negative *t*-value) in some areas, while increasing (reds and yellows; positive *t*-value) in others.

Additional Resources

National Research Council (US) and Institute of Medicine (US) Committee on the Mathematics and Physics of Emerging Dynamic Biomedical Imaging. Single photon

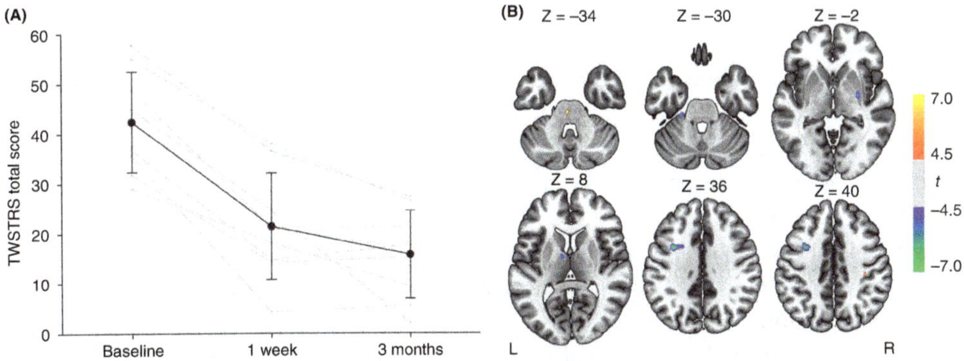

Figure 3.18 A SPECT scan. Source: Park S, Jeong H, Chung YA, et al. Changes of regional cerebral blood flow after deep brain stimulation in cervical dystonia. *EJNMMI Res.* 2022; 12:47. http://creativecommons.org/licenses/by/4.0/.

emission computed tomography. *Mathematics and Physics of Emerging Biomedical Imaging*, Chapter 5. Washington, DC: National Academies Press (US); 1996. www.ncbi.nlm.nih.gov/books/NBK232492/.

3.7 Electroencephalogram (EEG)

Background Information

The **electroencephalogram** (**EEG**) is a method for studying the neural activity of ensembles of neurons primarily in the cortex. An array of electrodes is placed on the scalp (**surface EEG**) which detects the changes in electrical potentials of the neurons closest to the electrodes. Populations of cortical neurons sometimes synchronize their activity, firing at roughly the same frequency. When they do, the collective change in electrical potential is large enough to be detected by the EEG. Because the electrical signal must be detected through several obstructions such as the hair, scalp, skull, and meninges, signals are typically small, usually on the order of microvolts (μV). This has added a source of race-based disparity, since hair type affects the strength of the signal.

The EEG has excellent temporal resolution capable of collecting information as quickly as 2,000 hertz (which means that 2,000 data points are collected each second). This frequency is called the **sampling rate**. Because a typical action potential lasts for a few milliseconds, this high temporal resolution allows for data collection at the speed of neuronal communication. EEG can differentiate between different frequency bands of neural oscillations using a mathematical process called the **fast Fourier transformation** (**FFT**):

1. **Gamma** (> 25 Hz) are the highest-frequency events. Special interest is given to the 40 Hz band, which is associated with peak concentration on heavy cognitive tasks.
2. **Beta** (12–25 Hz) are at their strongest during focused attention.
3. **Alpha** (8–12 Hz) is the frequency that dominates during relaxation.
4. **Theta** (4–8 Hz) is most prominent during stage 2 sleep.
5. **Delta** (< 4 Hz) is the main frequency band during deep sleep.

On the other hand, the EEG has poor spatial resolution, meaning that it cannot precisely identify which population of cells is being observed by each electrode. Usually, the degree of spatial resolution is as broad as identifying the anterior, middle, or posterior part of the lobe. Furthermore, the standard scalp surface EEG has a difficult time detecting signals from brain structures deeper than the cortex.

EEGs are cheap compared to other imaging strategies, since the equipment used is easy to manufacture and does not require large pieces of heavy machinery. It is completely noninvasive and poses no risks to the participant. It is also sensitive and can detect signals on the order of microvolts.

EEG is used for both clinical and research purposes. Common applications for EEG include monitoring anesthesia, recording atypical brain activity in epilepsy, and diagnosing sleep disorders.

Both panels of Figure 3.19 show raw EEG traces. Each row represents the readings between different pairs of electrodes (labeled on the far left) over the course of 10 seconds. Colors indicate brain hemisphere: red is right hemisphere, blue is left hemisphere, and green indicates electrodes along the midline. The bottom row, labeled ECG, shows heart rate as measured by electrocardiogram. Figure 19a is an EEG from a person with epilepsy, whose brain is showing atypical activity. Figure 19b is an EEG from a healthy awake brain.

Other measures that rely on the principles of EEG include:

- **Quantitative EEG (qEEG)**, where numerical information can be extracted from EEG traces. Ratios between different frequency bands, total EEG power, and power value analysis are all strengthened by qEEG. These measurements may be useful for diagnosing potential biomarkers for many different types of neurological conditions, ranging from generalized anxiety disorder to chronic fatigue syndrome.
- **Electrocorticogram (ECoG**; also called **intracranial EEG** or **iEEG)**, where a grid of electrodes is placed directly onto the cortex. Because the detection probes are closer to the neurons, which are the origin of the signal, the threshold for detecting events is lower, and the ECoG can detect events that are much smaller. Also, the electrodes can be placed closer together, offering superior spatial resolution compared to standard EEG. This implantation is highly invasive and requires a **craniotomy**, the surgical opening of the skull. The procedure is therefore reserved for nonhumans and rare clinical cases.

  Figure 3.20 illustrates how an ECoG offers spatial resolution at the millimeter level (right side of image), compared to much lower resolution from a standard EEG, and can accurately identify the origins of epileptic activity.
- **Electromyogram (EMG)**, a measure of the depolarization produced by motor neuron activation of skeletal muscle (or **electrocardiogram**, **ECG** or **EKG**, when measuring heart muscle). EMG placement is identified by the muscle under the electrode. For example, an anterior tibialis EMG is placed above the shin muscle, and may be useful in diagnosing restless leg syndrome or periodic limb movement disorder, while an **extraocular muscle EMG (EOM-EMG)** is placed around the eyes for diagnosing isolated nerve damage. Signals from skeletal muscle are orders of magnitude larger (millivolts) than signals detected from the brain by scalp EEG (microvolts).
- **Electrooculogram (EOG)** measures potential differences from the cornea to the retina, which is useful for diagnosing eye disease or quantifying eye movements.
- **Electrocochleogram (ECochG**, sometimes abbreviated as **ECoG**, not to be confused with electrocorticogram) measures electrical signals in the cochlea and is used in studies of hearing loss.

Additional Resources

Britton JW, Frey LC, Hopp JL, et al. *Electroencephalography (EEG): An introductory text and atlas of normal and abnormal findings in adults, children, and infants*. St. Louis EK, Frey LC, editors. Chicago: American Epilepsy Society; 2016. PMID: 27748095.

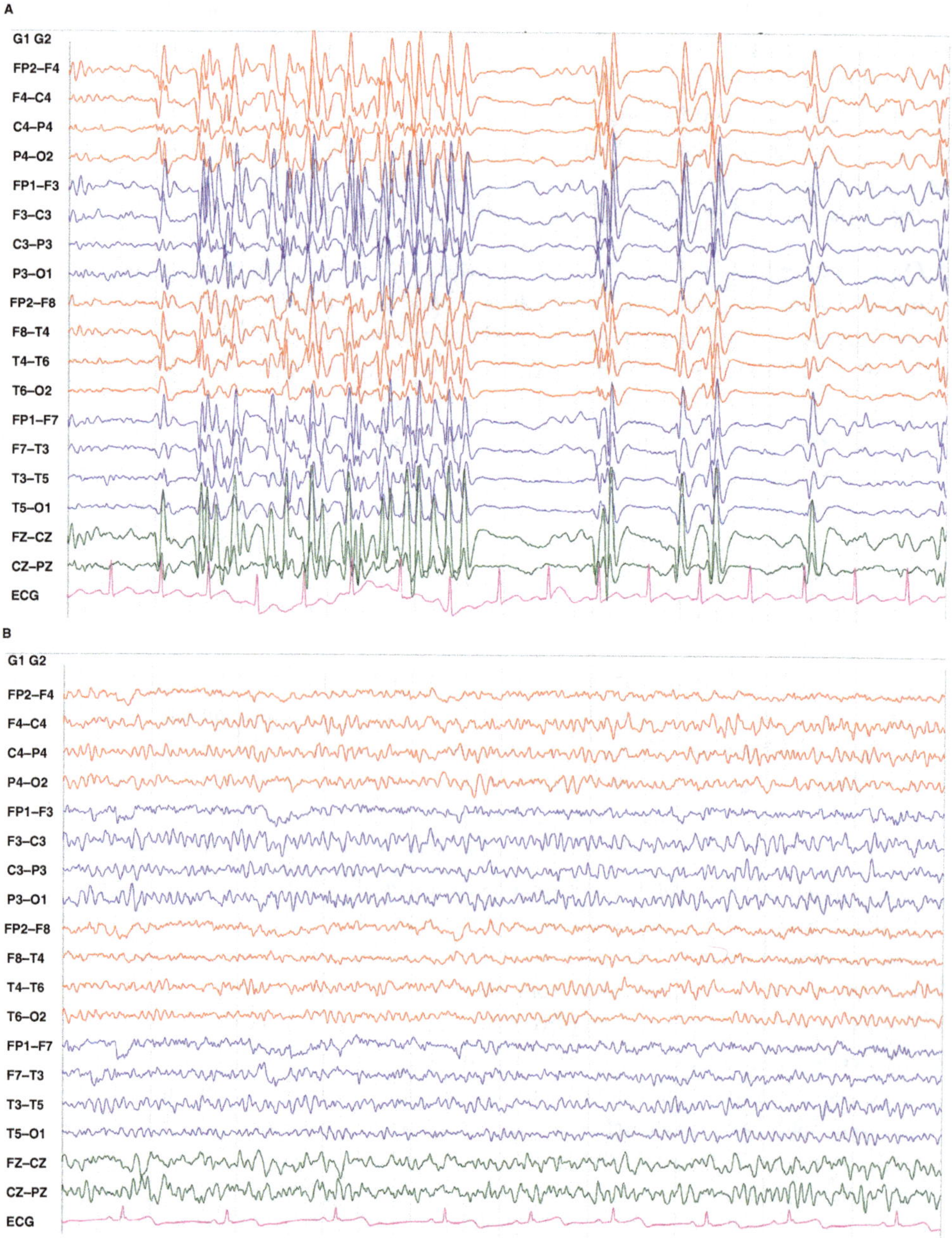

Figure 3.19 EEG traces. Source: Fasil OK, Rajesh R, Ravindren RK. Scalp EEG recordings of pediatric epilepsy patients: A dataset for automatic detection of interictal epileptiform discharges from routine EEG. *Data Brief.* 2021 Dec 4; 39:107680. http://creativecommons.org/licenses/by/4.0/.

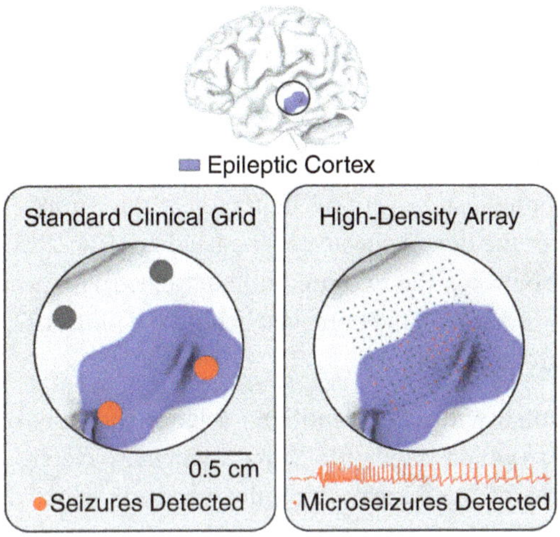

Figure 3.20 An array of electrodes for ECoG. Source: Sun J, Barth K, Qiao S, et al. Intraoperative microseizure detection using a high-density micro-electrocorticography electrode array. *Brain Commun.* 2022 May 27; 4(3):fcac122. https://creativecommons.org/licenses/by/4.0/.

Choy T, Baker E, Stavropoulos K. Systemic racism in EEG Research: Considerations and potential solutions. *Affec Sci.* 2022; 3:14–20.

Nayak CS, Anilkumar AC. *EEG normal waveforms*. StatPearls. Treasure Island, FL: StatPearls Publishing; 2023 Jan 21. www.ncbi.nlm.nih.gov/books/NBK539805/.

3.7.1 EEG Electrode Placement Map/Topographic Maps

Background Information

EEG electrode placement maps are used to inform the reader where the electrodes have been placed in an experiment. Alone, they show only experimental protocol, but they may be combined with the collected data to show which particular set of electrodes is most active under different conditions, such as when shown alongside measures of **event-related potentials** (**ERPs**, discussed in Section 3.7.2).

Reading the Images

These images show a top-down cartoon representation of the head. Usually, anterior (or **rostral**, the front of the head) is upwards, indicated by a triangular shape that represents the nose.

The **international 10-20 system** is the standard placement of electrodes of an EEG cap, named for the intervals across the head where the electrodes are placed: electrodes are placed at distances representing 10% and 20% of the length across the head. Placement is in relationship to specific anatomical landmarks of the head, including:

- **Nasion** (or **Nz**), the space between the eyes where the deepest depression of the skull is found.
- **Inion** (or **Iz**), the bulge at the base of the skull at the back of the head. Drawing a line from N to I traces the midline of the brain. Between N and I, electrodes are placed at 10%, 20%, 20%, 20%, 20%, and 10% of the distance.
- **Pre-auricular**, the bone just in front of the tragus of the ear lobe. Electrodes are placed from left to right over the dorsal surface of the head at 10%, 20%, 20%, 20%, 20%, and 10% of the distance between the two pre-auricular electrodes.
- **Auricle** (**A**, or **M** for **mastoid**), the bone just behind the pinna of the ear. Commonly, this is the reference or ground electrode.

Electrodes may be named with two identifiers: a letter (or pairs of letters), followed by a number or the letter **z** (which stands for "zero", which are electrodes along the midline). Letters indicate the area of the cortex which the electrode is placed above. From N to I, abbreviations are as follows.

- **Fp**: prefrontal lobe; Fpz is 10% of the distance between N and I along the midline, the anterior-most portion of the brain.
- **F**: frontal lobe; Fz is 30% of the N–I distance.
- **C**: central; perpendicular to the brain's midline, 50% of the N–I distance.
- **P**: parietal lobe; Pz is 70% of the N–I distance.
- **T**: temporal lobe, which is not along the midline. It is usually found at 50% and 70% of the N–I distance around the circumference of the head.
- **O**: occipital lobe; Oz is 90% of the N–I distance.

The numbers refer to the hemisphere of the patient's brain, with odd numbers placed above the left hemisphere and even numbers above the right. Smaller numbers are those closer to the midline, while larger numbers are those located more laterally.

Figure 3.21 gives an overhead view of electrode placement in an EEG cap. This representative person is facing upwards, indicated by the nose (triangle) at the top of the image.

In high spatial resolution systems containing more electrodes, pairs of letters may be used to identify junction sites between lobes. For example, FT refers to fronto-temporal area, and PO refers to parieto-occipital area. The numbering convention remains the same.

Interpreting the Data

Data may be shown as overlays on these diagrams as a two-dimensional topographic map. Each set of data may show the power (or intensity) of each specific band of signal (gamma, beta, etc.). Colors indicate F-values, the results of a statistical test that suggest differences between groups. The color spectrum may differ, but a guide is presented alongside the maps.

Figure 3.22 shows topographic maps of resting-state EEG data comparing healthy controls (HC) with stroke survivors without visuospatial neglect (Non-VSN) or with it

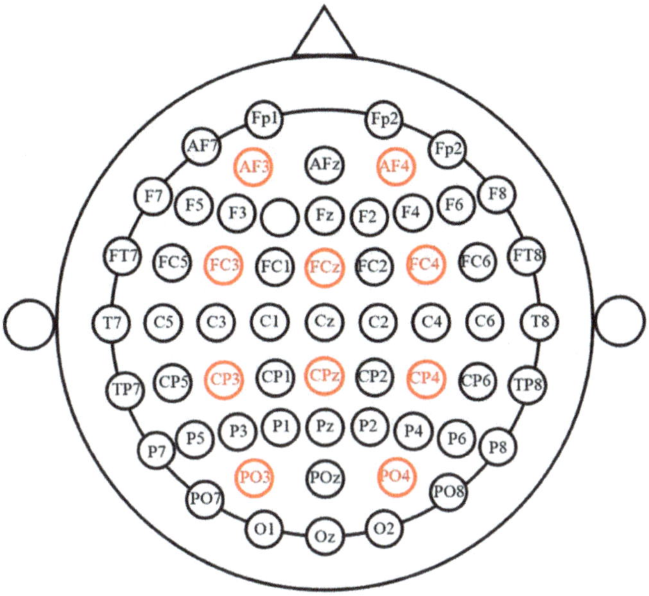

Figure 3.21 Placement of EEG electrodes. Source: Song C, Jeon S, Lee S, et al. Augmented reality-based electrode guidance system for reliable electroencephalography. *BioMed Eng OnLine*. 2018; 17:64. http://creativecommons.org/licenses/by/4.0/. Image cropped and text label removed.

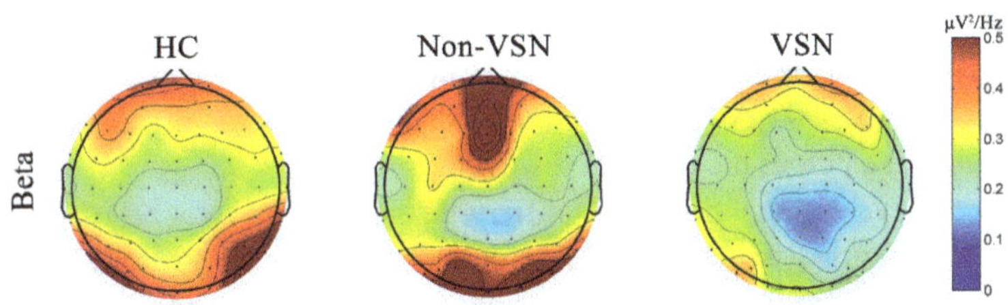

Figure 3.22 A resting state EEG experiment. Source: Zhang Y, Ye L, Cao L, Song W. Resting-state electroencephalography changes in poststroke patients with visuospatial neglect. *Front Neurosci.* 2022; 16:974712. http://creativecommons.org/licenses/by/4.0/. Image cropped and text label removed.

(VSN). The power of the beta activity band differs across the cortex and is notably lowest in the patients with VSN. Raw EEG traces were converted to a power measurement by an FFT to obtain the strength of the beta activity, and these data represent average activity over the course of 5 minutes. In these images, the spectrum ranges from dark red (highest beta strength) to dark blue (lowest beta strength).

Additional Resources

Sazgar M, Young MG. Overview of EEG, electrode placement, and montages. In *Absolute Epilepsy and EEG Rotation Review*. Cham: Springer; 2019. Chapter 5, 117–125.

3.7.2 Event-Related Potentials (ERPs)

Background Information

Using EEG, it is possible to observe changes in electrical activity in response to an event. These recordings are called event-related potentials (ERPs). The event could be the presentation of a visual, auditory, or tactile stimulus (stimulus-locked ERP), or a button press (response-locked ERP). ERPs are "locked" because the change in recorded potential occurs in a predictable time window following the event. Traces shown in figures typically average results of several participants over several trials, and different regions of interest may be targeted for analysis.

Clinically, **auditory-evoked potentials (AEPs)** are used in monitoring the depth of anesthesia. These events happen within the first 100 ms of sound presentation. They are first detected in the brainstem (BAEP) before the cortex. Generally, anesthesia increases the delay between the stimulus and the response (latency) and decreases the amplitude of the measured event.

Reading the Graphs

In sample traces, the x-axis plots time, generally in hundreds of milliseconds (ms). To the left is negative time, the data collected prior to the event, shown to demonstrate the stability of the baseline potential. It is typical to show at least 200 ms of baseline. Time zero represents the onset of the event; there may be a vertical line drawn here. Positive time may be analyzed as far out as 1,000 ms (1 second) and should eventually show a return to baseline potential.

The y-axis plots changes in potentials at the scalp as measured by the EEG, usually on the order of a few microvolts (μV). The zero point on the y-axis is arbitrary and may be set to the baseline average before the onset of the event.

Following the event, there are several different peaks (or **waveforms**) that are expected to appear. The direction (or polarity) of an event does not carry any real significance, since the direction of the event depends on the placement of electrodes compared to each other. However, by convention, downward deflections (valleys) are labeled as **P** for positive, while upward deflections (peaks) are labeled as **N** for negative. The number that follows indicates some number of milliseconds after the event when a peak is expected, but the precise value of the peak falls within a range of tens or hundreds of milliseconds.

In summary data, comparisons are often made between groups with respect to the amplitudes of each peak and the time after the event at which that specific peak appears. In a within-subject experimental design, ERP observations are compared before and after some element of cognition or behavior is manipulated.

Interpreting the Data

Several peaks and valleys in EEG waveforms may appear depending on the nature of the event. Some of the commonly analyzed events are described below, roughly divided into three categories:

1. **Early** (or **short latency**) **events** are peaks in the EEG that occur within the first 100 ms after the event. These are usually attributed to somatosensory (or **exogenous**) potentials. These may consist of:

    - A **P50 peak**, which corresponds to sensory "gating" phenomenon, which allows the person to isolate incoming stimuli and to block extraneous signals while focusing attention only to the most relevant.
    - An **N100 peak** (or **N1** or **vertex potential**), which appears after the presentation of an unpredictable stimulus, particularly auditory stimuli, which strongly evoke the N100 peak. This signal is strongest in the F-C pairs of electrodes. This peak appears later and smaller in patients with multiple sclerosis.
    - The **error-related negativity** (or **ERN**) is a response-locked event that peaks between 80 and 150 ms following an incorrect motor response.

2. **Middle latency events** are EEG peaks that occur between 100 and 200 ms after the event. These are usually associated with higher cognitive processes.

    - A **P200 peak** (or **P2**) is related to attentional processes. This signal is strongest in frontal lobe.
    - An **N200 peak** (or **N2**) is related to conscious awareness of stimuli.

3. **Late events** are peaks that appear more than 200 ms after the event. These are involved with cognitive processes, working memory, and feedback mechanisms. Notable late events include the following:

    - The **P300 peak** (or **P3**) is the most well-studied component of the ERP and is strongly associated with memory processes and mental workload. In response-locked events where a person makes an incorrect response, a similar peak called the error-related positivity (or **Pe**) is observed around 300 ms.
    - A **late positive potential** (or **LPP**) reaches a peak between 300 and 800 ms. This signal is correlated with emotional states.
    - The **N400 peak** is related to familiarity or recognition.
    - **Slow waves** typically peak around 800 ms after the event, and increase during working memory tasks.

Figure 3.23 shows results from a stimulus-locked ERP study. Data were collected by intracranially implanted EEG electrodes placed in four areas: amygdala (AM), hippocampus (HI), fusiform gyrus (FU), and parahippocampal gyrus (PH). Participants were shown either a face or a scrambled mosaic of that face, which served as the negative control for visual inputs. Two populations of people with epilepsy were compared, those with their seizure onset zones outside of the mesial temporal region (Group O column) and those with mesial temporal lobe onset (Group M column). Faces (blue traces) often evoked a larger ERP at the N240 and N360 peaks compared to a mosaic stimulus (black traces).

Not all peaks will appear in every ERP, and the peaks depend on the stimulus or task as well as on the placement of the electrodes being used. For example, a sensory evoked potential, such as an air puff, produces different peaks from a facial emotional processing task.

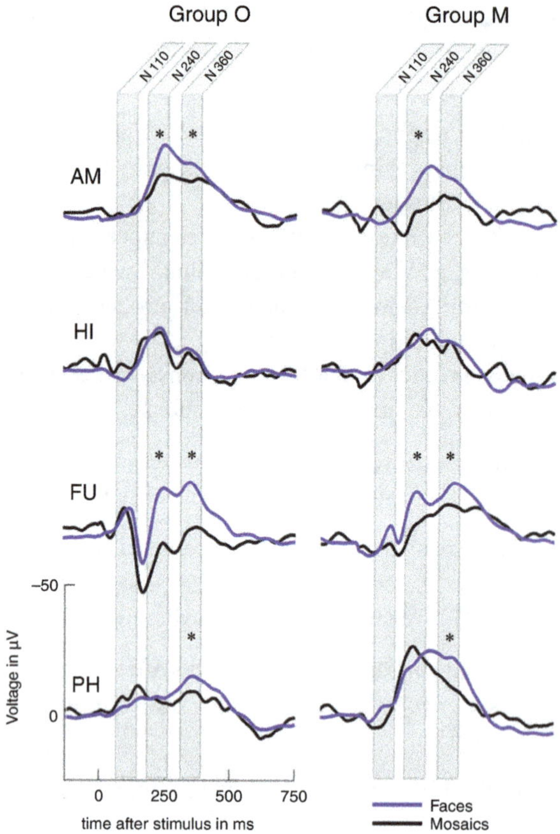

Figure 3.23 A stimulus-locked ERP experiment. Source: Kim JW, Brückner KE, Badenius C, et al. Face-induced gamma oscillations and event-related potentials in patients with epilepsy: An intracranial EEG study. *BMC Neurosci.* 2022; 23:36. http://creativecommons.org/licenses/by/4.0/. Image cropped and text labels removed.

Additional Resources

Sur S, Sinha VK. Event-related potential: An overview. *Ind Psychiatry J.* 2009 Jan; 18(1):70–3. DOI: 10.4103/0972-6748.57865. PMID: 21234168; PMCID: PMC3016705.

Summary

In this chapter, we have described the many techniques used to image the gross anatomical features of the brain. The figures that show these data are often representative images. It is also common to extract numerical data out of these techniques and then perform statistical analyses on those combined data.

As an important point of consideration, population-level neuroanatomical data has been collected with a disproportionate overrepresentation of white participants and a simultaneous underrecruitment of minoritized populations. This raises issues regarding the generalizability of imaging-related observations.

Although many of these anatomical imaging tools were originally designed for humans in clinical settings, some have been adopted for nonhumans and humans alike in research settings. Because of this, many of these strategies are less invasive than experimental techniques covered in future chapters.

It is also noted that each technique has a limit on its spatial and temporal resolution, and these limitations should be considered when interpreting data.

Additional Resources

Ricard JA, Parker TC, Dhamala E, et al. Confronting racially exclusionary practices in the acquisition and analyses of neuroimaging data. *Nat Neurosci*. 2023; 26:4–11.

Key Terms

- anisotropic diffusion
- anterior
- arterial spin labeling
- apparent diffusion coefficient
- autopsy
- axial
- axial diffusivity
- block design
- blood oxygenation level dependent (BOLD) signal
- bregma
- caudal
- cerebrospinal fluid
- connectome
- coronal
- cross section
- cryostat
- CT/CAT scan
- default mode network
- diffusion tensor imaging (DTI)
- diffusion weighted image
- dorsal
- electrocardiogram (ECG)
- electrocochleogram (ECochG)
- electrocorticogram (ECoG)
- electroencephalogram (EEG)
- electromyogram (EMG)

- electrooculogram (EOG)
- event-related design
- event-related potentials
- fixative
- Fluid-attenuated inversion recovery (FLAIR) image
- fluorodeoxyglucose
- fractional anisotropy
- frontal
- functional magnetic resonance imaging (fMRI)
- gamma radiation
- horizontal
- hyperdense
- hypodense
- inferior
- interaural midpoint
- international 10-20 system
- intracranial EEG
- isotropic diffusion
- lambda
- laminar imaging
- lateral
- lesion
- magnetic resonance imaging
- mass effect
- mean diffusivity
- medial
- microtome
- midline
- midline shift
- midsagittal
- nondisplaceable binding potential
- oblique
- occupancy study
- parasagittal
- PET scan
- planes of imaging
- post-mortem dissection
- posterior
- quantitative EEG
- radial diffusivity
- radioligand
- radiotracer

- regional cerebral blood flow
- resting state fMRI
- rostral
- single photon emission computed tomography (SPECT)
- spatial resolution
- standard uptake value ratio
- stereotaxic surgery
- superior
- T1-weighted image
- T2-weighted image
- task-based design
- temporal resolution
- tesla
- time activity curve
- tomography
- total volume of distribution
- ventral

CHAPTER FOUR

Cellular Imaging

4.1 Introduction to Cellular Imaging

Although surgical dissection or other imaging strategies allow for gathering information at the millimeter level of resolution, it may be more meaningful to try to visualize the nervous system at a higher magnification, down to the level of micrometers. For example, if we were to try to analyze information about the shapes and structures of neurons, we would need to use tools that can provide a higher level of zoom than previously described.

This chapter explains these tools, including microscopy and the various methods used in conjunction with microscopy to image micron-level features of the nervous system.

Learning Objectives

By the end of this chapter, you will be able to:

- Understand the principles of microscopy for visualizing cellular anatomy and organelles.
- Understand the tools used to analyze the cells of the nervous system, including distinguishing cell populations, the direction of axonal projections, and changes to the structures of cells (microanatomy).

4.1.1 Neuronal Microanatomy

A neuron can be thought of as having three major domains, through which information typically flows.

1. **Dendrites** are the heavily branched parts of neurons that represent the input sites of a neuron. There may be small (on the order of a micron or less) protrusions of cell membrane on dendrites called **spines**. Spines often represent the postsynaptic component of excitatory inputs, and may contain an accumulation of transmembrane proteins, collectively called the **postsynaptic density**. Dendrites may be classified based on their orientation, which is particularly relevant for pyramidal cells. **Apical dendrites** are longer and start at the peak of the neuron, while **basal dendrites** are shorter and originate at the base.
2. The **soma** (plural: **somata**; also called the **cell body**) is where the nucleus and many organelles of the neuron are found. Some cells may form synapses with the soma instead of with the dendrites. Anatomically speaking, **gray matter** are areas of the nervous

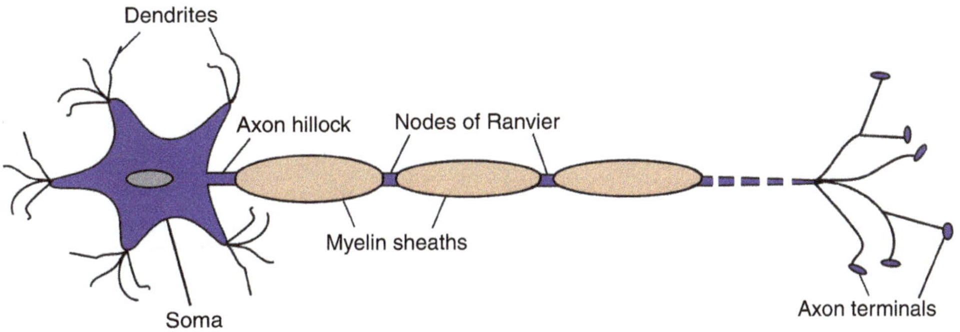

Figure 4.1 A cartoon neuron. Source: Adapted from Pixabay (https://pixabay.com/vectors/motor-neurone-neuron-neurone-nerve-2040692/) and modified by author.

system containing several somata, and a **ganglion** (plural: ganglia) is a clump of somata in the peripheral nervous system.

3. The **axon** is a single extension from the soma, but it may send offshoots in different directions. Axons are usually thinner than dendrites. The junction site between the cell body and the axon is called the **axon hillock**. Immediately following is an area called the **axon initial segment** (**AIS**), which is the origin of the **action potential**, the temporary change in membrane potentials that are the main communicative element of the nervous system. Axons may be wrapped in layers of lipids called **myelin** (or a **myelin sheath**), a cellular modification that increases the speed of action potentials. In between sections of myelinated axons are exposed areas of axonal membrane called **nodes of Ranvier**. Anatomically, heavily myelinated sections of tissue are called **white matter**, which appear white due to the lipids found in myelin that reflect light. The **axon terminal** (or **terminal bouton**, sometimes **button**) is the output site of the neuron, containing specialized structures necessary for the release of neurotransmitter. In between an axon and the neighboring cell is the **synapse**, a short distance (20–40 nanometers) of extracellular space.

Figure 4.1 is a cartoon schematic illustrating neuronal microanatomy. The figure is not to scale: axons are usually thinner than dendrites, and myelin sheaths and the swellings of axonal terminals are not visible at this level of magnification.

4.1.2 Glia

In addition to neurons, the nervous system contains other populations of cells called **glia**. Contrary to the origin of their name ("glia" means glue), they carry out a much wider variety of functions than holding neurons together. Figure 4.2 shows cartoon representations of the morphologies of different glial cell types based on their location, along with a short description of their functions. Some glial populations include the following:

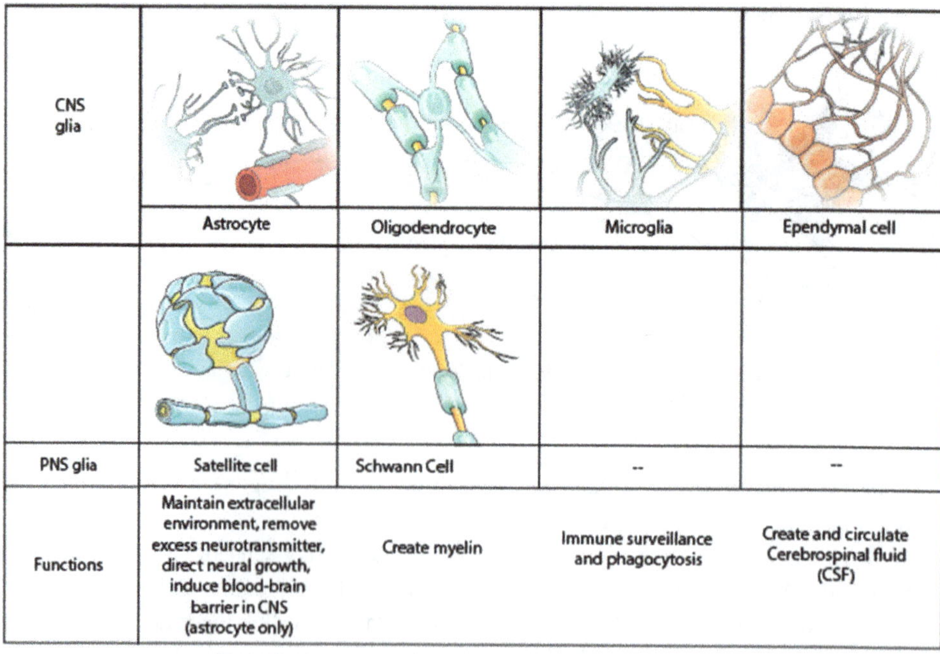

Figure 4.2 Cartoons of glia and their functions. Source: Biga LM, Bronson S, Dawson S, et al. *Anatomy & Physiology*. Oregon State Open Educational Resources; 2019. https://creativecommons.org/licenses/by-sa/4.0/. Image cropped.

- **Astrocytes** are star-shaped cells that regulate extracellular ion concentration, modulate neurotransmission at the tripartite synapse, produce nutrition for neurons, and help maintain the blood–brain barrier. A related population of cells called **satellite** cells exist in the peripheral nervous system, where they carry out similar functions, except for the maintenance of the blood–brain barrier.
- **Oligodendrocytes** produce myelin and secrete chemical factors. They are exclusive to the brain and spinal cord.
- **Schwann cells** also produce myelin and chemical factors. They also contribute to repair of axons. They are only found in the peripheral nervous system.
- **Microglia** are immune-derived cells that become activated in response to waste products that accumulate in the brain. They also contribute to plasticity.
- **Ependymal cells** produce CSF and are found in the choroid plexus of the ventricles and central canal.

4.1.3 Cellular Organelles

Both neurons and glia have **organelles**, just like many of the other cells of our body. Visualizing organelles may be called **subcellular imaging**. These organelles carry out important cellular functions, and disruptions of organelles may be the root of the pathology in neurodegenerative disorders. Common organelles of relevance to neuroscience include the following:

- The **nucleus** houses the cell's DNA and is contained in the cell body.
- The **endoplasmic reticulum** is made up of nuclear membrane and may contain ribosomes on its surface. It also is a repository for intracellular calcium.
- **Ribosomes** are responsible for synthesizing proteins.
- **Mitochondria** are the site of cellular respiration and produce energy for the cells.
- The **Golgi apparatus** (or **Golgi body**) packages and prepares proteins for transport throughout the cell. In neurons, it is usually close to the nucleus. Similar structures called Golgi outposts can be found in some dendrites.
- **Lysosomes** are highly acidic membrane-bound organelles which function as recycling centers to break down molecules. They are mostly found in the soma, but some can be found in dendrites.
- **Neurofilaments** are the molecular tracks along which proteins are sent.

Figure 4.3 shows fluorescent images of different organelles from genetically modified cell cultures. Left: The endoplasmic reticulum (green) is mostly found continuously near the nucleus. Middle: Mitochondria (red) have a more punctate appearance. Right: The merged image shows the location of both organelles in relationship to one another.

Additional Resources

Koppers M, Farías GG. Organelle distribution in neurons: Logistics behind polarized transport. *Curr Opin Cell Biol.* 2021 Aug; 71:46–54.

4.2 Microscopy

Microscopy encompasses a variety of tools used for visualizing objects smaller than the unaided eye can see (less than a tenth of a millimeter). Microscopes (informally, **scopes**) are therefore necessary for identifying individual cellular structures (such as neurons and glia)

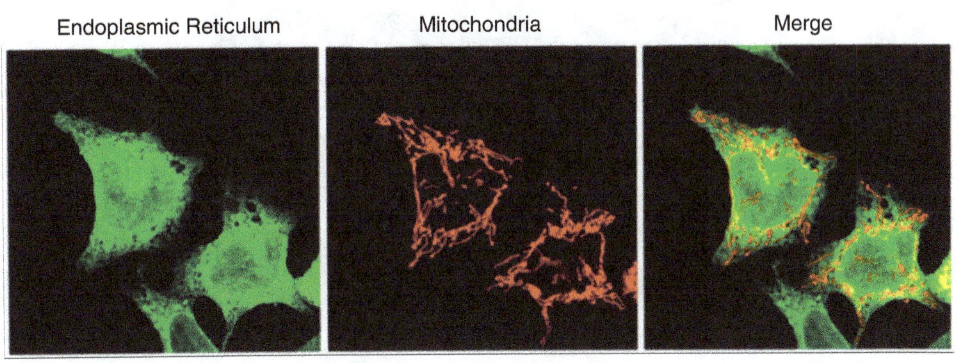

Figure 4.3 Fluorescence microscope images of organelles. Source: Guardia-Laguarta C, Area-Gomez E, Schon EA, Przedborski S. Novel subcellular localization for α-synuclein: possible functional consequences. *Front Neuroanat.* 2015; 9(17). http://creativecommons.org/licenses/by/4.0/.

and organelles (such as the nucleus or the synapse). The degree of magnification is usually written out as a number and the letter x (representing a multiplication symbol), approximately translated as "times magnified".

Microscopes are often used even when no representative images are needed, such as when isolating small samples of tissue, when placing electrodes in patch-clamp electrophysiology, when viewing cells in a culture dish, or when looking to verify placement of injection sites. However, microscopes are essential in conjunction with many other techniques for producing images. All of the image-making techniques described in this chapter rely on using some form of microscopy.

Some microscopy strategies allow for three-dimensional imaging. In these images, the ***z*-axis** refers to visualizing cells within the tissue (perpendicular to the direction of the passing beam of light). A series of these images is called a ***z*-stack**.

Figure 4.4 shows fluorescent microscope images of a neural stem cell. The left image shows the *z*-stack at 1 micron between images, while the right image shows a "flattening" of the cell. The *z*-stack can be thought of as images taken parallel to the plane of the image.

4.2.1 Light Microscopy (Bright-Field and Fluorescence)

Background Information

Light microscopes use visible light (380–750 nanometer wavelength) to see samples. There are two major types of light microscopes used in neuroscience research: bright-field microscopes and fluorescence microscopes.

A **bright-field microscope** is the simplest tool, and most likely what you imagine when you think of a microscope. At the highest end, bright-field microscopes offer magnification at the level of around 1,000x, which allows for resolution of objects about a few microns apart: cells can be seen, but subcellular structures such as organelles, synapses, and vesicles cannot be distinguished. A bright-field microscope can be used for visualizing living

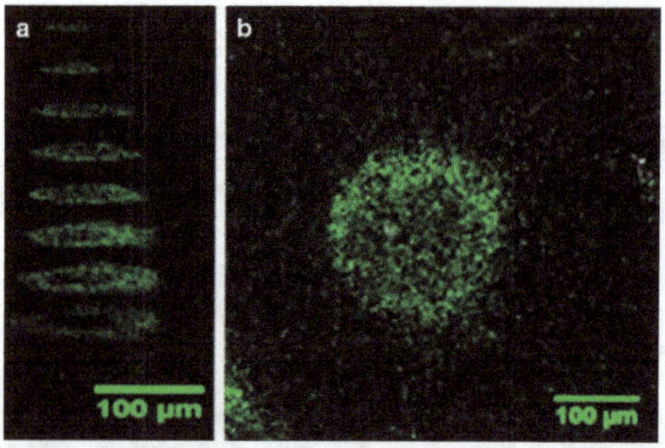

Figure 4.4 Fluorescence microscope images of a *z*-stack. Source: Kravets V, Almemar Z, Jiang K, et al. Imaging of biological cells using luminescent silver nanoparticles. *Nanoscale Res Lett.* 2016; 11(30). http://creativecommons.org/licenses/by/4.0/.

samples in real time, such as when counting cells in a culture dish or when looking at a slice of living tissue.

In a standard bright-field microscope, the pathway of light is a straight line originating from some light source, such as an incandescent bulb or LED which emits broad-spectrum white light. That light is focused by a **condenser**, a lens that captures the rays of light and focuses them into a narrow beam on the sample, and a **diaphragm**, a window of adjustable diameter that regulates the amount of light that passes through. The light passes through the sample and then through the **objective lens**, which provides the main magnification power and is placed closest to the sample. Multiple objective lenses may be mounted on a revolving turret, each lens offering a different degree of magnification, usually between 4x and 100x. Low-power lenses can function with air between the sample and the lens. However, high-power lenses must use a solution in contact with both the sample and the lens, such as water, artificial cerebrospinal fluid, glycerol, or oil. These solutions have a higher **index of refraction** than air, closer to that of glass, allowing more light to be captured by the lens. These types of lenses are called **immersion lenses**. Lastly, light passes through the **eyepiece lens** (also called the **ocular lens**), which adds magnification power before finally entering the eye or camera. Generally, these will provide an additional 10x or 20x magnification. Eyepiece lenses may be printed with a scale bar or a pointer.

A **fluorescence microscope** uses specific wavelengths of light to excite molecules in the sample which then emit light, and that emitted light is then detected. Fluorescence microscopy offers higher spatial resolution than bright-field, often down to the level of hundreds of nanometers. However, it still cannot precisely visualize synapses or vesicles.

Fluorescence microscopy uses the activation of molecules called **fluorophores** (also called **fluorochromes**). Fluorophores reach a higher energy state when exposed to light of specific wavelengths. The wavelength that most strongly activates the fluorophore is called the **absorption** or **excitation peak**, and these are unique to each fluorophore. After this excitation event, the fluorophore gives off photons at a longer wavelength, and the wavelength of these new photons is called the **emission peak**. As an example, the most common fluorophore is **green fluorescent protein** (**GFP**). GFP absorbs light at ~470 nm (blue) and emits light at ~500 nm (green). This difference between absorption and emission may be described as a **rightward shift** (or **red shift**), since green is closer to the red end of the color spectrum than blue. Typically, the difference in wavelengths between the excitation and emission peaks (also called the **Stokes shift**) is less than 100 nanometers. Many fluorophores are named based on the color emitted, such as yellow fluorescent protein (YFP) or cyan fluorescent protein (CFP), while others may have names that hint at their color, such as TdTomato, mCherry, or Citrine. Keep in mind that the names of the fluorophores refer to the colors emitted.

Figure 4.5 shows microscope images of dorsal root ganglion neurons in a culture dish. Left: Neurons visualized by phase-contrast microscopy, a modification of the bright-field method. Visible are three healthy cells which have formed processes. Right: Those same neurons which express green fluorescent protein under fluorescent microscopy.

The pathway of light is more complex in a fluorescent microscope than in a bright-field one. First is the light source, which may include a broad-spectrum mercury or xenon arc

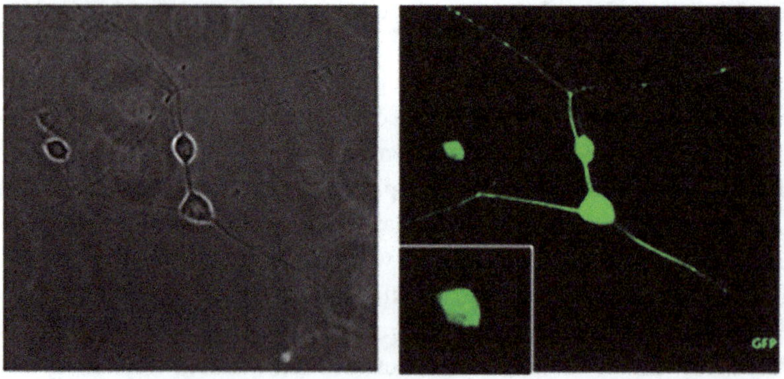

Figure 4.5 Microscope images of cultured neurons. Source: Yu L, Reynaud F, Falk J, et al. Highly efficient method for gene delivery into mouse dorsal root ganglia neurons. *Front Mol Neurosci.* 2015; 8(2). http://creativecommons.org/licenses/by/4.0/. Image cropped.

lamp, an LED of specific wavelengths, or a laser. The intensity of light in a fluorescence scope are typically higher than that needed for imaging with bright-field microscopy. Broad-spectrum light passes through an **excitation filter**, a piece of tinted glass that blocks wavelengths of light outside of the absorption wavelengths. That light is reflected through a **dichroic mirror** (or **dichromatic beamsplitter**), which reflects only certain wavelengths, while allowing other wavelengths to pass. It is angled to reflect the light onto the sample. As light then passes through the sample, it activates fluorophores, which emit light that passes through the dichroic mirror a second time. Now, light at the longer wavelength passes through the mirror rather than being reflected. Then, the **emission filter** (or **barrier filter**) allows the emitted wavelengths of light to pass while blocking other wavelengths, such as that coming from ambient light sources. For example, green fluorescent protein (GFP) would use an excitation filter that passes 450–490 nm blue light, a dichroic mirror that reflects anything shorter than 495 nm but passes anything longer, and an emission filter that passes 500–550 nm green light. Finally, there is the eyepiece lens for direct viewing or some acquisition software for storage and analysis. When high-resolution imagery from a low light signal is necessary, the emitted photons may be passed through a **photomultiplier tube** (**PMT**). This captures incoming photons which displace electrons, and running variable voltage through the PMT accelerates and increases the number of electrons, thereby amplifying a small signal so it can be more easily detected.

Figure 4.6 shows representative fluorescence microscope images of rat intracardiac autonomic ganglia. The researchers were curious as to whether the glucocorticoid receptor (GR) is found in the cholinergic cells, identified by the presence of the protein vesicular acetylcholine transporter (VAChT). Neurons containing GR are red (left), while neurons containing VAChT are green (middle). Also, the nuclei of the neurons are stained by **DAPI**, a fluorescent DNA stain that appears blue. The three colors are overlaid (right). The appearance of some yellow (red light plus green light) indicates that some neurons contain both GR and VAChT, while the appearance of red alone suggests that other neurons have

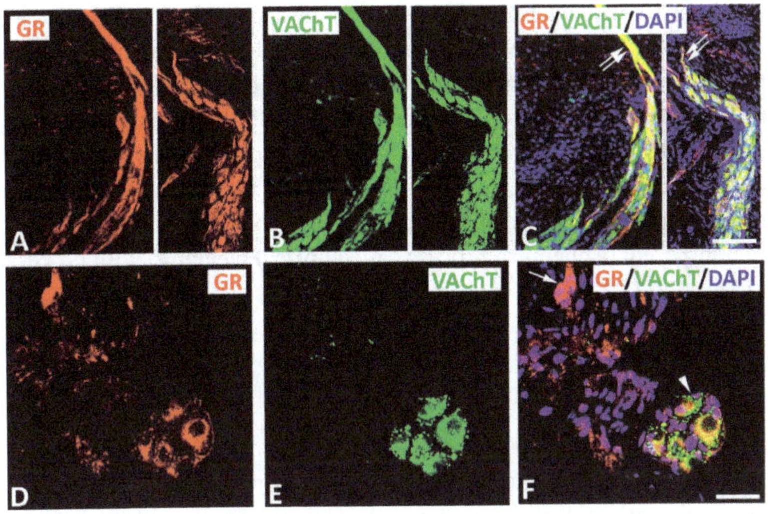

Figure 4.6 Fluorescence microscopy images showing co-expression. Source: Mousa SA, Dehe L, Aboryag N, et al. Identification of glucocorticoid receptors as potential modulators of parasympathetic and sympathetic neurons within rat intracardiac ganglia. *Front Neuroanat.* 2022; 16:902738.

only GR but no VAChT. Neurons are visible through immunohistochemical methods (discussed in Section 5.4 of this book).

There are several types of microscopes that use the principles of fluorescence microscopy. These include the following:

- **Epifluorescence** (also called **wide-field fluorescence**) **microscopes** are the simplest form of fluorescence microscope, where both the excitation and emission light pass through the same objective lens. An epifluorescence microscope floods the entire sample with light and cannot accurately capture three-dimensional information. These are best used for quickly identifying whether a cell contains a fluorescence tag or not, such as in a patch-clamp electrophysiology experiment.
- A **confocal microscope** uses light that is focused at only one point at a time, which is then scanned across the entire sample while collecting fluorescence emission information. Confocal imaging uses a small-diameter **pinhole** that eliminates extraneous light, such as out-of-focus emission signals. Using this technique, it is possible to perform **optical sectioning**, adding together information collected during the scanning process. Confocal imaging is useful for collecting three-dimensional images in the *z* dimension. These scopes can be used for creating reconstructions of fluorescent signals across a few cells at a time.
- A **two-photon microscope** delivers two high-wavelength photons (at the near infrared range, for example) to excite fluorophores. The two-photon technique allows for deep tissue penetration, which is useful when trying to visualize *ex vivo* slices. It also exposes the sample to less light overall, so photobleaching is minimized.

- A **spinning disk confocal microscope** uses a disk perforated with several pinholes, which spins at a high rate, allowing for more rapid collection of confocal information. It also minimizes photoexcitation caused during scanning.
- A **light-sheet microscope** uses a laser focused into a flat sheet as the source of illumination. Like confocal microscopes, light-sheet microscopy is also used for capturing three-dimensional images. But it can perform this function much more rapidly, making it ideal for analyzing large volumes such as whole brain preparations that have been rendered optically transparent (a chemical process called **optical clearing**) with processes such as CLARITY or iDISCO.

Reading and Interpreting the Images

Although the bright-field microscope can accurately and meaningfully capture information about color, images shown in publications may appear grayscale since most mammalian cells are not particularly colorful (compared to some plant cells with their vibrant hues of green) and it is often cheaper to publish figures in grayscale.

Representative images of fluorescence microscopy will have a dark background, since most wavelengths of ambient light are blocked by the emission filter. Images of cell cultures tend to have a "**cleaner**" signal (an informal term referring to images with bright fluorescence against a dark background) compared to images of tissue, partially because biological molecules sometimes exhibit **autofluorescence**, the emission of photons even in the absence of fluorophore.

Representative images from fluorescence microscopy may be used to illustrate **coexpression**, a qualitative observation asking if two different proteins are expressed on the same cell. For example, one experiment might ask whether a population of opioid receptors is found in the same cells that express the enzyme choline acetyltransferase (ChAT). In these experiments, the experimenter might use immunochemistry with fluorophores of two different colors, such as a red fluorescent signal for the opioid receptor and a green fluorescent signal of ChAT. In a representative high-magnification image, three panels may be shown: a red neuron indicating opioid receptor expression, that same green neuron indicating ChAT expression, and a third panel showing an **overlay** of the two images with the neuron in a yellowish tint.

A **colocalization** study can also be performed in this manner, which might ask whether the different proteins are found in the same part of the cell. For example, the protein Nav1.1 is found at the nodes of Ranvier, while the protein Kv1.2 is found on the axonal membrane underneath the myelin. Here, the overlay will show two distinct areas with different colors, demonstrating no colocalization. Typically, panels will have text indicating which target is being observed; text may be shown in the color of the emission fluorescence. Colocalization or coexpression can also be quantified; data may be represented as a stacked bar chart or pie chart showing percentages of cells in a defined region expressing a receptor, for example.

There are limitations to colocalization studies in fluorescence microscopy, however. Since fluorescence imaging relies on light, it is difficult to resolve two signals that are closer than a few hundred nanometers, such as proteins found on the presynaptic versus the postsynaptic membranes (electron microscopy, discussed in the next section, is capable of this level of spatial resolution).

Additional Resources

Goodwin PC. A primer on the fundamental principles of light microscopy: Optimizing magnification, resolution, and contrast. *Mol Reprod Dev.* 2015; 82:502–507.

Rah JC, Choi JH. Finding needles in a haystack with light: Resolving the microcircuitry of the brain with fluorescence microscopy. *Mol Cells*. 2022 Feb 28; 45(2):84–92.

4.2.2 Electron Microscopy

Background Information

Electron microscopy (EM) is a technique useful for imaging **subcellular structures**, components smaller than the wavelength of visible light (hundreds of microns). EM relies on using electrons emitted by an electron gun pointed at the sample and detectors which sense the location of those electrons after they interact with the sample. Electrons oscillate at a much higher frequency than visible photons, so EM offers higher spatial resolution compared to light microscopy. Some example applications of EM include measuring morphological changes in cells and organelles, assessing the severity of demyelination in degeneration, and reconstructing the network of neurons.

There are mainly two types of electron microscopes:

- In a **scanning electron microscope (SEM)**, the sample is coated in a substance that responds to electrons, while the detector collects the electrons and calculates the way they interact with the sample. This produces a 3D image.
- A **transmission electron microscope (TEM)** shoots electrons through a sample, and then the detector senses the electrons that have passed through. For electrons to pass through the sample in TEM, **ultrathin** slices (less than 100 nanometers each) must be collected. TEM can only produce 2D images. To overcome this shortcoming, multiple sequential images can be combined to make a three-dimensional rendering of the tissue. Between SEM and TEM, TEM images are more common in neuroscience publications.

The major advantage is that EM offers a magnification of around 1,000,000x. The lower limit of resolution for an SEM is around 10 nanometers; for a TEM it is under 1 nanometer. This high magnification allows for visualization of organelles, vesicles, synapses, myelin, and protein densities.

There is currently no way to use EM in living biological samples. All EM must be performed in a vacuum, since electrons can interact with molecules of air and bounce off them in unexpected ways. Additionally, samples must be treated with a cocktail of toxic chemicals, some of which include lead and uranium.

Reading the Images

Usually, sample images are shown when EM is used. Images produced by EM are black and white. The denser the material being imaged, the darker the color. The background is usually a very light gray in TEM, or completely black or white in SEM. EM can be used in conjunction with immunohistochemistry. Here, the secondary antibody is conjugated with an electron-dense particle such as gold nanoparticles, which appear as dark.

Some visual features of neuronal structures are as follows:

- Cell membranes are denser and thus darker than cytosol or extracellular space.
- Synaptic vesicles are circular and bounded in cell membranes, typically 40 nm in diameter. Enclosed areas containing several synaptic vesicles are usually the axon terminal of the presynaptic neuron. There can be several synaptic vesicles (10 to hundreds) in a single presynaptic terminal. Another type of vesicle, called dense-core vesicles, are larger in diameter (up to 250 nm), appear darker, and can be found in cytosolic areas outside of the axon terminal.
- Close to the presynaptic membrane is the postsynaptic cell, which is most often a dendrite or soma. The postsynaptic cell is identified as having a dark band around 60 nm thick on the inside of the cell opposite from the presynaptic cell called the postsynaptic density (PSD), which contains several proteins including receptors, enzymes such as CaMKII, and scaffolding proteins.
- EM can be used to differentiate asymmetric from symmetric synapses. **Asymmetric synapses** (historically called **Gray type I**) are formed between an axon terminal and a dendritic spine or shaft, a connection called an **axodendritic synapse**. They feature a prominent PSD. A **symmetric synapse (Gray type II)** does not feature a prominent PSD. Asymmetric synapses make up most synapses and are usually glutamatergic and therefore excitatory. Symmetric synapses tend to form between the axon and a soma, called an axosomatic synapse. The axon terminals of symmetric synapses often produce and release GABA and are usually inhibitory.
- Myelin is made up of several layers of cell membranes and therefore appears as dark circular bands of uniform thickness. Myelin thickness differs across populations of axons; some myelin may be up to a micron thick. At higher magnification, it may be possible to see the individual layers of myelin, which appear as several concentric circles.

Glia can also be identified in EM images.

- Astrocytes have cytosol that is lighter in color, but still contains a few gray dark spots. Astrocyte identification is useful for studying tripartite synapses.
- Oligodendrocyte cytosol is darker and may contain some regions of densities.
- Microglia cytosol is also denser than astrocytic cytosol. They are also smaller than neurons.

Organelles can be identified by EM.

- Endoplasmic reticulum (ER) are membranes that are continuous with the nuclear membrane, and predominantly found in the soma. They are wavy with membranes close to each other, and roughly concentric to the outer membrane of the nucleus.
- Ribosomes appear as small (~20 nm) dark round dots, all roughly similar in size. They can be free in the cytoplasm or attached to the ER. It is possible to see up to a hundred ribosomes in some EM images.
- Mitochondria are oval-shaped organelles that can be found in neuronal dendrites, somata, and axons. Mitochondria have two layers of membrane around them and are denser than the surrounding cytosol, so they appear darker. The inside of the mitochondria has several (fewer than twenty visible) stacks of folded membrane called **cristae**. These cristae can be seen in EM as a series of wavy double lines, typically perpendicular to the long axis of the mitochondria.
- Vacuoles tend to be small, light-colored round shapes.

Figure 4.7 shows two electron microscope images. Left: an excitatory synapse with the presynaptic (axonal) terminal on top, as determined by the presence of several round spheres, which are the synaptic vesicles. The site of the postsynaptic component (dendrites, or spines) is indicated by the slightly darker postsynaptic density (PSD). Here, the scale bar represents 0.1 μm. Right: an image highlighting myelin, made up of several concentric circles wrapped around the axon of a neuron.

EM images may also be pseudocolored, where arbitrary colors are overlaid by the computer after the EM image is collected. This may be useful to help illustrate differences in areas between two groups, to identify pre- versus post-synaptic components, or to highlight continuities between structures across multiple serial slices, commonly shown alongside a similarly colored 3D reconstruction.

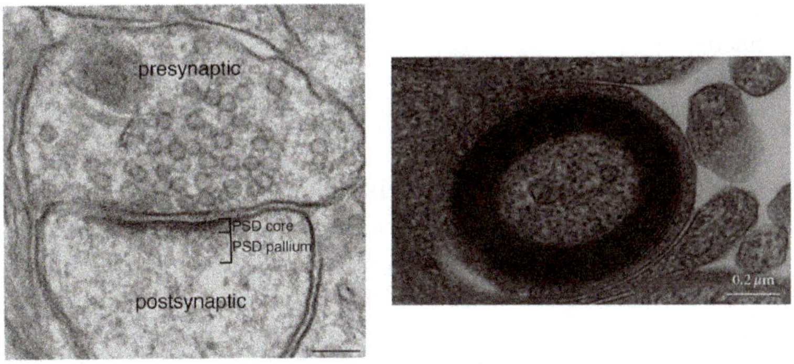

Figure 4.7 Electron microscope images. Source of left image: Dosemeci A, Weinberg RJ, Reese TS, Tao-Cheng J-H. The postsynaptic density: There is more than meets the eye. *Front Synaptic Neurosci.* 2016; 8(23). http://creativecommons.org/licenses/by/4.0/. Source of right image: Kazunori S, Yanagisawa H, Takaku S, Kawakami E, Watabe K. Immortalized adult rodent Schwann cells as in vitro models to study diabetic neuropathy. *J Diabetes Res.* 2011; 2011:374943. https://creativecommons.org/licenses/by/3.0/.

Various features seen on an EM can be quantified and plotted on a graph. Commonly, different groups are plotted across the *x*-axis. The *y*-axis may plot density, quantified as number per unit area or volume, such as symmetric synapse density or mitochondrial density. Since each EM image is essentially capturing a random section of tissue, several samples (hundreds to tens of thousands) are ideally taken. Because the tissue samples are so thin, some groups will assume they are two-dimensional images and will normalize to area rather than volume.

Alternatively, morphological features may be quantified and plotted on the *y*-axis. Some possible measures might include mitochondrial perimeter, synapse length, or thickness of PSD, all of which are usually on the order of nanometers to micrometers.

Additional Resources

Nahirney PC, Tremblay M-E. Brain ultrastructure: Putting the pieces together. *Front Cell Dev Biol*. 2021; 9:629503. DOI: 10.3389/fcell.2021.629503.

4.3 Unbiased Stereology

Background Information

Unbiased stereology refers to methods used to systematically sample and quantify features of cells in three-dimensional space before extrapolating those data to bigger samples. The most common application of stereology in neuroscience is to count cells, measure lengths, or calculate areas and volumes. These values can then be compared across experimental conditions or treatments. For example, cell counts may change in neurodegeneration, toxin exposure, genetic conditions, or disease diagnosis/models.

Stereology is often done in conjunction with other cellular and molecular imaging strategies, such as staining or immunochemistry. Images are usually collected using light or confocal microscopy.

Reading and Interpreting the Graphs

Stereological methods may show representative photographs or cartoon drawings of the tissue being analyzed. There may be both a macro-level image (of a brain slice, for example) and a micro-level image (showing neurons, for example). In obvious cases, a difference in cell counts can be observed in the micro-level image without formal quantification.

Accompanying data graphs are typically group averages, representing data from different conditions or manipulations on the *x*-axis. The *y*-axis may plot the total number of cells, such as when counting cells in a particular region as defined by distinct anatomical borders (for example white matter tracts in the corpus callosum). Because stereology is often done by computer, it is possible to quickly collect very large numbers counts, sometimes more than tens of millions. A single sample of tissue can be stained with different agents or with immunochemistry techniques, so both neurons and glia in the same region can be counted, for example. These values may also be represented as percentages, where they may be represented in a stacked bar chart or a pie chart.

Cell count can be normalized to volume, usually reported in number per cubic millimeter. These numbers are a measurement of cell density and may range up to tens of thousands per cubic millimeter.

In the experiment illustrated in Figure 4.8, researchers were curious about the location of neurons expressing the neuregulin 1 gene in different subregions of the hippocampus. They used CRISPR to create a genetically modified mouse that has a red fluorescent tag on neurons containing neuregulin 1. Panel A is a schematic of the mouse brain showing a parasagittal slice and a half coronal slice. The vertical line on the parasagittal slice shows the location of the coronal slice. The box on the coronal slice highlights the hippocampus. Panel B is a fluorescence microscope image of the hippocampus, the region of interest. Dotted lines indicate the approximate boundaries between subregions. In panel C, unbiased stereology was used to count the number of red cells (and therefore neuregulin-1-positive cells) in different areas of the hippocampus. Data are summarized in the bar graph as a percentage of total cells counted within the area of interest. They conclude that most neuregulin-1-positive cells are found in the dentate gyrus (DG), with significantly fewer cells in the fasciola cinereum (FC), subiculum (Sub), CA1, CA2, or CA3 regions.

Additional Resources

Kneynsberg A, Collier TJ, Manfredsson FP, Kanaan NM. Quantitative and semi-quantitative measurements of axonal degeneration in tissue and primary neuron cultures. *J Neurosci Methods*. 2016 Jun 15; 266:32–41.

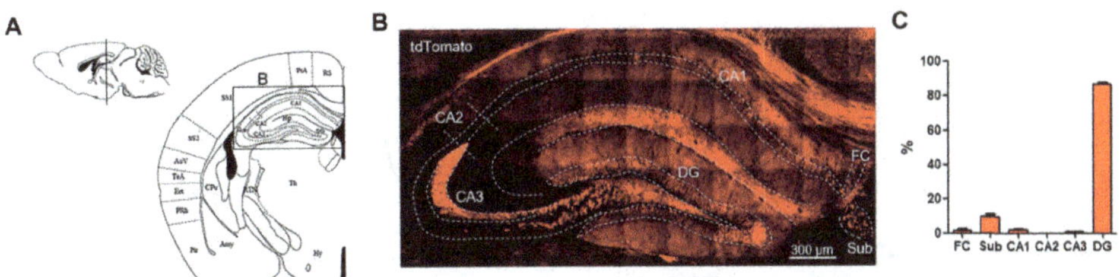

Figure 4.8 Fluorescence microscope images used for unbiased stereology. Source: Ding CY, Ding YT, Ji H, et al. Genetic labeling reveals spatial and cellular expression pattern of neuregulin 1 in mouse brain. *Cell Biosci.* 2023; 13(79). http://creativecommons.org/licenses/by/4.0/. Image cropped.

4.4 Fluorescence Recovery After Photobleaching (FRAP)

Background Information

Fluorescence recovery after photobleaching (FRAP) relies on the observation that fluorophores lose their ability to emit fluorescence after exposure to high-intensity excitation (**photobleaching**). If a small number of fluorophores are bleached by strong light exposure, the recovery of the fluorescent signal in that area can be tracked over time. With FRAP, you can track the movement of molecules, such as those found in synaptic vesicles or in lipid rafts within the cell membrane. For example, consider a genetically modified animal with a fluorescent tag bound to a population of receptors. A focused beam of high-intensity light can be shined onto the receptors, causing the fluorescence to bleach. Over time, those bleached receptors become internalized and new receptors with active fluorescent tags are trafficked to the surface, which gives an estimate of the time needed for receptor turnover.

Figure 4.9 is a cartoon representation of a FRAP experiment at four different time points. In this neuron, GFP is bound to the molecule actin, a cytoskeletal structural protein. Pre-bleach serves as the baseline, where actin and the GFP signal are found throughout the spine. A single spine is targeted for precision photobleaching, after which the GFP signal is lost in the spine, but not in the dendrite. As actin is a protein that regularly moves around, GFP-labeled actin from the dendrite eventually enters the spine, displacing the bleached actin from the spine head first until the entire spine recovers from photobleaching.

Reading the Graphs

Representative images of the same field of view are shown over time. Time is indicated with "t =" where negative t is the baseline fluorescence before photobleaching, t =0 is immediately after the photobleaching paradigm, and positive t indicates elapsed time after photobleaching. A black-and-white image conveys the same information as a color image, since fluorophore brightness is typically the only feature being observed.

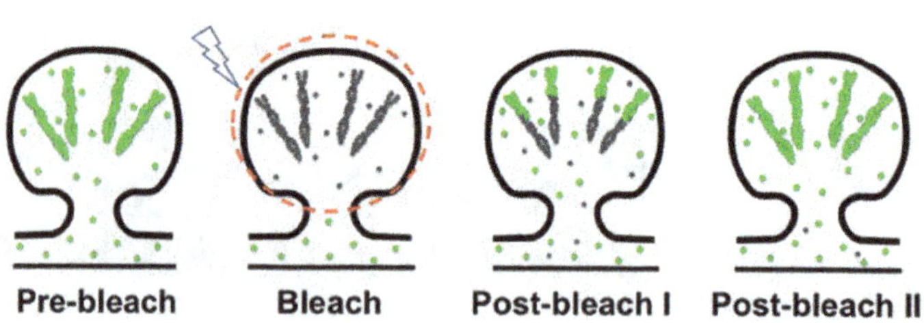

Figure 4.9 Cartoon showing the steps of FRAP. Source: George J, Soares C, Montersino A, Beique JC, Thomas GM. Palmitoylation of LIM Kinase-1 ensures spine-specific actin polymerization and morphological plasticity. *Elife.* 2015 Apr 17; 4:e06327. http://creativecommons.org/licenses/by/4.0/. Image cropped.

In graphs of group data, the x-axis plots time (seconds to hours) while the y-axis may plot fluorescence intensity, sometimes measured in arbitrary units (a.u.). The y-axis might alternatively plot maximum fluorescence recovery, which can be represented as a fraction or percentage. These graphs typically have the same approximate shape: flat baseline before photobleaching, a sudden decrease of fluorescence during photobleaching, then a logarithmic curve eventually reaching a plateau.

Figure 4.10 illustrates a FRAP experiment focused on axonal fluorescence of the molecule SEP. Panel A shows sample fluorescence microscopy images of axons. The region in the box has been photobleached and its brightness signal tracked over 15 minutes. Without Schwann cells, the fluorescence recovers the fastest (left column). By contrast, the nodes are the most stable regions (least mobile) since there is almost no recovery after 15 minutes. Panel B shows group averages of the time course of FRAP. On average, nodes show very little recovery, even up to 800 seconds after photobleaching. Here, because fluorescence is normalized to intensity pre-bleach, a baseline signal is not plotted.

Interpreting the Data

Plateau fluorescence is the main dependent variable. An upward-shifted curve suggests a higher plateau fluorescence, meaning that the fluorescence signal is more mobile (or less stable). The **stable** (or **immobile**) **fraction** may be presented, which is the baseline fluorescence minus the plateau value. This value represents the amount of fluorescence that did not recover after photobleaching. A higher stable fraction (lower plateau) means the fluorescent particles are less mobile. Measures of time to recovery may be quantified using $\tau_{1/2}$ (**recovery halftime**; pronounced tau), which is the time it takes for the fluorescence

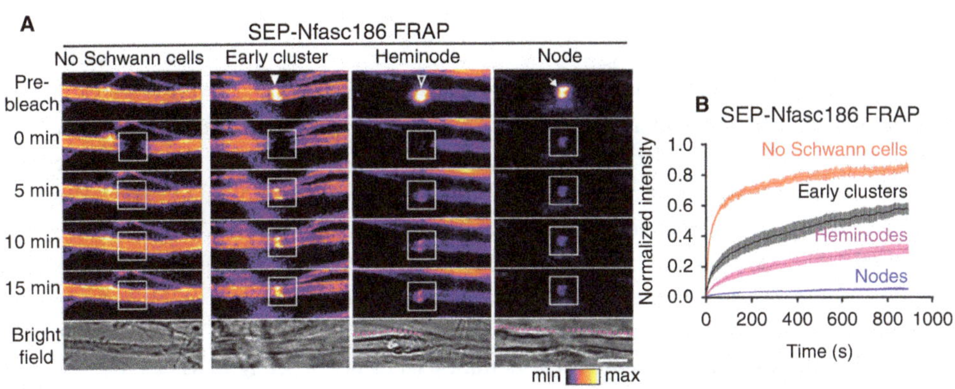

Figure 4.10 Fluorescence microscope images showing results of a FRAP experiment. Source: Malavasi ELV, Ghosh A, Booth DG, et al. Dynamic early clusters of nodal proteins contribute to node of Ranvier assembly during myelination of peripheral neurons. *eLife*. 2021; 10:e68089. http://creativecommons.org/licenses/by/4.0/. Image cropped.

signal to return to half plateau. A shorter $\tau_{1/2}$ is reflected by a leftward-shifted curve and it indicates that fluorescent particles move faster.

Data from various control experiments may also be plotted on the same graph.

- The pre-bleached condition (negative time) is a measurement of the fluorescence at baseline and is the most common internal control. It is necessary for calculating the fraction of recovery.
- To control for autofluorescence, a background control may also be measured by looking at a section of the image without the intended fluorescent signal. This background fluorescence is subtracted from the region of interest. Autofluorescence signal is brighter in tissue compared to cell cultures and is not observed using two-photon excitation.
- With two-photon excitation, precisely targeted light can bleach individual spines, while leaving adjacent spines unbleached. Measuring fluorescence of a nearby, size-matched dendritic spine before and after the photobleaching protocol is a within-cell but between-spine negative control. Both the unbleached spine and the dark-background controls are expected to be unchanged by the light exposure protocol. The unbleached spine control should remain high, while the background should be low.
- In addition to these methodological controls, data from experimental controls may also be plotted (wild type or saline-treated mice, for example).

Additional Resources

Lippincott-Schwartz J, Snapp EL, Phair RD. The development and enhancement of FRAP as a key tool for investigating protein dynamics. *Biophys J.* 2018 Oct 2; 115(7):1146–1155.

4.5 Flow Cytometry (FCM)

Background Information

Flow cytometry is a tool for counting and analyzing cells based on characteristics such as size, granularity, or receptor expression. The sample is a suspension of cells in solution which flows through a narrow funnel so that only one cell passes at a time. A laser is shined at each cell as it passes, and an array of detectors sense how that light responds after hitting the cell. Based on these properties, the FCM can differentiate the cells as they flow through the machine.

Figure 4.11 is a cartoon schematic of the flow cytometry process. The blend of cells is passed through a narrow funnel. The sensor detects different properties of the passing cells, ranging from size to fluorescence expression (Markers A, B, or C). Then, a dot plot is formed that shows which cells are more common (those expressing marker C).

Forward scatter (**FSC**, also called **low** or **small angle light scatter**) helps differentiate cells based on size. These detectors are placed directly across from the source of the laser and detect the light that passes through the cell. That light is diffracted when it hits cell membranes, so the greater the diffraction, the larger the cell.

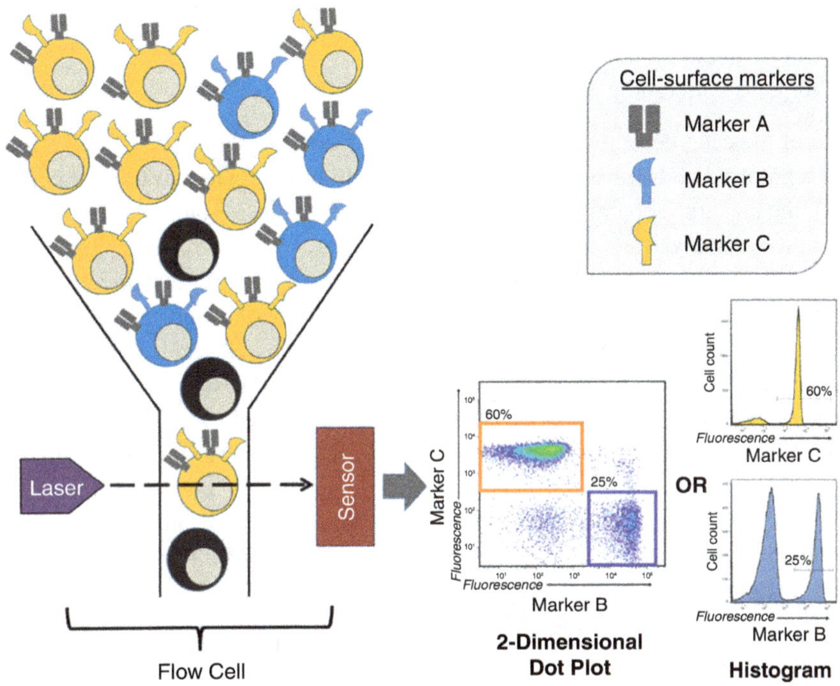

Figure 4.11 Cartoon showing the principles behind flow cytometry. Source: Verschoor CP, Lelic A, Bramson JL, Bowdish DME. An introduction to automated flow cytometry gating tools and their implementation. *Front Immunol.* 2015; 6:380. http://creativecommons.org/licenses/by/4.0/. Image cropped, images reorganized, and text changed.

Side scatter (**SSC**, or **wide angle light scatter**) helps distinguish cells based on **granularity**, the internal complexity of the cell. When light strikes an organelle, such as the nucleus or ribosomes, that light bounces off at a steep angle and strikes detectors located perpendicular to the beam of light. More side-scatter fluorescence detected suggests more granularity but does not give absolute information about the number of organelles or the types of organelles contained in the cell.

Based on size and granularity alone, it is possible to distinguish certain cell types. But the cell suspension can be exposed to fluorophore-conjugated antibodies (immunochemistry, discussed in Section 5.4 of this book), a process called **immunophenotyping**. This allows for detecting cell surface proteins expressed on each cell. For example, immunophenotyping allows the researcher to count the number of GluR3-expressing cells in a particular brain area.

Common markers for identifying nonneuronal cell types relevant for neuroscience research include:

- GLAST or GFAP for astrocytes
- CD11b for microglia

- A2B5 or O4 for oligodendrocyte precursor cells
- Annexin V for apoptotic cells
- EdU for cells undergoing the cell cycle

The fate of the cells depends on the machine being used. In standard flow cytometry, the sample is not used after it passes through the laser. In **fluorescence-activated cell sorting (FACS)**, the machine separates the cells based on the signal, automatically separating the cells for further analysis.

As an advantage of the technique, flow cytometry is a high-throughput method of analysis, capable of scanning tens of thousands of cells per second. Samples often have cell counts as high as millions of cells. It also offers single-cell resolution, which may be preferable over techniques which use a mix of cells such as Western blotting.

In neuroscience research, flow cytometry is most often used for the identification and study of glial cells, but it can target neurons as well. Results are mostly descriptive and exploratory rather than experimental. Research interests that may use flow cytometry include looking to see if certain receptor populations are found on different cell types, which populations of immune cells are involved in spinal cord injury, and how apoptosis proceeds under different conditions.

Reading the Graphs

Data from flow cytometry may show a hierarchy of gates, representative data, and group data.

Gates are screening measures used to separate genuine fluorescent signals from false positive events, and then later for distinguishing specific cell populations based on their fluorescent properties. Each gate excludes some number of cells, leaving a smaller number of events to be analyzed in the next step.

Graphs of gates are **two-parameter plots**, representing a combination of two histograms, one for the variable described on the *x*-axis and one for the *y*-axis. These graphs are shown as **dot plots**, **density** (or **pseudocolor**) **plots**, or **contour plots**, all of which can be used to represent the same set of data. Dot plots show each individual cell as a single dot. Density plots use different colors to represent where more points are clustered. Typically, "warmer" colors (reds, oranges, and yellows) indicate more cells than "cooler" colors (blues and greens). Contour plots will show concentric shapes, like a topographic map. More shapes that enclose a particular area on the plot indicate a higher number of counts.

Common gates may include:

- A **light scatter gate**, which plots FSC on the *x*-axis and SSC on the *y*-axis. Events that are too small (left half of the plot) or of too low complexity (bottom half of the plot) are likely debris not useful for analysis, such as fragments of cell membrane or free organelles remaining after cell rupture.
- A **viability gate**, which plots SSC on the *x*-axis versus propidium iodide (PI), 7-AAD, Trypan blue, or DAPI on the *y*-axis. Many of these dyes bind to DNA, so they will increase in fluorescence only if the cell membrane has been compromised, as in dead or dying cells. Low signal indicates viable cells, so only the bottom cells are included in the next step.

- A **multiplet exclusion gate**, which plots front scatter area (FSC-A) or width (FSC-W) against the height (FSC-H). This process eliminates a false positive signal called **multiplets** (or **aggregates**), which happen when two or more cells stick together during the flow process. Singlets may be identified by a diagonally shaped polygon drawn around the upper left portion of this plot.
- The remaining gates depend on the population and question of interest, such as fluorescence signals against certain cell markers or transmembrane proteins.

In Figure 4.12, representative dot plots present a sample series of sequentially applied gates to show which cells have been included for analysis. In all graphs, dots represent the properties of individual cells. Color represents where the cells "overlap" with their properties: warmer colors indicate more cells have those properties. Only the cells contained within specific boundaries (ovals or rectangles) were included for the gates used in this experiment. Panels A and C: cells based on size and complexity. Panel B: cells eliminated if they are multiplets. Panel D: cells included only if they expressed microglial markers. Panel E: differentiation of microglial type, whether they had high CD45 and positive CD11c, had low CD45 and positive CD11c, or were CD11c-negative.

The output variables are fluorescence, quantified as **mean** (or **median**) **fluorescence intensity** (**MFI**). These units are arbitrary and unitless. Because the values often cover

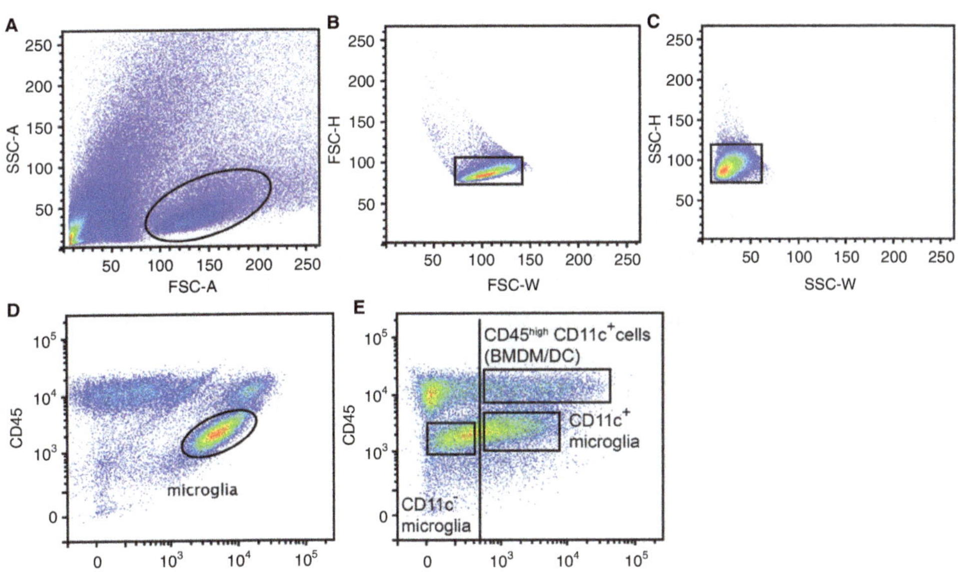

Figure 4.12 Dot plots showing scatter gates in a flow cytometry experiment. Source: Wlodarczyk A, Cédile O, Jensen KN, et al. Pathologic and protective roles for microglial subsets and bone marrow- and blood-derived myeloid cells in central nervous system inflammation. *Front Immunol.* 2015; 6:463. DOI: 10.3389/fimmu.2015.00463. https://creativecommons.org/licenses/by/4.0/.

several orders of magnitude, the axes are often on a logarithmic scale usually ranging from 0 to 10^5, but this range of values will depend on the software and the machine.

Sometimes, representative data may be shown as a single-parameter (or univariate) histogram. These plot log fluorescence intensity on the *x*-axis and number of cells on the *y*-axis. In single parameter histograms, there is often a bar which indicates the cutoff point between positive (on the right side of the graph) or negative expression (on the left side of the graph, or all cells that do not fall within the inclusion criteria).

Group data may plot the different experimental conditions or manipulations on the *x*-axis and the percentage of cells having some characteristic (or maybe stacked bar graphs) on the *y*-axis.

Interpreting the Data

Plots of gates and representative data are often marked into quadrants of unequal size with boundaries drawn around clumps of data points. There may be numbers in each quadrant, which typically represent the percentage cells that have those characteristics. Alternatively, polygons may be drawn around certain populations of cells.

There may be two or more representative plots, one showing the control data and the others being experimental groups. The plots will sometimes have a quadrant of interest, or a boundary highlighted. The relevant statistic of interest may be the percentage of cells in the region of interest after the manipulation. The average of these data points may then be presented in a summary graph.

In antibody-mediated fluorescence experiments, more fluorescence suggests stronger expression of that receptor. It may be challenging to clearly identify the boundary between cells that have a positive expression (denoted with a superscript +, such as in $CD11c^{+}$) versus negative expression (a superscript −; $CD11c^{-}$).

If a measure of apoptosis is shown on the axes, higher fluorescence indicates more cell death.

Figure 4.13 illustrates flow cytometry used to measure cell viability. Populations of cultured neurons were exposed to seven different conditions. A: Flow cytometry results for the seven different conditions. High fluorescence of Annexin-V-FITC and PI (upper right quadrant for each graph) suggests dead cells. When cells were exposed to oxygen-glucose deprivation (OGD), more cells died compared to the control condition. Exposure to the chemicals DEX, 3-MA, or both decreased the number of dead cells, showing a partial reversal of effect. RAPA does not reverse the cell death caused by OGD, but adding DEX does. B and C: Bar graphs to quantify group data.

Additional Resources

Herzenberg L, Tung J, Moore W, et al. Interpreting flow cytometry data: A guide for the perplexed. *Nat Immunol.* 2006; 7:681–685.

FlowJo. Software package for analyzing flow cytometry data. https://docs.flowjo.com/flowjo/.

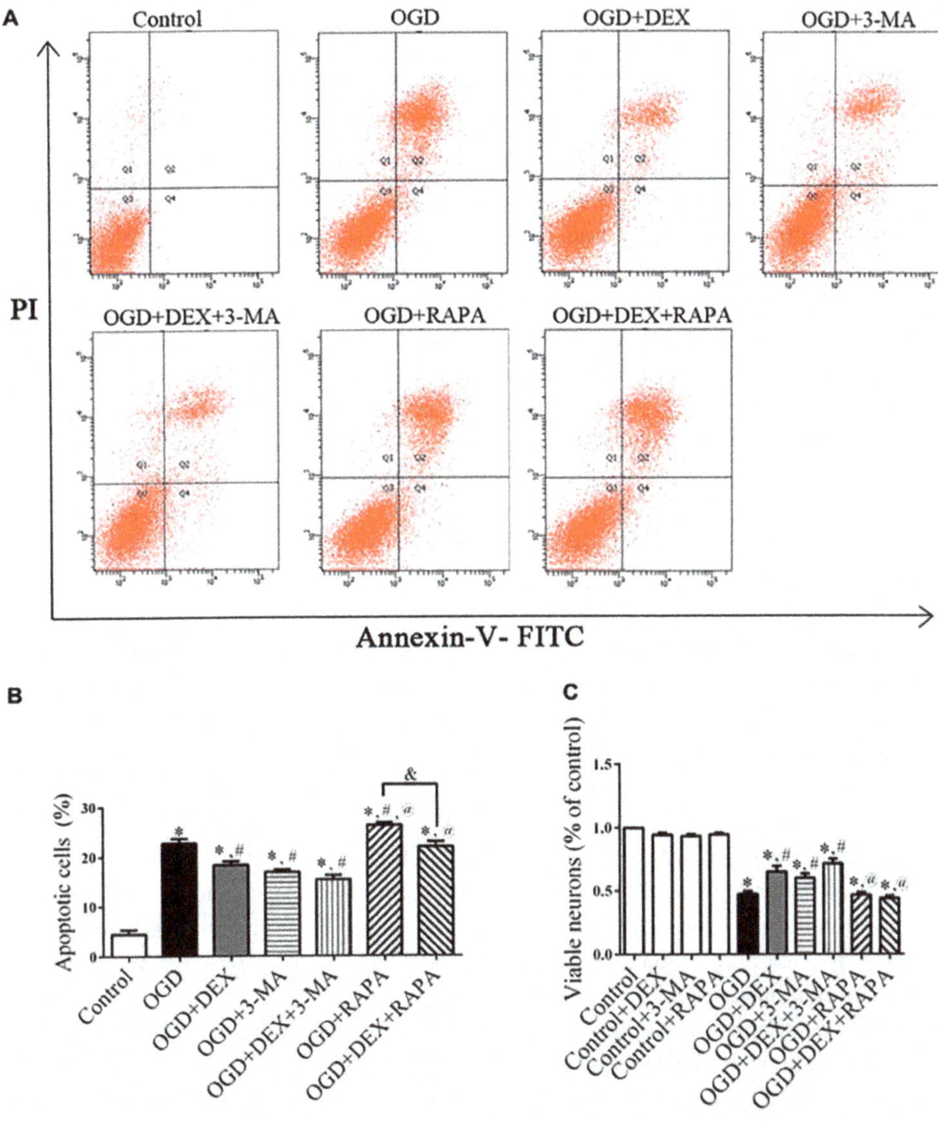

Figure 4.13 Dot plots showing results of a flow cytometry experiment to quantify cell viability. Source: Luo C, Ouyang M-W, Fang Y-Y, et al. Dexmedetomidine protects mouse brain from ischemia-reperfusion injury via inhibiting neuronal autophagy through up-regulating HIF-1α. *Front Cell Neurosci.* 2017; 11:197. http://creativecommons.org/licenses/by/4.0/.

4.6 Stains, Dyes, and Tracers

A **stain** or a **dye** is a chemical treatment that allows for visualization of parts of cells. Typically, stains are observed under bright-field or fluorescence light microscopy. Stains themselves can be acidic or basic. Acidic dyes are salts where the colored ion has a negative charge, and these often stain cytoplasmic proteins. On the other hand, the colored ion of basic dyes has a positive charge. These often stain nuclear material.

Many different stains are used in neuroscience research, and representative images are often shown alongside group data.

- **Golgi stain** (or the derivative **Golgi-Cox stain**) is used to map out the morphology of neurons. This stain causes the entire cell to be filled, even at the level of the dendritic spines. But it sparsely labels cells in tissue, only targeting about 1% of neurons. Originally called the "**black reaction**," cells labeled by the Golgi stain appear black on a light-gray or yellow-tinted background. Golgi stained cells can be used for quantifying neuronal complexity (**Sholl analysis**; see Section 4.6.1) or dendritic spines (Section 4.6.2).
- **Cresyl violet** (**CV**, or **Nissl**) **stain** is a basic dye that targets RNA, found densely in the rough endoplasmic reticulum (rER). Representative images of tissue stained with cresyl violet are in shades of purple, with gray matter being darker than white matter since most of the rER is found in the dendrites and the soma (axons contain little rER). CV stains can be used to compare differences in numbers of neurons or sizes of certain brain structures with distinct gray/white matter differences, such as the corpus callosum, retinal layers, or hippocampus, for example. Decreases in numbers of cresyl-violet-stained neurons suggests cell death.
- **Luxol fast blue (LFB) stain** is a myelin stain. Sections of tissue are shades of blue, where areas of more myelin will appear darker and areas with less myelin are pale. LFB is useful for determining the degree of demyelination after injury or in models of multiple sclerosis, for example.
- **Propidium iodide** (**PI**) and **DAPI** are fluorescent stains that are useful for identifying DNA. Because PI is not membrane-permeable, it produces signal only when the cell membrane integrity is weakened, or the cell has died.
- **Hematoxylin and eosin** (**H&E** or **HE**) **stain** is a pair of stains, one acidic and one basic, used commonly in histopathological analysis useful for detecting cell loss. The result is grayish-pinkish-purple images of tissue. Cell nuclei will show up dark purple against a lighter pink background.
- Terminal deoxynucleotidyl transferase (TdT) dUTP nick end labeling, abbreviated the **TUNEL stain**, is used for assaying the degree of apoptosis in a section of tissue. During apoptosis, the DNA breaks apart. The enzyme TdT adds nucleotides to the broken sections of DNA, which increases the intensity of the TUNEL stain. Under light microscopy, TUNEL-positive cells appear as reddish-brown, but the TUNEL stain can also be conjugated with a fluorophore, which can be seen with fluorescence microscopy. More TUNEL-positive cells means more cell loss, so a manipulation that causes cell death, such as ischemia, will result in increased TUNEL signal.

Figure 4.14 shows stained brain tissue slices. Left two figures: Golgi-Cox stained samples from the cortex of an adult rat. In this stain, neurons appear dark against a light-gray background. At high magnification, this stain allows for quantification of spines. Scale bar represents 100 μm at low power (left) and 10 μm at high power (right). Right two figures: Cresyl violet stained tissue samples showing the cortex of an adult mouse. Certain

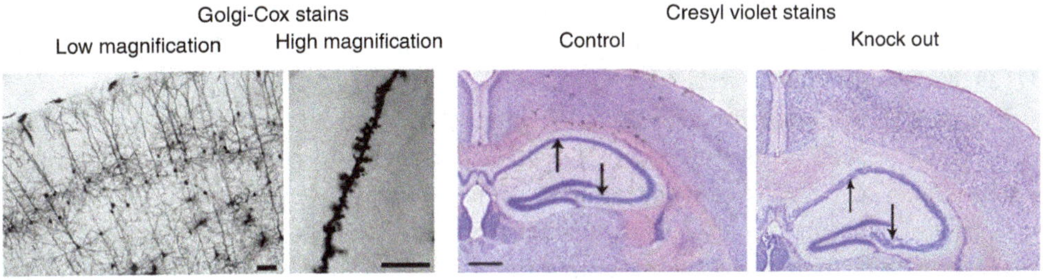

Figure 4.14 Tissue that has been stained. Source: Zhong F, Liu L, Wei J-L, Dai R-P. Step by step Golgi-Cox staining for cryosection. *Front Neuroanat.* 2019; 13:62. Zhang B, McDaniel SS, Rensing NR, Wong M. Vigabatrin inhibits seizures and mTOR pathway activation in a mouse model of tuberous sclerosis complex. *PLOS One.* 2013; 8(2):e57445. http://creativecommons.org/licenses/by/4.0/. Images have been cropped and text labels removed.

structures of the hippocampus, such as the layers of pyramidal cells (arrows), appear as darker shades of purple. In wild type control mice (left), the layers are neatly organized. Among conditional knockouts of the Tsc1^{GFAP} gene, these neurons appeared disorganized. Scale bar represents 500 µm.

To identify different cell parts or types in the same tissue, it can be treated with two stains, a process called **counterstaining**. For example, counterstaining with cresyl violet and Luxol fast blue will target gray matter in violet and white matter in blue.

While stains and dyes are useful for identifying parts of cells, **tracers** are chemical substances that are used to examine the connections of the nervous system. They help in identifying the afferent (incoming) and efferent (outgoing) connections in an area, a strategy called **tract-tracing**. Studies using tracers are generally exploratory and may provide ideas for new hypothesis to test using functional methods such as electrophysiology.

Conventional tracers are compounds that are put directly into a region of interest. A microsyringe filled with the tracer is placed in the region of interest, and then positive physical pressure may be applied (injection) or electrical current may be passed (**iontophoresis**), which causes the tracer to diffuse through the brain tissue. The tracers are then taken up into cells through a process of endocytosis. Some commonly used tracers include **wheat germ agglutinin (WGA)**, **horseradish peroxidase (HRP)** and **biotinylated dextran amine (BDA)**. These tracers may be conjugated with fluorophores for visualization.

Viral-mediated tracers use viruses containing specific DNA sequences to deliver the tracer molecule to the cells. The researcher injects the virus into the region of interest, and then the virus delivers the DNA of the tracer into the adjacent cells in a process called **transduction** (not to be confused with transfection, which doesn't utilize viruses). The DNA typically codes for fluorophore such as GFP. Viral-mediated tract tracing in genetically modified animals (such as Cre lines of mice) offers the option of selecting for cell type, which is a major advantage in regions that are a heterogenous mix of cell populations. For example, the striatum contains two very similar types of spiny projection neurons that differ in their receptor expression patterns. Using viral-mediated tracers and genetically modified

Cre mice, we can target these two populations differently. Examples of commonly used viral vectors for tract-tracing include **adeno-associated virus 2 (AAV2)**, **herpes simplex H129**, and **rabies virus**.

Figure 4.15 is an experimental protocol figure showing how three viral vectors (CAV, AAV, and Rbv) can be used to trace afferents and efferents of a theoretical brain area of interest, locus X. CAVCre is injected into the putative output site of locus X, which causes both anterograde and retrograde signal (blue). For CAVCre, cells in the output site as well as those that send their axons into the output site, such as cells in locus X, will signal in blue. When AAV is injected into locus X, there is a local signal (red), and only cells in locus X will appear red. When Rbv is injected into locus X, there is both a local and a retrograde signal (green), so neurons in locus X as well as neurons that project into locus X appear green.

After being taken up by the neurons, tracers may move in two different directions. **Anterograde tracers** are taken up by the cell bodies in the injection area and show

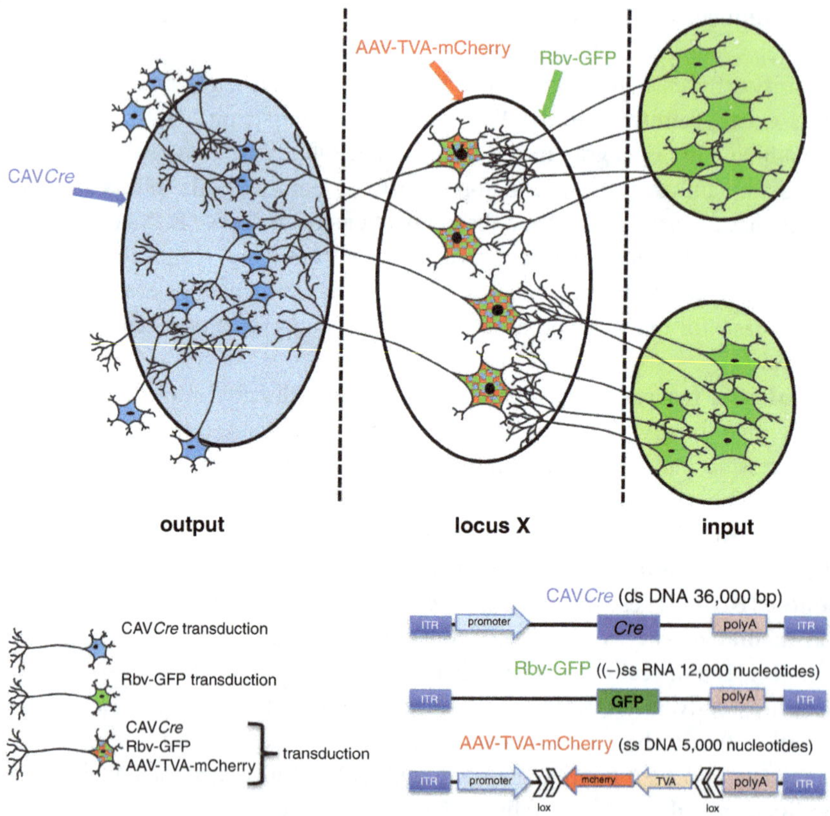

Figure 4.15 Cartoon representation of an experiment using tracers. Source: del Rio D, Beucher B, Lavigne M, et al. CAV-2 vector development and gene transfer in the central and peripheral nervous systems. *Front Mol Neurosci.* 2019; 12:71. http://creativecommons.org/licenses/by/4.0/.

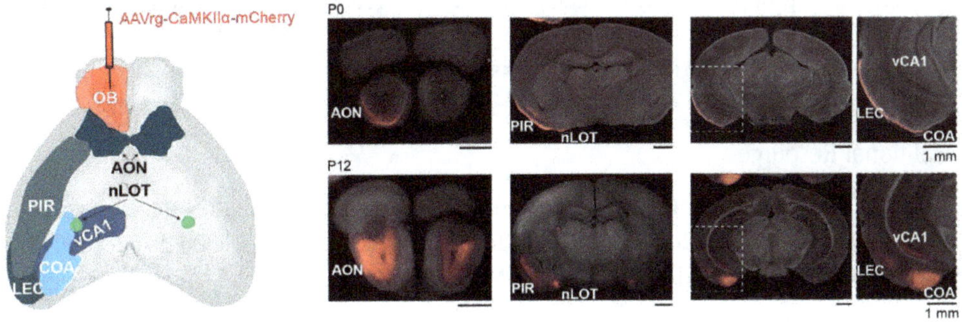

Figure 4.16 Results from a retrograde tracing experiment. Source: Kostka JK, Bitzenhofer SH. Postnatal development of centrifugal inputs to the olfactory bulb. *Front Neurosci.* 2022; 16:815282. http://creativecommons.org/licenses/by/4.0/. Image cropped and figures rearranged.

where these neurons send their axonal projections. A **retrograde tracer** is taken up by axons in the area and then moves toward the cell bodies, showing which areas send projections. Some tracers are **transsynaptic** and can even "hop" across synapses.

Figure 4.16 shows results from a viral mediated retrograde tracer experiment in mice. Experimenters were curious as to which areas of the brain send axonal projections into the olfactory bulb, and whether this pattern changes during the first two weeks of development. The image on the left shows a horizontal slice of the mouse brain with the anterior direction facing upwards. Highlighted in red is the site of viral injection, the olfactory bulb (OB). The virus delivered is a retrograde AAV (AAVrg), so it will be taken up by the axons of neurons that send their projections into the OB. Virus was injected at two different time points during mouse development, some at birth (or postnatal day 0, P0) and others 12 days after birth (P12). Depending on the animal's age during injection, different brain structures took up the red AAV signal; those regions are shown in the four pairs of images on the right, which are coronal brain slices overlaid with red wherever the signal appeared. There were no contralateral connections at age P0. Some areas that contain cell bodies that send projections into the olfactory bulb include the anterior olfactory nucleus (AON), piriform cortex (PIR), nucleus of the lateral olfactory tract (nLOT), lateral entorhinal cortex (LEC), cortical amygdala (COA), and ventral CA1 of the hippocampus (vCA1).

Reading the Images

Representative images are typically photomicrographs of transmission bright-field microscopy for stains and fluorescence microscopy images for tract tracing. Overlaid on these images may be defined brain areas or boundaries. In three-dimensional reconstructions of the whole brain, axes may be added to indicate the dorsal/ventral, medial/lateral, or anterior/posterior direction. In tract tracing studies, illustrations are sometimes drawn to show injection sites or tracings of individual neurons of different colors, which may be helpful since multiple tracers can be used in the same experiment.

Quantifiable group data may include percentage of area with positive stain signal, optical density of signal, number of cells with a certain marker per area, Sholl analysis (discussed in Section 4.6.1), or dendritic spine analysis (Section 4.6.2).

Additional Resources

Lanciego JL, Wouterlood FG. Neuroanatomical tract-tracing techniques that did go viral. *Brain Struct Funct.* 2020 May; 225(4):1193–1224. DOI: 10.1007/s00429-020-02041-6. Epub 2020 Feb 15. PMID: 32062721; PMCID: PMC7271020.

4.6.1 Sholl Analysis

Background Information

The Sholl analysis is used to quantify the complexity of neuronal processes (or neurites), which includes both dendrites and axons. This analysis can also be applied to glial cells with branched processes.

First, the target cells must be stained so that the phenomenon can be visualized using techniques such as a Golgi stain or immunochemistry. Then, a series of concentric circles with progressively larger radii are drawn (called **shells**), with their centers at the middle of the soma. The number of intersections between each shell and the cell are counted.

Sholl analysis is typically performed on "flattened" images of cells, which reduces the fluorescence signal from the third dimension into two. But a three-dimensional Sholl analysis can also be done, in which case the shells are concentric spheres.

Reading the Graph

Images of representative cells or a traced reconstruction may be shown. The shells may be overlaid, and each intersection between the cell and a shell may be indicated.

In a group summary graph, the radius of each shell is plotted on the x-axis, usually in intervals of 5 or 10 micrometers (μm). The number of intersections (or **crossings**) is plotted on the y-axis. For each of the shells (each unit on the x-axis), the number of intersections is counted. The x-axis values may go as high as the length of the longest process, which may be as large as 800 μm. Even in cells with extensive branching, the y-values do not often exceed 25.

Data will appear as an **inverted U**. At lower x-axis values (smaller shells), there may be no overlap with dendritic process since this represents the cell body. At large shells, there are no longer any neurites to intersect. Therefore, intermediate values will have the greatest number of intersections.

Figure 4.17 represents Sholl analysis performed on hippocampal astrocytes from guinea pigs. Four different conditions were tested: a control condition (CT), and conditions where animals were given either bicuculline methiodide (BMI) alone, BMI plus a dosage of h-recombinant albumin (BMI+h-ALB), or BMI+hALB followed by a final dose of BMI

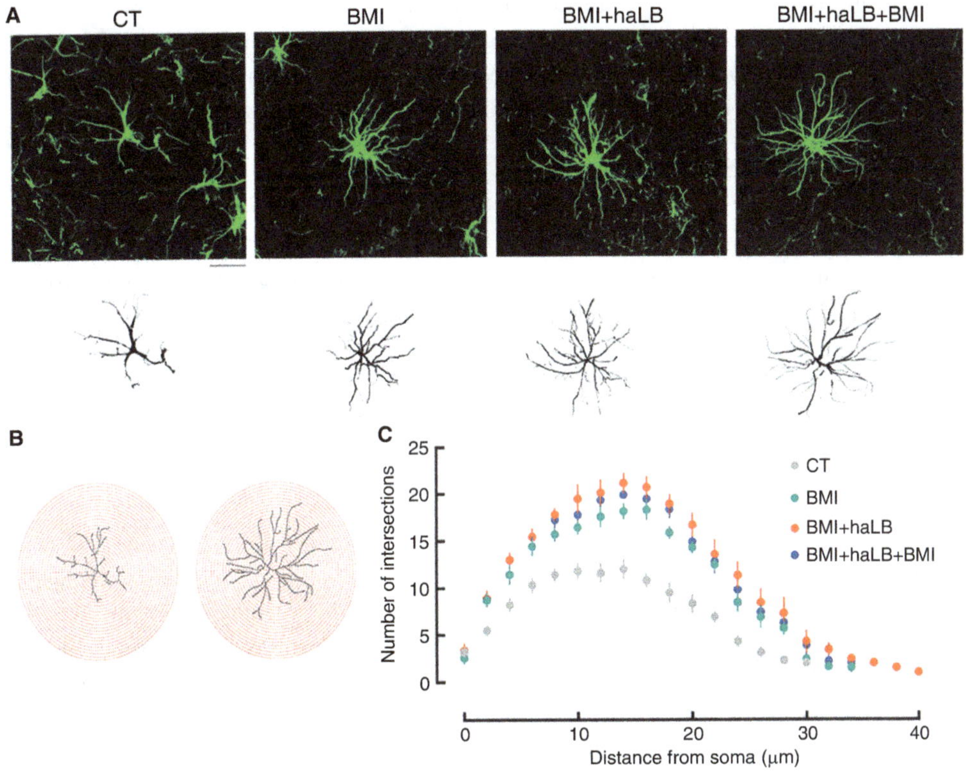

Figure 4.17 Results of a Sholl analysis. Source: Vila Verde D, de Curtis M, Librizzi L. Seizure-induced acute glial activation in the in vitro isolated guinea pig brain. *Front Neurol.* 2021; 12:607603. http://creativecommons.org/licenses/by/4.0/. Image cropped.

(BMI+hALB+BMI). Panel A: representative fluorescent images (top) and 3D reconstructions using confocal microscopy (bottom). Panel B: concentric rings are drawn overlaying two representative astrocyte reconstructions showing astrocytes from control (left) and BMI+hALB+BMI (right) conditions. Panel C: group average data quantifying the number of intersections (*y*-axis) at progressively farther distances from the center (*x*-axis). In this experiment, astrocytic complexity increases in all three experimental conditions.

Interpreting the Data

Increases in complexity (upward shifts in the curve) suggest a greater potential for communication, as the cell has more dendrites to receive inputs or axonal branches to send outputs. On the other hand, a downward shift suggests potential decrease in communication.

A limitation of Sholl analysis is that it only approximates neurite length, especially in analysis of a two-dimensional compressed *z*-stack. The neurite may extend into the *z*-stack, so its length is therefore underestimated in a Sholl analysis. Even in a 3D Sholl analysis, neurites are likely to curve and weave through space. Imagine a neurite that extends away from the soma but doubles back like a looped hairpin. The length of this neurite will be much longer than the number of intersections counted by a Sholl analysis.

Additional Resources

Wilson MD, Sethi S, Lein PJ, Keil KP. Valid statistical approaches for analyzing sholl data: Mixed effects versus simple linear models. *J Neurosci Methods*. 2017 Mar 1; 279:33–43. DOI: 10.1016/j.jneumeth.2017.01.003. Epub 2017 Jan 16. PMID: 28104486; PMCID: PMC5346342.

4.6.2 Dendritic Spine Analysis

Background Information

Dendritic spines are small (~1 micron) protrusions of some neurons that extend from dendrites. Changes in spines represent one form of **plasticity**, a long-lasting change in the communication between neurons that is likely to underlie learning and memory.

Spines shapes are named based roughly on their morphology. Typically, spines have at least two obvious components, the **neck** which branches off the dendrite, and the **head** which is the end of the spine. Three common quantifiable characteristics of spines include spine length (L), neck diameter (ND; also neck width WN), and head diameter (HD; also head width, WH). The relationships between these values are used to classify spines into categories.

- **Mushroom** spines are spines where the ratio of head diameter to neck diameter is larger than 1, like a top-heavy mushroom cap. Sometimes, these are also called **mature** spines.
- **Thin** (or **long**) spines have a length greater than 0.75 μm, but shorter than 3 μm. The diameter of the head and neck should be similar.
- **Stubby** spines have a length shorter than 0.75 μm.
- **Multiheaded** spines have two or more heads.
- **Filopodia** have lengths greater than 3 μm. In filopodia, the HD and ND are the same. Filopodia tend to be the most plastic of the dendritic spines, and some may be immature spines in the process of finding long-term synapses.

Instead of shape, head diameter alone may be used to distinguish spines. A size-based system may categorize spines as small (<0.3 μm), medium, or large (>0.5 μm), or may analyze them as continuous variables.

Visualizing spines can be done in either fixed tissue or live tissue. Fixed-tissue imaging methods only allow us to capture a snapshot of the spines, meaning that analyses are between-subject comparisons, since changes cannot be observed over time for the same set of spines. Fixed-tissue methods commonly used in spine analysis include:

- Golgi staining with bright-field (light) microscopy.

- Immunostaining and fluorescence microscopy. Specific antibodies may be used with reactivity against proteins that are found only in dendritic spines, such as filamentous actin (F-actin) or Drebrin (developmentally regulated brain protein). Alternatively, a neuron in a slice can be filled using a patch pipette such as biocytin, which can be later identified with immunohistochemistry.
- Electron microscopy (EM). Since it has higher resolution than light microscopy, it can provide more accurate estimations of measurements, as long as several ultrathin sections can be analyzed.

In live-tissue imaging, the same set of dendritic spines can be tracked over a time course of tens of minutes up to days, allowing for within-subject comparisons. Techniques include the following:

- Acute brain slices with individual neurons injected with a fluorescent dye such as Lucifer Yellow (LY). This can be done alongside electrophysiological experiments, since a patch pipette can be used to diffuse the dye throughout the cell. However, the time course of imaging is limited on the timescale of hours, since slices lose viability over time.
- Genetically encoded fluorescence. The sequence for fluorescent proteins (informally: **markers** or **tags**) are introduced into the genes of specific animal proteins and can be visualized with microscopy. The marker is identified by animal strain, typically described in the methods section of the publication. Spines can be observed using two-photon imaging and a **thin skull preparation**, where the researcher uses a drill to shave away the outer layers of the skull directly above the region of interest (also called **transcranial imaging**), allowing light to pass through the skull. (Markers can also be visualized in fixed tissue.)

Reading the Figures

Representative images usually show a straight section of a single dendrite with several spines. The cell and spines may be darker than the background (Golgi-Cox stain) or lighter than the background (fluorescent imaging).

In group data, different measures may be analyzed and plotted, including:

- Number of spines, possibly normalized to a set distance of dendrite (dendritic spine density, DSD). Typical numbers may range from 0.1 spines per micron in spinal cord to 1 spine per micron in the brain.
- Spine or head volume, typically on the order of tenths of a micron cubed.
- Length of spine, typically a few microns.
- Some measure of spine redistribution, including whether there are more spines closer to the soma or more along the apical dendrites.

In live-tissue imaging, a plot may show time on the x-axis and some dependent variable measurement on the y-axis.

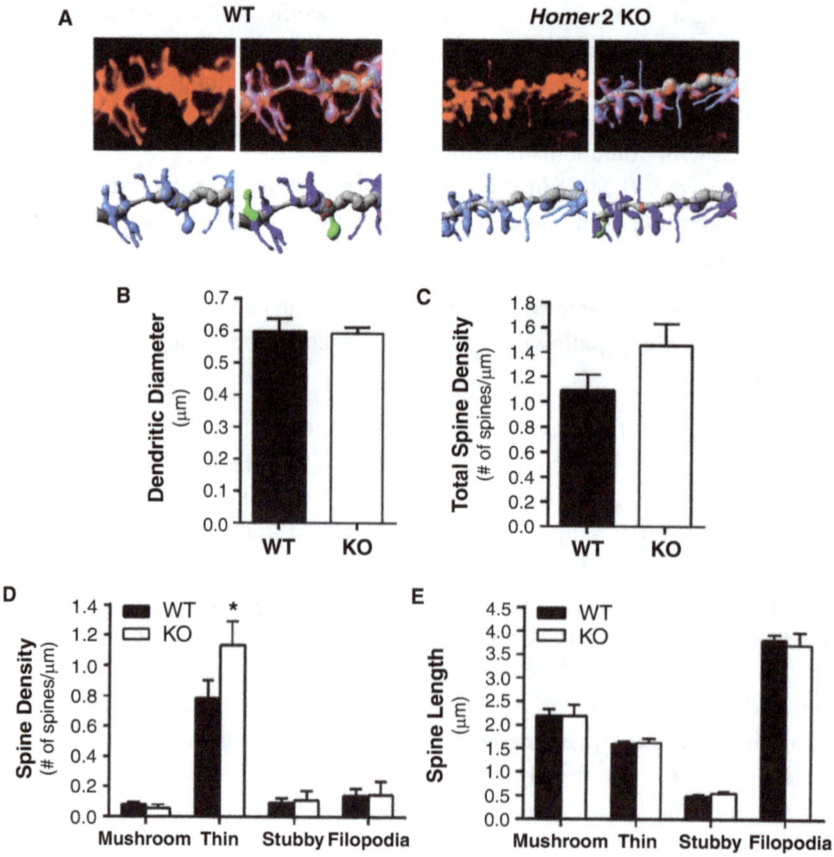

Figure 4.18 Quantification of dendritic spines. Source: McGuier NS, Padula AE, Mulholland PJ, Chandler LJ. Homer2 deletion alters dendritic spine morphology but not alcohol-associated adaptations in GluN2B-containing N-methyl-D-aspartate receptors in the nucleus accumbens. *Front Pharmacol.* 2015; 6:28. http://creativecommons.org/licenses/by/4.0/.

Figure 4.18 represents an analysis of dendritic spines of medium spiny neurons from the nucleus accumbens core comparing between WT mice and those with a knockout of the Homer2 gene. Panel A: representative fluorescent confocal microscope images and corresponding digital reconstructions. In reconstructions, gray shows dendritic shaft while light blue represents spines. Other colors are used to show spines based on their morphology: dark blue are long thin spines, pink are filopodia, red are stubby, and green are mushroom spines. Panels B, C, D, and E: Bar graphs showing averages of group data, each plotting different quantifiable measures. Dendritic diameter, total spine density, and spine length were unchanged in the knockout mice. Only the density of thin spines was increased among the knockout mice.

Interpreting the Data

Spines may change their properties in response to manipulations, throughout development, and in aging. Since spines often represent the postsynaptic site for the excitatory neurotransmitter glutamate, increases in spine number or volume/surface area may indicate potentiation since more receptors may be present. Spine changes proximal to the soma may have a greater impact on cell excitability compared to distal changes.

Additional Resources

Meldolesi J. Post-synapses in the brain: Role of dendritic and spine structures. *Biomedicines*. 2022 Aug 2; 10(8):1859. DOI: 10.3390/biomedicines10081859. PMID: 36009405; PMCID: PMC9405724.

Minegishi T, Kastian RF, Inagaki N. Mechanical regulation of synapse formation and plasticity. *Semin Cell Dev Biol*. 2023 May 15; 140:82–89. DOI: 10.1016/j.semcdb.2022.05.017. Epub 2022 Jun 1. PMID: 35659473.

Summary

This chapter has introduced the tools used in analyzing the nervous system at the level of neurons and glia. Since these cells in mammals are on the scale of tens of microns or smaller, specialized imaging strategies, such as microscopy, are necessary. We have described three microscopy techniques, including their applications and limitations: bright-field microscopy, fluorescence microscopy, and electron microscopy.

These microscopy techniques are often used in conjunction with other techniques for cellular level analysis, including:

- Unbiased stereology for quantifying three-dimensional aspects of cells
- FRAP for measuring movement of fluorescently labeled particles
- Flow cytometry for rapidly identifying unique cell populations
- Stains, dyes, and tracers for assessing cell morphology and projections.

The next chapter looks at techniques used for understanding molecules, particles even smaller than cells.

Key Terms

- action potential
- anterograde tracer
- astrocyte
- autofluorescence
- axon
- axon hillock
- axon terminal

- bright-field microscope
- cell body
- coexpression
- colocalization
- confocal microscope
- conventional tracer
- counterstain
- cresyl violet
- DAPI
- dendrite
- dichromatic beamsplitter
- dye
- electron microscopy
- emission filter
- endoplasmic reticulum
- ependymal cell
- excitation filter
- FACS
- filopodia
- flow cytometry
- fluorescence-activated cell sorting
- fluorescence microscope
- fluorescence recovery after photobleaching (FRAP)
- fluorophore
- forward scatter
- ganglion
- gate
- glia
- Golgi apparatus
- Golgi stain
- granularity
- hematoxylin and eosin stain
- immunophenotyping
- index of refraction
- light-sheet microscope
- Luxol fast blue
- lysosome
- microglia
- mitochondria
- multiheaded
- multiplet
- mushroom

- myelin
- Nissl stain
- node of Ranvier
- nucleus
- neurofilament
- oligodendrocyte
- optical clearing
- organelle
- photobleaching
- postsynaptic density
- propidium iodide
- recovery halftime
- retrograde tracer
- ribosome
- scanning electron microscope
- Schwann cell
- shells
- Sholl analysis
- side scatter
- soma
- spine
- spinning disk confocal microscope
- stable fraction
- stubby
- synapse
- thin
- thin skull preparation
- tracers
- transmission electron microscope
- transsynaptic tracer
- TUNEL stain
- two-parameter plot
- two-photon microscope
- ultrathin slice
- unbiased stereology
- viral-mediated tracer
- *z*-stack

CHAPTER FIVE

Molecular Methods

5.1 Introduction to Molecular Methods

Compared to understanding whole organisms (Chapters 2 and 3) or cellular structures (Chapter 4), the biggest challenges in molecular biology are about visualization. Molecules operate at a tiny scale, sometimes on the order of angstroms (abbreviated as Å, equivalent to 0.1 nanometers; to provide some context of scale, the atomic radius of a hydrogen atom is about 0.5 angstroms). Because of this, methods of studying molecules rely on indirect tools and strategies that allow for subcellular observations. This chapter focuses on some of these techniques.

Since the **central dogma of molecular biology** in the late 1950s, science has made great strides in understanding the process of molecular action. According to this framework, genetic material is stored in the form of a double-stranded molecule called **deoxyribonucleic acid (DNA)**, which is contained in the nucleus. During a closely regulated process called **transcription**, DNA is made accessible to enzymes. These synthesize molecules called messenger ribonucleic acid (**mRNA**), which are single-stranded pieces of genetic material. This mRNA exits the nucleus, where nearby ribosomes coordinate with molecules of **transfer RNA (tRNA)** to create **proteins** in a process called **translation**. Proteins are molecules made up of amino acid residues.

A protein's structure can be described at four levels – primary, secondary, tertiary, and quaternary – as illustrated in Figure 5.1.

1. **Primary structure** is the sequence of amino acids, usually written out as a string of capital letters where each letter represents a specific amino acid. The primary structure can always be predicted based on the sequence of the mRNA.
2. **Secondary structure** describes the protein's shape after considering bonds between nonadjacent amino acids. Common shapes found in secondary structures include the alpha helix, beta sheet, and beta barrel.
3. **Tertiary structure** is the complete three-dimensional structure of the protein, including amino-acid-to-amino-acid-residue interactions such as disulfide bridges and hydrophobic interactions. Predicting tertiary structures from the primary structure requires tremendous computational power and is one of the major challenges in biochemistry.
4. **Quaternary structure** is how the protein interacts with other similar proteins. For example, the nicotinic acetylcholine receptor is made up of five related proteins which interact with one another to form the receptor and the pore across the cell membrane. Not all proteins will have a quaternary structure.

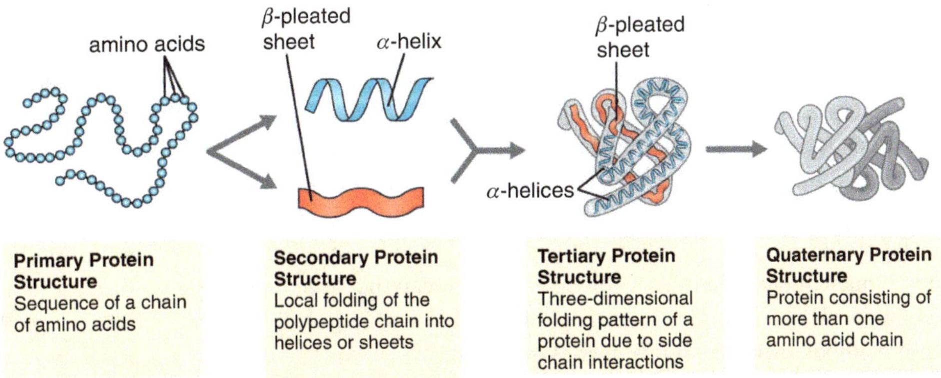

Figure 5.1 Cartoons showing the four levels of protein structure. Source: OpenStax Microbiology. Provided by: OpenStax CNX. https://openstax.org/books/microbiology/pages/1-introduction. License: CC BY: Attribution. https://creativecommons.org/licenses/by/4.0/. License terms: Download for free at http://cnx.org/contents/e42bd376-624b-4c0f-972f-e0c57998e765@4.2.

Protein structure is critically important in neuroscience. Gene mutations cause differences in protein structure, which has been implicated in many diseases of the nervous system ranging from prion diseases such as Creutzfeldt-Jakob disease and mad cow disease to neurodegenerative conditions such as Parkinson's and Alzheimer's diseases.

Learning Objectives

By the end of this chapter, you will be able to:

- Describe the theory and principles behind some of the techniques used to study molecular structure, location, or interaction between molecules.
- Explain the advantages and limitations of each of the techniques, understanding that each technique is best suited for a particular type of research question.
- Describe the figures that represent results collected using these methods.

Additional Resources

Kuhlman B, Bradley P. Advances in protein structure prediction and design. *Nat Rev Mol Cell Biol*. 2019; 20: 681–697.

5.2 *In Situ* Hybridization

Background Information

***In situ* hybridization** (*in situ* means "in place") is used to identify the location of specific sequences of mRNA or DNA. A single-stranded molecule of genetic material called a **probe** is designed to interact with a sequence of interest. The **antisense probe** (also called a **complementary RNA (cRNA)** probe, or **riboprobe**) is washed over a slice of fixed tissue, binding to its complementary sequence wherever it is found by forming bonds across nucleotide pairs (this process is hybridization). The exact sequence of interest is often identified by an **accession number**, which can be found in the NCBI database, or is provided in the text or table. Probes can range in length from 20 to more than a thousand nucleic acids long.

The probes are tagged with a molecule used for visualization. Some probes use radioactive nucleotides, such as S35-UTP, which can be seen using x-ray film or with a computer-based detection system. However, because radioactivity emits a diffuse signal, these methods suffer from low spatial resolution.

A technique with higher spatial resolution is **fluorescence *in situ* hybridization (FISH)**. FISH uses riboprobes tagged with a marker such as biotin or digoxin (DIG) followed by secondary treatment with antibodies tagged with a fluorophore (an approach called **immunochemistry**; see Section 5.4). Fluorescence microscopy allows for visualization.

These techniques are common in research for nonhuman samples but can also be done using human tissue slices. They are performed on fixed tissue, so they can only provide information about a single instance.

Reading the Figures

Representative images at both low- and high-power magnification may be shown. Low-magnification images show patterns of RNA levels across several brain structures, while high magnification offers subcellular level resolution, able to identify RNA location with respect to organelles.

Images of radiography using bright-field microscopy will appear in grayscale with a mostly gray background. A positive signal will appear darker compared to the background. In dark-field microscopy, the opposite is true: the image is mostly dark, while lighter areas indicate the presence of a positive signal. FISH produces fluorescence microscope images with a black background and various colors indicating the presence of mRNA hybridized signal.

Sample tissue may be counterstained (described in Section 4.6) to help identify brain regions or cellular structures and organelles. For example, counterstaining with DAPI identifies that the mRNA signal is near the nucleus, and counterstaining with Luxol fast blue can show if mRNA is in a white matter tract (low magnification) or in the axon (high magnification).

Figure 5.2 shows representative data of coronal slices from an mRNA *in situ* hybridization study in a person with diabetes. Panel A shows Nissl stain at low magnification, useful to show major anatomical landmarks which have been labeled by abbreviations. The box indicates the location of the zoomed-in panels that follow. Panels B, C, and D show *in situ* hybridizations against mRNA for oxytocin (panel B) and GLP-1R (panels C and D). Panel D is the same slice from C shown using dark-field radiography. These data show that, for this

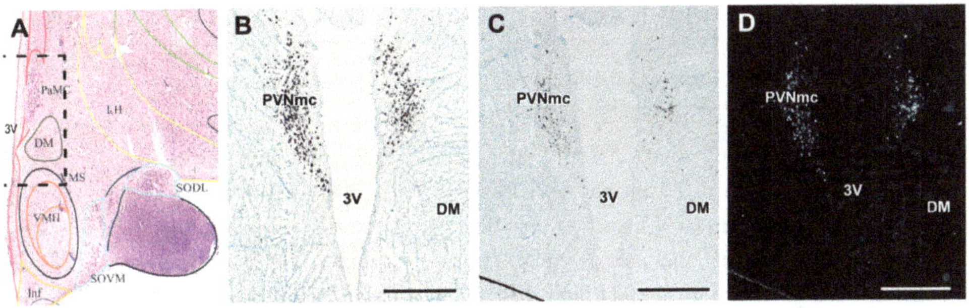

Figure 5.2 Results of an *in situ* hybridization experiment. Source: Renner É, Dóra F, Oszwald E, Dobolyi Á, Palkovits M. Elevated glucagon-like peptide-1 receptor level in the paraventricular hypothalamic nucleus of type 2 diabetes mellitus patients. *Int J Mol Sci.* 2022; 23(24):15945. https://creativecommons.org/licenses/by/4.0/.

person, mRNA levels for both oxytocin and GLP-1R were highest in the paraventricular nucleus of the hypothalamus (PVNmc) but low or absent in the adjacent brain areas. The scale bar represents 2 mm.

Sometimes, *in situ* hybridization data can be quantified by plotting:

- A measure of brightness intensity, which may be represented as arbitrary units (a.u.), intensity compared to background, or mean gray value, which assigns the signal of each pixel as a binary white or black and then averages the values detected in a certain brain area. In all cases, higher values suggest greater mRNA levels.
- A number or percentage of cells in an area with a positive mRNA signal.
- A ***z*-score**, which is the number of standard deviations a given signal changes compared to the baseline or control condition. Positive *z*-scores indicate increases in mRNA levels, while negative *z*-scores indicate decreases.

Interpreting the Data

A strong mRNA signal does not always mean that mRNA is actively being translated into functional protein. Furthermore, *in situ* hybridization provides only a relative measure, and does not give information about absolute values of mRNA concentration.

Sometimes, data from exposure to a **sense probe** is shown. This has the same sequence as the sequence of interest, so exposing the tissue to the sense probe is a negative control, causing no signal.

Additional Resources

Young AP, Jackson DJ, Wyeth RC. A technical review and guide to RNA fluorescence in situ hybridization. *PeerJ*. 2020 Mar 19; 8:e8806.

5.3 RNA-Sequencing (RNA-seq)

Background Information

Stains and microscopy can differentiate cells based on their structure or shape. Electrophysiology can differentiate cells based on action potential firing rate or connections. **RNA-sequencing** (RNA-seq) excels because it can differentiate cells based on their **transcriptomic profiles**, the sum of mRNA transcripts that the cells make. This allows for further subcategorization of cells than otherwise possible: for example, where microscopy and electrophysiology could distinguish stellate from basket cells in the molecular layer of the cerebellum, RNA-seq might discover that there are several cell types based on transcriptional activity.

RNA-seq is a high-throughput strategy that can process thousands or millions of cells in a single experiment, even if the sample begins as a jumbled blend of cells. It relies on similar principles as cell sorting (see Section 4.5).

A few variations of RNA-seq exist. Single cell RNA-sequencing (scRNA-seq) captures transcript information from entire cells. Single nucleus RNA-sequencing (snRNA-seq) looks only at RNAs found in the nuclei of the cells, ignoring cytoplasmic transcripts.

RNA-seq provides a snapshot of information from each data point, and RNA transcripts from the same sample cannot be tracked over time. Between-subject comparisons are made when studying the timing of when genes turn on or off during development, for example.

Reading the Graphs

Transcriptional profiles differ across many different dimensions. Plots are used to reduce these dimensions down onto only two axes, where distinct clusters of cells suggest transcriptomic heterogeneity. Some of these analysis methods include a **principal component analysis (PCA)**, a **uniform manifold approximation and projection (UMAP)** plot, or a **t-distributed stochastic neighbor embedding (t-SNE)** approach. In these graphs, each dot represents a single data point (cell or nucleus). The *x*- and *y*-axes are given numerical values, and these indicate how "different" each cell is from the others. Similar cells will appear in clusters, which may be denoted by using different colors or drawn polygons that represent population boundaries.

RNA-seq data may also be presented in a **hierarchical cluster analysis**. These figures are helpful for identifying whether there are "families" of genes that are closely related. Each space on the grid has a color from a binary spectrum (for example, red to white to blue) that denotes the *z*-score which represents decreases or increases where the neutral color indicates no change. The genes are usually shown as being clumped together so the patterns can be visibly apparent.

Figure 5.3 shows an RNA-seq analysis of retinal neurons. Two mouse populations were compared: the control, healthy mice (wild type, WT), and mice with a genetic mutation leading to retinal degeneration (*rd1*). Neurons were studied at three different ages, marked

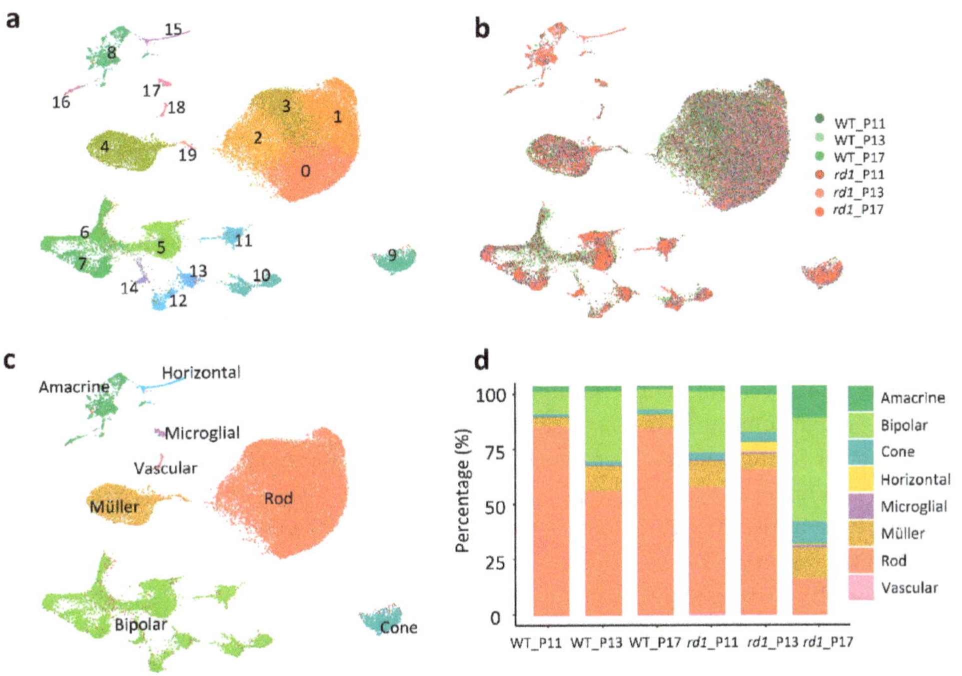

Figure 5.3 Results of an RNA-seq experiment. Source: Chen Y, Dong Y, Yan J, Wang L, Yu S, Jiao K, Paquet-Durand F. Single-cell transcriptomic profiling in inherited retinal degeneration reveals distinct metabolic pathways in rod and cone photoreceptors. *Int J Mol Sci.* 2022; 23(20):12170. https://doi.org/10.3390/ijms232012170. https://creativecommons.org/licenses/by/4.0/.

as days postnatal (P11, P13, and P17). In panel a, each dot represents one of 43,979 cells, which have been divided into twenty clusters based on RNA-seq data cell. In panel b, different clusters are more prominent depending on genotype and time points. In panel c, clusters of cells have been identified by cell type. The stacked bar graph in panel d shows the relative percentage of each cell type. The results suggest that the *rd1* mice lose many of their rod cells at age postnatal day 17 (*rd1*_P17, far right column) compared to their age-matched wild type controls (WT_P17, third column).

Interpreting the Data

RNA-seq techniques are largely descriptive, acting as a screen rather than an experiment, and can lead to the development of hypotheses which can be tested experimentally. For example, an RNA-seq study of cortical samples from people with bipolar disorder (BD) may find that certain genes are upregulated in BD. Then, an experiment may choose to knock out those specific genes in mice to see if it changes their BD-like symptoms.

Additional Resources

Hedlund E, Deng Q. Single-cell RNA sequencing: Technical advancements and biological applications. *Mol Aspects Med*. 2017. http://dx.doi.org/10.1016/j.mam.2017.07.003
Olsen TK, Baryawno N. Introduction to single-cell RNA sequencing. *Curr Protoc Mol Biol*. 2018; 122(1):e57.

5.4 Immunochemistry (Immunohistochemistry and Immunocytochemistry)

Background Information

Immunochemistry (informally, **immunostaining**) involves exposing a sample to **antibodies**, protein complexes that bind selectively to **epitopes**. Epitopes are specific regions of targets of interest, such as enzymes, receptors, and transporters. Depending on the sample, two different words may be used: immuno**histo**chemistry (IHC) is for working with sections of tissue, such as slice of brain or spinal cord, while immuno**cyto**chemistry (ICC) is for working with cell cultures.

Immunochemistry is done in **fixed** tissue or cells. After fixation, the sample may be permeabilized by a **detergent**, a chemical (such as sodium dodecyl sulfate (SDS) Triton-X, or Tween) that punches holes in the cell membranes, allowing the antibodies to access the intracellular component. The sample is then exposed to the **primary antibody** (abbreviated 1o), which binds to the target of interest. Then, a different antibody (the **secondary antibody**, or 2o) is washed onto the sample. The target of the secondary antibody is an epitope on the primary antibody. This secondary antibody may be conjugated with a **fluorophore**, a light-sensitive and light-emitting molecule that allows for visualization by fluorescence microscopy. Fluorophores are indicated by a number and will fluoresce maximally when exposed to light at that wavelength (see Section 4.2.1).

Between steps, samples are **rinsed** (or **washed**), the process of physically covering and agitating the tissue with various solutions to dilute the previous solution or remove unbound antibody. There are also **blocking** steps, which are rinses using solutions such as milk or bovine serum albumin (BSA) that prevent antibodies from binding to the wrong targets.

Example applications of immunochemistry include:

- Identifying which areas of the brain express a protein, or quantifying the proportion of cells in such an area. For example, experiments may be done to see which layer of the hippocampus has the greatest density of CB1 receptors.
- Determining whether a specific population of cells expresses multiple receptors, or quantifying the proportion of cells in a certain area that express multiple receptors. These designs are also called **coexpression** or **colocalization** studies. For example, a study might look to see if the cells that express opioid receptors also express GABA receptors.
- Quantifying relative changes in target levels across two different conditions. For example, males may have more oxytocin immunoreactivity than females, suggesting higher receptor levels.

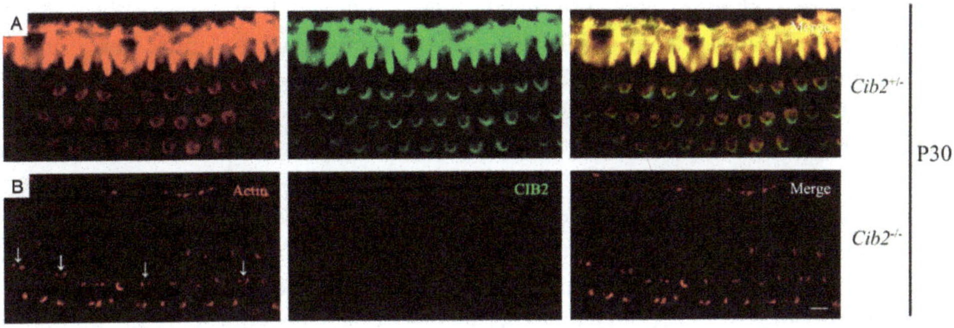

Figure 5.4 Results of an immunohistochemistry experiment. Source: Wang Y, Li J, Yao X, Li W, Du H, Tang M, Xiong W, Chai R, Xu Z. Loss of CIB2 causes profound hearing loss and abolishes mechanoelectrical transduction in mice. *Front Mol Neurosci.* 2017; 10:401. http://creativecommons.org/licenses/by/4.0/. Image cropped and text labels changed.

Figure 5.4 shows representative images of immunostaining results from the cochlea of a 30-day-old (P30) mouse. The experimenters were curious about how the Cib2 gene is involved with hair cell development, so they compared the hair cell morphology of a control mouse (panel A: $Cib2^{+/-}$, top) with a knockout mouse (panel B: $Cib2^{-/-}$, bottom). In the left two images, red fluorescence shows actin, a protein important for cytoskeletal structure. In the control mouse (top), you expect to see normal cochlear development. However, the Cib2 knockouts (bottom) had abnormal actin development. In the middle two images, green fluorescence shows location of CIB2 protein, which is completely missing in the knockout mouse (bottom). In the right two images, merged images show where both actin and CIB2 are localized.

Antibodies are often created in nonhuman animals, including rat, mouse, cow (bovine), goat, chicken, donkey, or rabbit. Antibodies are identified by the animal they are isolated from, as well as their antigen-seeking component, written as "anti-[target]". Some antibodies might also be labeled with the conjugated fluorophore. For example, consider an experiment to identify where the enzyme choline acetyltransferase (ChAT) is located in a rat. An appropriate primary antibody might be "Goat anti-ChAT", which was synthesized in goat, and will bind to an epitope on the enzyme ChAT. An appropriate secondary antibody could be "rabbit anti-goat-488", which was synthesized in a rabbit and will bind to the goat epitope present on the primary antibody.

Sometimes, nonanimal binding pairs may be used, such as fluorescently labeled **avidin** (or **streptavidin**), which binds to a protein called **biotin** that has been conjugated with the secondary antibody. Secondary antibodies can also be conjugated with nanoparticles such as colloidal gold for higher-resolution imaging using electron microscopy.

Reading the Figures

Representative images under low magnification are used to show anatomical features in the "big picture." For example, these images may be used to show that CB1 are expressed at different layers of the hippocampus. Another experiment may show a cross-section of the spinal cord, with more labeled astrocytes on the injured half of the cord compared to the healthy half. High magnification allows for cellular-level resolution. For example, immunochemistry can show the location and density of the cytoskeletal protein actin before and after plasticity. It may also show that the expression of certain proteins, such as PSD-95, is restricted to the synaptic adjacent components of neurons and not found in the soma.

The limits of visualization are determined by the imaging tool: fluorophores are visualized with fluorescence microscopy (resolution on the scale of hundreds of nanometers) while nanoparticles are seen with electron microscopy (nanometers).

Figure 5.5 shows the results of experiments to see how introduction of human oligomeric tau (oTau) changes cells in a culture preparation. On the left are representative immunocytochemical images of cells from a control group (Ctrl; top row) and cells exposed to a model of toxic tau accumulation (oTau; bottom row). Each set of images is taken of the same sample under four different fluorescent excitation wavelengths. The oTau group had increased fluorescent binding by the anti-AT8 antibody (red). Other protein levels may have also changed in the oTau group, including decreased MAP-2 (purple) and increased GFAP (green). DAPI (blue) is used as a marker for neuronal nuclei. The Merge panels show the combined fluorescent signal from all four colors. On the right of the figure, group data are represented by a bar graph with individual data points for quantifying fluorescence intensity of the red signal (AT-8) as a fraction of the purple signal (MAP-2).

Additional Resources

Ramos-Vara JA. Principles and methods of immunohistochemistry. *Methods Mol Biol.* 2011; 691:83–96.

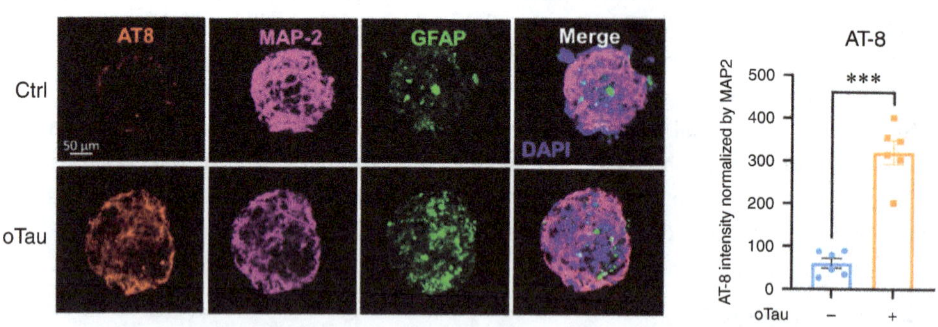

Figure 5.5 Results of an immunocytochemistry experiment. Source: Rickner HD, Jiang L, Hong R, et al. Single cell transcriptomic profiling of a neuron-astrocyte assembloid tauopathy model. *Nat Commun.* 2022; 13:6275. https://doi.org/10.1038/s41467-022-34005-1. http://creativecommons.org/licenses/by/4.0/. Text labels have been removed.

5.4.1 Western Blot

Background Information

A **Western blot** uses immunochemistry principles to quantify changes in protein levels in samples of tissue under different experimental or treatment conditions. The tissue from multiple animals is dissected out anatomically according to defined volumes and coordinates from a standardized brain atlas. The cells are treated and homogenized until a slurry of cells remains. Next, samples undergo a three-step process. Figure 5.6 is a cartoon representation of the steps involved, from sample isolation (top) to bands (bottom).

1. **Gel electrophoresis**. The sample is treated with sodium dodecyl sulfate (SDS) at high temperatures (< 100°C), which denatures the protein and adds a predictable negative charge on each amino acid. The experimenters make a **gel**, usually made of polyacrylamide. The gel is liquid after warming but thickens at room temperature. The liquid gel is poured into a **case**, which serves as a mold for the final gel. As the gel is being poured, the liquid fills around a tool called a **comb** made up of several teeth. After the gel hardens, removing the comb forms **wells**, small indentations in the gel into which the samples are **loaded** using a micropipette. An electrical current is passed through the gel, causing the negatively charged proteins to move from the anode (negative electrode, usually colored with black wires) to the cathode (positive electrode, usually colored with red wires). This is what it means for the gel to be **run**. The smaller molecular weight proteins move through the gel quicker and will end up farther from the wells; larger molecular weight proteins move more slowly, and therefore stay closer to the wells. The combination of protein denaturation and polyacrylamide gel electrophoresis is abbreviated as **SDS-PAGE**.
2. **Membrane transfer**. A "sandwich" is created, made up of several layers of sponges, filter papers, the gel (which contains the protein sample), and a **blot**, which is a nitrocellulose or polyvinylidine fluoride (PDVF) membrane. Electrical current is then passed through the sandwich causing the proteins to migrate from the gel onto the blot.
3. **Immunochemistry** and visualization. Finally, the blot is subjected to immunochemistry techniques: exposure to primary and secondary antibodies. Visualization is then performed using chemiluminescence, fluorescence, or radiography, usually with help from a computerized system or film. The signals that appear are called **bands**, and these are what is typically shown in figures.

Since Western blots can be quantified to compare between groups, it is important to compare against control proteins to ensure that there are similar levels of proteins to start with. Typical positive controls used for comparison are **housekeeping proteins** (**HKPs**), proteins that are stably expressed robustly across many cell types. Common housekeeping proteins and their weight in **kilodaltons** (**kDa**) include:

- GAPDH (36 kDa), a glycolytic protein used in glucose metabolism.
- Beta-actin (42 kDa), a structural protein that helps maintain the shape of cells.

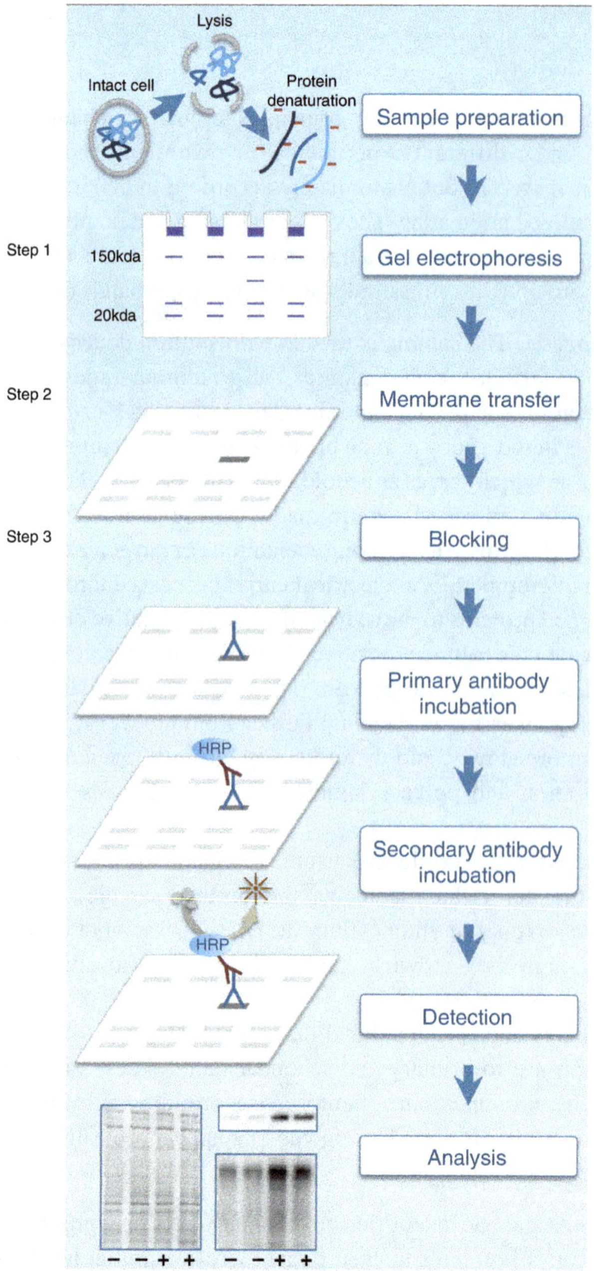

Figure 5.6 Cartoon representation of steps of a Western blot. Source: Bass JJ, Wilkinson DJ, Rankin D, et al. An overview of technical considerations for Western blotting applications to physiological research. *Scand J Med Sci Sports*. 2017 Jan; 27(1):4–25. https://creativecommons.org/licenses/by/4.0/. Image cropped.

- Beta-tubulin (55 kDa), a structural protein that makes up microtubules, which function in the maintenance of cell shape and intracellular transport.
- Vinculin (117 kDa), a cytoskeletal protein that interacts closely with actin.

However, HKP levels may change in certain conditions (e.g. brain injury, schizophrenia, or Alzheimer's disease), across different developmental stages, and in different cell types, sometimes making them inappropriate normalization factors. To overcome this challenge, researchers are more often normalizing to total protein instead of to an HKP.

Reading the Figures

Representative blots are grayscale images. In most presentations of representative blots, the background color will be set to white or very light gray. The darker the band, the more protein is present. Images are often heavily cropped, showing only thin horizontal strips of blots, each band corresponding to protein levels for different samples. Proteins are usually identified by name and by weight in kilodaltons (kDa). When presented in figures, the order of the rows is not usually important, even though the location of the band in gel electrophoresis is used for identification based on weight (for example, the control protein may be shown at the bottom row even though its weight might be larger than other proteins of interest).

Each column (or **lane**) shows bands from different conditions. If some manipulation is applied differentially across samples, labels of + and − might be used, with the + columns indicating samples taken in the presence of the manipulation and the − columns representing the negative control. Other controls may appear, including the housekeeping protein control or a **ladder** or protein **standard** (or a marker) as a positive control. These samples contain proteins of known weight which allow comparisons to proteins of interest.

Representative data from a time series may be shown. For example, we may be curious about how protein levels change in the hours and days following a head injury. It would be possible to injure several animals on the same day, then harvest tissue 1 hour, 6 hours, 1 day, and 3 days after the injury. Samples from each of these time points will be loaded in sequential wells with each time point indicated above the image of the corresponding blots. Relatedly, dose-response experiments can also be performed to assess how different doses of drug (or intensity of manipulation) affects protein levels.

In graphs of group data, different groups are plotted across the *x*-axis. The quantity of protein, assessed by the intensity of the signal, may be plotted on the *y*-axis. Intensity may be reported as the **optical density** (**OD**; also called **relative density**) as a percentage (or ratio) of the values in the control condition or compared to housekeeping protein (or total protein) intensity.

Figure 5.7 shows Western blots of hippocampal tissue from mice. Researchers were curious about how expression of the serotonin receptor 6 (HTR6) changes in response to different diets. On the left of the image are representative Western blots from 10 mice, five of which are given unlimited access to food (left, AL for *ad libitum*) and five of which are under dietary restriction (right, DR). Immunostaining against serotonin receptor type 6

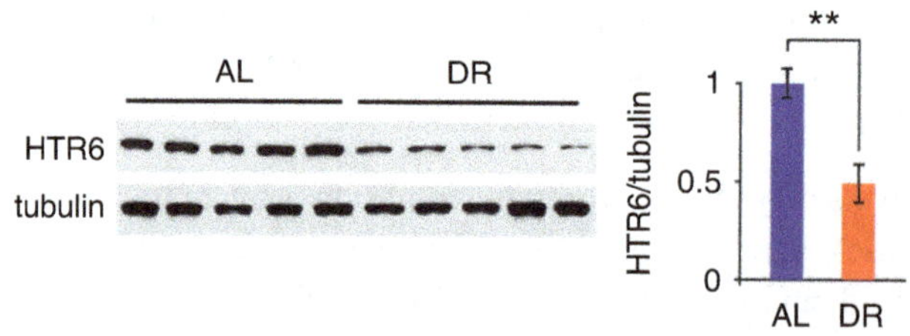

Figure 5.7 Results of a Western blot experiment. Source: Teng L-L, Lu G-L, Chiou L-C, et al. Serotonin receptor HTR6-mediated mTORC1 signaling regulates dietary restriction-induced memory enhancement. PLoS Biol. 2019; 17(3): e2007097. http://creativecommons.org/licenses/by/4.0/. Text labels removed and figures rearranged.

(HTR6) on blots are shown to decrease under DR compared to the AL condition. Staining against the housekeeping protein tubulin is a control experiment and did not change across conditions. The bar graphs on the right show HTR6 signal intensity as a percentage relative to tubulin intensity. The researchers concluded that DR decreases hippocampal HTR6 expression.

Interpreting the Data

The important limitation of the Western blot technique is that intensity quantification is not a measure of absolute protein levels, but rather only a comparison between samples containing similar protein levels. Intensity of the signal depends on gel homogeneity, blocking efficiency, antibody exposure duration and binding, fluorophore intensity, and many other factors that do not allow for comparison between blots.

In quantifications of optical density, proteins of interest with averages greater than 100 (as a percentage) or 1 (as a ratio) indicate an upregulation of that protein; averages lower than 100 or 1 indicate downregulation. The control condition value average will be at 100 or 1.

Phosphorylation is a posttranslational modification of a protein which functions as a molecular "switch." For many proteins, the phosphorylated form of the protein (often designated with the prefix **phospho-** or just **p-**) indicates the active version of that protein. Phosphorylated protein can also be detected and differentiated from the nonphosphorylated protein using antibodies. Changes in phosphorylated proteins may indicate differences in enzymatic activity: increases suggest more kinase activity or decreased phosphorylase activity. Increased levels of phosphorylated protein suggest that protein has been activated under the given condition.

The housekeeping or total protein (positive control) is expected to be the same across all groups. Differences in relative levels of housekeeping proteins, while unexpected, may be scientifically meaningful.

Figure 5.8 shows Western blot results from a study examining isolated rat hippocampi. Researchers were curious as to whether rats born to older mothers (advanced maternal age,

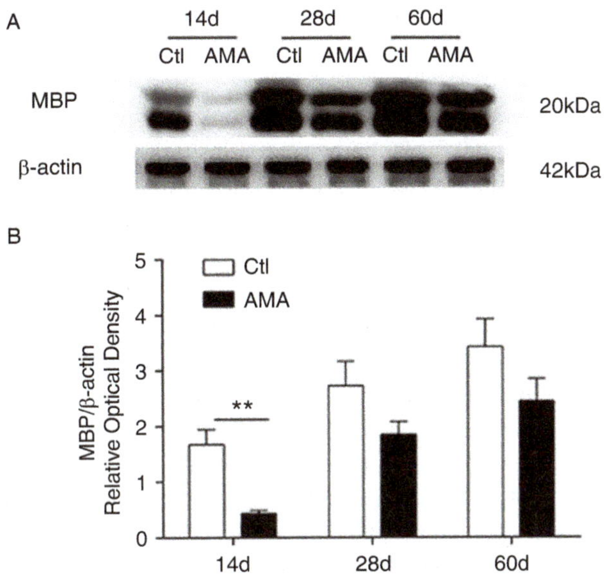

Figure 5.8 More results of a different Western blot experiment. Source: Han W, Pan Y, Han Z, Cheng L, Jiang L. Advanced maternal age impairs myelination in offspring rats. *Front Pediatr.* 2022; 10:850213. http://creativecommons.org/licenses/by/4.0/.

AMA group) had deficits in hippocampal myelin as quantified by the presence of myelin basic protein (MBP) compared to rats born to younger mothers (controls, Ctl). They wanted to see if there is a developmental difference, so offspring were studied at three different ages: 14 days old (14d), 28 days old (28d), and 60 days old (60d). In panel A, representative Western blot results show bands under the three time points and both conditions. The sizes of the proteins have been indicated by the label on the right (20 kilodaltons corresponds to MBP, and 42 kilodaltons corresponds to β-actin). In all cases, the MBP bands from the AMA group look lighter in intensity, suggesting less MBP. β-actin is run as the housekeeping control. Note that, on the gel electrophoresis, you would normally expect to see the smaller MBP band lower on the gel since it is smaller and therefore will run faster. Here, since MBP is the protein of interest, it has been put on top. Panel B shows group bar graphs quantifying the signal intensity of the MBP band as a fraction of the β-actin band (y-axis). They report a statistically significant decrease in MBP levels at 14 days old among animals born to mothers with AMA.

Additional Resources

Kurien BT, Scofield, RH. *Western Blotting: An Introduction*. Methods in Molecular Biology, vol. 1312. Clifton, NJ: Springer; 2015. https://doi.org/10.1007/978-1-4939-2694-7_5.

Mahmood T, Yang PC. Western blot: Technique, theory, and trouble shooting. *N Am J Med Sci*. 2012; 4(9):429–434. https://doi.org/10.4103/1947-2714.100998.

5.4.2 Affinity Capture (Pull-Down Assays and Co-immunoprecipitation)

Background Information

Affinity capture techniques determine whether two proteins interact with one another. A pull-down assay uses known proteins to capture proteins of interest, while co-immunoprecipitation (co-IP) uses antibodies. RNA interactions can be detected using RNA immunoprecipitation (RIP). Consider an example experiment based on the observation that genetic mutations are found in the gene that codes for the protein PRRT2 in various forms of epilepsy, a disease characterized by unexpected neuronal activity. Researchers may become curious as to whether PRRT2 interacts with a specific subunit of the voltage-gated calcium channel, which is one modifier of cell excitability. Affinity capture can determine whether there is an interaction between these two proteins.

In a **pull-down assay**, the cells are lysed using chemical treatments and centrifugation until only a slurry of protein isolates (called the **lysate**) remain. The lysate is then passed through a **column**, which contains particles such as agarose that are physically attached to the column. These molecules have been modified to carry some affinity ligand, such as a molecule of glutathione. One of the proteins of interest (this protein is called the **bait**) will have a tag, such as a molecule of glutathione-S-transferase (GST), which will bind to the glutathione on the column (another pair of interacting molecules is a cobalt ion and a histidine (His) tag). The technique is called **co-immunoprecipitation** when one of the binding pairs is an antibody. Then, the lysate will be passed through the column. Only the molecules that interact with the bait (called the **prey**) will bind to its partner and remain in the column. Then, the molecules will be **eluted**, the process of causing the molecules to unbind from the column. This flow-through is then collected, run on an SDS-PAGE, transferred to a Western blot, and then imaged using immunochemistry.

Co-immunoprecipitation can also be performed without the column. The antibody can be incubated with the sample slurry. Then, agarose beads may be added to the mixture. The beads bind to the antibody-protein complex, increasing their mass, which allows for separation by centrifugation. As with column affinity separation, the remaining complex can be eluted then analyzed through SDS-PAGE, Western blot, and immunochemistry.

Reading the Graphs

Typically, figures show sections of Western blot results, where darker bands indicate more interaction between the proteins.

Co-immunoprecipitation experiments may use two different antibodies. The antibody used in the affinity immunoprecipitation step is usually labeled as IP, while the antibody used to identify the protein in the Western blot will be labeled as WB. The big question behind these experiments is to see if two proteins, for example Protein A and Protein B, interact with one another. If the anti-Protein A on the IP and anti-Protein B on the WB show a band, and the anti-Protein B on the IP and anti-Protein A on the WB also show a band, then the interaction is confirmed.

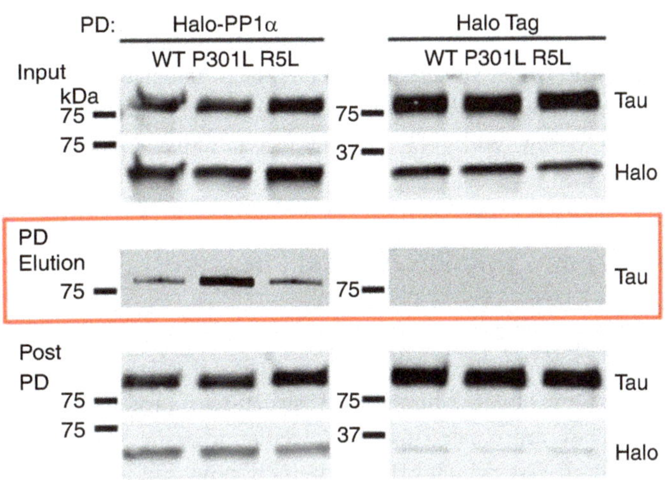

Figure 5.9 Results of a pull-down assay. Source: Combs B, Christensen KR, Richards C, et al. Frontotemporal lobar dementia mutant tau impairs axonal transport through a protein phosphatase 1γ-dependent mechanism. *J Neurosci.* 2021; 41(45):9431–9451. DOI: 10.1523/JNEUROSCI.1914-20.2021. https://creativecommons.org/licenses/by/4.0/. Text labels removed.

Many controls are often run on the same blots across different lanes. Addition of a sample is denoted by +; when the sample is not loaded, that is indicated by −. The sample labeled lysate (or **input**) is a positive control, which is the Western blot of all the lysate that goes into the affinity process. All of these blots should have strong bands upon exposure to their corresponding antibody in the Western blot. A negative control is to run both prey proteins through the column separately (without a bait) to ensure that the protein does not interact with the tag on the column.

An IgG serves as a negative control to eliminate the possibility of nonspecific binding. The lane loaded with the IgG should have no band corresponding to the protein targeted by the WB antibody.

Figure 5.9 represents a pull-down assay demonstrating interaction between the prey protein tau and the bait enzyme PP1α (left blots). Mutant tau (P301L; middle band) interacts more strongly with PP1α compared to the WT or R5L mutant. Tau does not interact with HaloTag alone (right blots), which serves as the negative control.

Interpreting the Data

Since affinity capture experiments provide qualitative evidence about whether two proteins interact or not, results from Western blots are generally not summarized in graphs, but sometimes relative measures of intensity may be quantified across different conditions.

Affinity capture may be helpful in identifying whether a protein modifies the activity of various ion channels, which can directly influence cellular excitation. Many transcription factors are also proteins with robust interactions that may regulate their activity, and affinity capture can help confirm the nature of these interactions.

Additional Resources

Louche A, Salcedo SP, Bigot S. (2017). Protein–protein interactions: Pull-down assays. In Journet L, Cascales E, editors. *Bacterial Protein Secretion Systems*. Methods in Molecular Biology, vol. 1615. New York, NY: Humana Press. https://doi.org/10.1007/978-1-4939-7033-9_20.

5.5 Ribbon Diagrams (Models, Crystal Structures)

Background Information

Ribbon diagrams show the three-dimensional structure of proteins (**tertiary** and **quaternary structure**). They are created using molecular imaging techniques such as x-ray crystallography or cryo-EM, which offers extremely powerful levels of resolution, down to the order of angstroms. In neuroscience, ribbon diagrams are commonly used to show the structures of ion channels, enzymes, transporters, or other proteins. Ribbon diagrams also contain functional information, such as ion- or ligand-binding sites, the diameter of the pore, the mutated shapes of proteins that may increase aggregation risk, or the biomechanics of ion channel opening, closing, inactivation, and deactivation.

Reading the Graphs

Ribbon diagrams may show different views of the protein. These views matter most for transmembrane proteins, which may be shown from three perspectives: extracellular, intracellular (or cytosolic), and from the side. In a side view, the lipid bilayer of the cell membrane may be illustrated, and the extracellular space may be differentiated from the intracellular space. These views are generally the "zoomed out" view, and a scale bar may be on the order of hundreds of angstroms or more.

In a more "zoomed in" view, a diagram may show the locations of specific amino acid residues, which are abbreviated as a letter and a number. The letter identifies the amino acid and the number indicates the position on the primary structure of the protein from N-terminus to C-terminus.

In ribbon diagrams showing quaternary structure, each individual subunit may be illustrated in shades of different colors. For example, enzymes such as the receptor tyrosine kinases are commonly made up of two subunit proteins (**dimers**) while voltage-gated potassium channels have four identical protein subunit units (**tetramers**). If all the subunits are identical they are called **homomers**, while proteins made up of different subunits are called **heteromers**. For example, nicotinic acetylcholine receptors are made up of five protein subunits (**pentamers**). The alpha7 types are homopentamers, while different combinations of alpha4 and beta2 receptors make up heteropentamers.

Transmembrane (TM) sections are parts of the protein that span the cell membrane. Sometimes, these sections are abbreviated with the letter S. Proteins may contain multiple

TM sections, so these are typically numbered in ascending order from the N-terminus to C-terminus. TM sections are often made up of hydrophobic amino acid residues in an alpha-helical or beta-sheet formation, since these structural orientations are most stable in the cell membrane. Metabotropic (G-protein coupled) receptors are also called "7 transmembrane receptors" because their protein structure contains seven TM sections.

Proteins may be divided into **motifs**, which are elements of the secondary structure of the protein that are seen commonly across many different types of proteins. Relatedly, **domains** represent a "functional unit" of the protein. Domains may be given Greek letters to differentiate them (not to be confused with structural components of proteins, such as the alpha helix or beta sheet), and sometimes are distinguished by different colors. Motifs provide small-scale structural information, while domains provide functional information.

Motifs described in ribbon diagrams include the following:

- An EF hand is a pair of alpha helices connected by a short loop. EF hands complex with a Ca^{2+} ion, and are found in proteins such as calmodulin and DAG kinase.
- P-loops bind to phosphate molecules and are found in ATP- or GTP-binding proteins, such as adenylate cyclase.
- Ankyrin repeats are two short alpha helices with a loop. These are found in TRP receptors.
- Axon-targeting motifs are sequences that help direct other proteins into the axonal compartment.
- Some motifs are named based on the combination of secondary protein structures, such as an alpha-loop-alpha motif or a beta-hairpin.
- Some motifs are named based on an amino acid sequence that appears, such as a DRF motif found in chemokine receptors.

Domains that may appear in a ribbon diagram include the following:

- **Ligand binding domains** (LBD) are areas that interact closely with some other molecule. In receptors, this may be an extracellular ligand such as a molecule of glutamate, or an intracellular ligand like a cyclic nucleotide.
- **Pore forming domains** (PD, or the ion conduction pore) are the parts of ion channel proteins that help form the transmembrane region.
- **Voltage sensing domains** (VSD, or the gate domain) are found on the intracellular sides of certain ion channels. These domains are typically rich in charged amino acid residues, and are important for state transitions (such as closed to open, or open to inactivate) in voltage-gated sodium channels, for example.
- The **amino terminal domain** (ATD) and **carboxy terminal domain** (CTD) are used to indicate the direction of the protein.

Figure 5.10 is a ribbon diagram showing the tertiary structure of human β-actin, a cytosolic protein. Monomeric actin can polymerize into a stable filament when a molecule of ATP is bound to the structure. The image on the left labels features of actin, including the four subdomains (1–4), two clefts which can bind to nucleotides or hydrophobic components, a sensor loop containing the amino acid residue histidine at position 73 (H73), and the site of

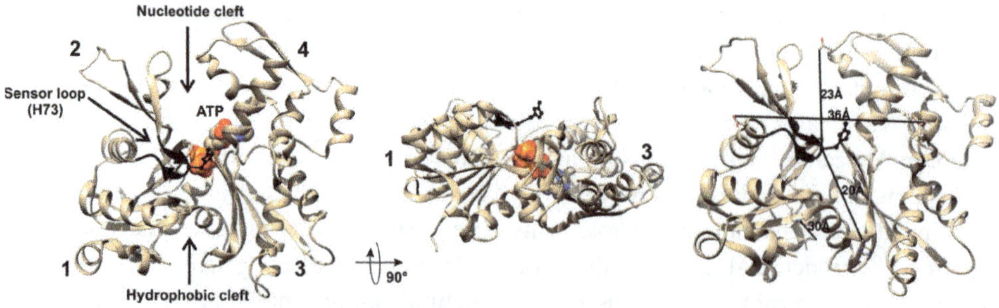

Figure 5.10 A ribbon diagram of a protein. Source: Kwiatkowski S, Seliga AK, Vertommen D, et al. SETD3 protein is the actin-specific histidine N-methyltransferase. *Elife*. 2018 Dec 11; 7:e37921. http://creative commons.org/licenses/by/4.0/. Image cropped and text removed.

ATP binding. Several alpha helix segments are shown. The middle image is a 90-degree rotation to show the protein from a different angle. On the right, residue distances between segments of the protein are indicated by measurements in angstroms (Å).

Interpreting the Data

Most ribbon diagrams are descriptive studies used to illustrate protein shape. They may help form hypotheses about mutations, especially when key amino acid residues, such as the ones adjacent to the pore forming or ligand binding domains, are identified. Mutations in genes that code for these amino acids may account for differences in ion conductivity or ligand-receptor affinity. For example, differences in the structure of the androgen receptor affect its ability to bind the hormone testosterone and are common among intersex people.

In analyzing pore forming proteins such as ion channels, one measure of interest is the location of the pore at its smallest diameter. Some graphs may plot pore diameter on the *x*-axis and distance along the transmembrane region on the *y*-axis. These graphs are usually placed next to the side view of the protein, which helps the reader visualize differences in pore diameter along the distance of the transmembrane region.

The ribbon diagrams in Figure 5.11 show the three-dimensional structure of a human voltage-gated sodium channel. Panel a is a side view with the extracellular side on top (left) and after a 90-degree rotation to see through the pore (right). Panel b shows two regions that make up the pore (left) and a graph quantifying pore radius as a function of distance along ion path (right).

Additional Resources

Stollar EJ, Smith DP. Uncovering protein structure. *Essays Biochem*. 2020 Oct 8; 64(4):649–680. DOI: 10.1042/EBC20190042. Erratum in *Essays Biochem*. 2021 Jul 26; 65(2):407.

Wang Y, Zhang H, Zhong H, Xue Z. Protein domain identification methods and online resources. *Comput Struct Biotechnol J*. 2021 Feb 2; 19:1145–1153.

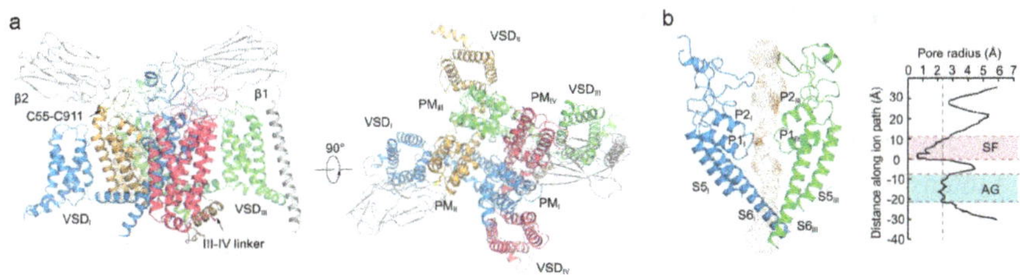

Figure 5.11 More ribbon diagrams. Source: Li X, Xu F, Xu H, et al. Structural basis for modulation of human $Na_V1.3$ by clinical drug and selective antagonist. *Nat Commun.* 2022; 13:1286. https://doi.org/10.1038/s41467-022-28808-5. https://creativecommons.org/licenses/by/4.0/. Figures have been rearranged and new text labels added.

5.6 Genetically Encoded Fluorescent Biosensors

Background Information

A **genetically encoded fluorescent biosensor** is a fusion molecule that contains a fluorescence protein that produces a signal when a certain molecular condition is met, such as changes in calcium or neurotransmitter concentration. The biosensor may be a transmembrane protein with the sensor components on the intracellular side. The intensity of the fluorescence signal can then be tracked over time with fluorescence microscopy. These tools offer many advantages over similar assays:

- Temporal resolution on the order of milliseconds. However, some fluorescent signals do not **quench** (or **decay**) as rapidly as the underlying signal changes.
- Ability to visualize hundreds or more cells simultaneously.
- Ability to distinguish individual neurons from adjacent cells. Unlike with EEG or an implanted array of electrodes, which record the sum of several (up to millions) cells altogether, single neurons can be pinpointed. This offers an advantage over the previously used **voltage sensitive dyes (VSDs)**, which do not offer high spatial resolution.
- Cell type selectivity using genetic manipulations such as a Cre-lox system, allowing the sensors to be put into a specific cell population within a brain area that contains a blend of cell types. For example, genetically encoded sensors have been put into only the 1% of acetylcholine-synthesizing neurons of the striatum, while sparing the other 99% of neurons.
- Noninvasiveness on the cellular scale. Certain types of electrophysiological methods offer the same level of spatial and temporal resolution as these biosensors. But they require a disruption of the cell membrane, which can cause intracellular signaling molecules to dialyze out of the neuron, changing physiological properties.

There are a variety of biosensors that allow for imaging of different molecular processes.

- **Calcium imaging** is a proxy measure of neural activity, since the concentration of calcium may increase by tenfold over the course of a few milliseconds during an action potential. A **genetically encoded calcium indicator (GECI)**, such as GCaMP, binds to intracellular Ca^{2+} and produces a fluorescence signal when bound.

- Neurotransmitter or neuromodulator sensors can detect neurochemical concentration during synaptic release events. For example, the iGluSnFR construct changes fluorescence intensity based on glutamate concentration, and the iGABASnFR does the same for GABA. For neuromodulators such as dopamine or serotonin, G-protein-coupled receptor-activator-based sensors (**GRAB sensors**) can be used.
- Changes in membrane voltage can be detected with **genetically encoded voltage indicators (GEVI)**. One such GEVI is ArcLight, which decreases in fluorescence intensity at depolarized potentials.
- Activation of second messenger molecules, which are downstream of G-protein coupled receptors (GPCR), can be detected by fluorescent reporters. After a GPCR is activated, a cascade of molecular events take place, some of which can influence cell excitability, gene transcription, or other processes. Certain second messenger molecules, such as cyclic AMP and protein kinase A (PKA), can be detected visually with a fluorescent molecule such as the A-kinase activity reporter (AKAR) or the exchange protein directly activated by cAMP (ePAC).
- Different elements of cellular metabolism can be visualized, such as ATP or glucose levels.

Figure 5.12 represents research on transgenic zebrafish with a GECI. Panel A shows representative fluorescent microscope images of larval brains. The control condition is exposed to

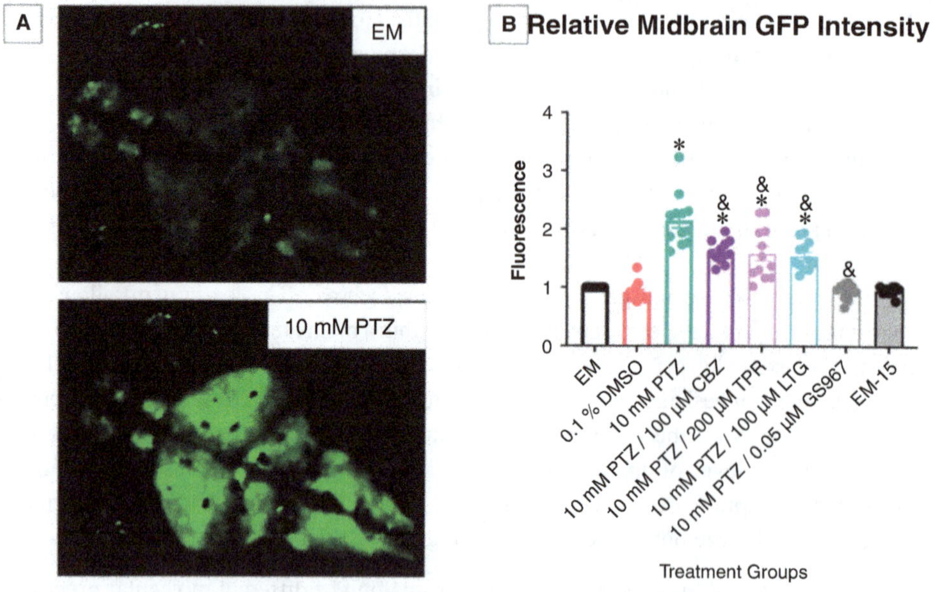

Figure 5.12 Results of a genetically encoded calcium indicator experiment. Source: Milder PC, Zybura AS, Cummins TR, Marrs JA. Neural activity correlates with behavior effects of anti-seizure drugs efficacy using the zebrafish pentylenetetrazol seizure model. *Front Pharmacol.* 2022; 13:836573. DOI: 10.3389/fphar.2022.836573. http://creativecommons.org/licenses/by/4.0/.

embryo medium (EM, top), while the experimental condition is exposed to the excitotoxin PTZ (bottom). Increased fluorescence suggests higher intracellular calcium levels. The group data in panel B shows quantification of those fluorescence results (y-axis) across different experimental conditions (x-axis). DMSO is a vehicle control and does not change fluorescence signal. As shown by the representative images, PTZ increases fluorescence. Other antiseizure agents, such as CBZ, TPR, and LRG, do not reverse the PTZ effect. A reversal of the PTZ effect is seen only with the compound GS967, suggesting this drug may be helpful to minimize the excitotoxic effect of PTZ. EM-15 is exposure to the embryo medium but 15 minutes later, to control for any time-dependent changes that may take place during drug administration.

These biosensors are powerful because they answer the same types of questions that electrophysiology does but can do so at a larger scale. Sometimes, use of GECIs and GEVIs to study neuronal activity may be called **optical electrophysiology**.

Reading the Graphs

Representative images are likely to show individual cells or groups of cells under fluorescence microscopy in different conditions, such as a before-and-after manipulation (within-cell comparison). In digital publications and presentations, videos of these representative data may be helpful.

In graphs showing individual traces or summaries of traces, time is plotted on the x-axis. The time scale may be as short as tens to hundreds of milliseconds, which takes advantage of the high temporal resolution offered by these biosensors. The y-axis may plot a measure of fluorescence, $\Delta F/F0$ (pronounced "delta F over F naught"). These values are essentially the change in fluorescence intensity compared to a baseline fluorescence. The baseline eliminates the influence of several variables, most importantly the concentration of background molecules before the manipulation. Absolute fluorescence intensity may be presented in arbitrary units (a.u.).

Some constructs (such as ArcLight, a GEVI) decrease in fluorescent brightness upon depolarization, so the positive values on the y-axis may represent negative $\Delta F/F0$, corresponding to more positive membrane potentials.

Figure 5.13 represents all-optical electrophysiology using a genetically encoded calcium indicator called GCaMP6s. Panel A is a representative image collected using two-photon microscopy. The fluorescence signal of three neurons (labeled by arrows) were tracked over time. Panel B shows changes in fluorescence signal and therefore intracellular calcium concentration for the three color-coded neurons over time. Each set of traces (top, middle, bottom) represents fluorescence signal several minutes apart.

Additional Resources

Bai L, Zhang Z, Ye L, et al. Volumetric imaging of neural activity by light field microscopy. *Neurosci Bull*. 2022; 38:1559–1568.

Day-Cooney J, Dalangin R, Zhong H, Mao T. Genetically encoded fluorescent sensors for imaging neuronal dynamics in vivo. *J Neurochem*. 2023 Feb; 164(3):284–308.

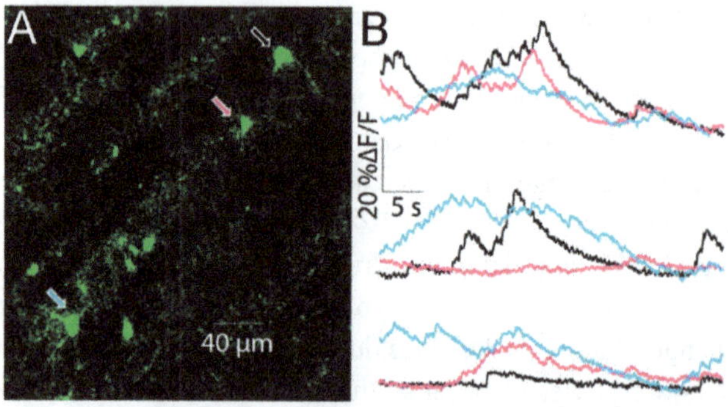

Figure 5.13 Results of an all-optical electrophysiology experiment. Source: Rehani R, Atamna Y, Tiroshi L, et al. Activity patterns in the neuropil of striatal cholinergic interneurons in freely moving mice represent their collective spiking dynamics. *eNeuro.* 2019; 6(1):ENEURO.0351-18.2018. DOI:10.1523/ENEURO.0351-18.2018. http://creativecommons.org/licenses/by/4.0/. Image cropped and text labels changed.

Jin L, Han Z, Platisa J, et al. Single action potentials and subthreshold electrical events imaged in neurons with a fluorescent protein voltage probe. *Neuron.* 2012 Sep 6; 75 (5):779–785.

5.7 Receptor Binding Assay (Autoradiography)

Background Information

The **receptor binding assay** (autoradiography) is a method for visualizing the location of and approximating the levels of certain proteins, such as receptors, transporters, or enzymes, based on the intensity of a radioactive signal. Autoradiography has largely been replaced by either receptor intensity PET scan, which has the advantage of being an *in vivo* imaging strategy that can capture information over time, or immunochemistry, which offers higher spatial resolution at the order of microns.

Autoradiography takes advantage of molecule–molecule interactions. Ligands interact closely with their substrate, for example in the way a neurotransmitter binds to its receptor or transporter protein. Autoradiography uses **radioligands**, artificially produced ligands that contain a radioactive substitution of one of the atoms of the ligand. ^{3}H and ^{11}C are commonly substituted isotopes used in radioligands. As an example, fallypride is an antagonist that binds to the D2/D3 dopamine receptors. The radioligand fallypride^{18}F substitutes the fluoride with a radioactive fluoride instead.

A sample of tissue, such as a brain slice, is fixed and exposed to the radioligand. Then, the sample is brought close to an x-ray film or a Phosphor screen that detects the radioactive signal and changes brightness in response. A computerized sensor or thin layer chromatography can also be used.

The technique was often used to answer questions about the approximate anatomical location of receptor expression. However, because radioactivity is a diffuse signal, it is difficult to precisely resolve where that signal originates from. Therefore, the technique suffers from low spatial resolution, generally at the level of tenths or hundredths of millimeters.

Reading the Graphs

Sample autoradiography images are grayscale images of brain slices. Usually, darker colors indicate more signal and therefore more binding, but this is reversed in **dark-field autoradiography**. Look to see if the background color is light or dark to identify what the absence of binding looks like.

Common anatomical landmarks may not be clearly identifiable in autoradiography images. Because of this shortcoming, slices may be **counterstained** with cresyl violet, which stains gray matter differently from white matter and is therefore good at identifying anatomical boundaries, helping to provide context to the location of the radiography signal.

Autoradiography data can also be quantified in a variety of ways:

- **Radiation intensity**, usually measured in units of nanocuries per gram (abbreviated nCi/g) or in disintegrations per minute per gram (abbreviated Dpm / g).
- **Optical density**, a measure of how dark the signal is compared to a background control area. Optical density is usually converted into a reading of receptor levels, which may be measured in units of femtomolar per milligram. These measures are commonly normalized against the brightness detected by a radioactive standard, such as ^{125}I or ^{14}C.
- **Competition of binding** is used when the same sample tissue is exposed to two different ligands, one of them being a radioligand. Different concentrations of the nonradiolabeled ligand may be applied, and the intensity of the radiolabeled ligand is measured. If the nonradiolabeled ligand outcompetes (has a stronger affinity for the receptor compared to) the radiolabeled ligand, the signal is less intense. This strategy may provide a measure of **dissociation constant** K_D where a low K_D means the ligand is "stickier" on the receptor.

Figure 5.14 shows the effect of female rat isolation following training on a female intruder test. Panel A shows quantification of a behavioral measurement of aggression. Here, researchers were curious as to whether isolated and trained female rats (IST) were more aggressive than group-housed (GH) control females. The data suggest they are. Panels B and C show quantification of autoradiography receptor binding where intensity is expressed as relative optical density (ROD). Among IST rats compared to GH rats, oxytocin receptor (OXTR) binding was increased but vasopressin 1A receptor (V1aR) binding was not. Panel D shows representative autoradiography images of coronal brain sections.

Additional Resources

Griem-Krey N, Klein AB, Herth M, Wellendorph P. Autoradiography as a simple and powerful method for visualization and characterization of pharmacological targets. *J Vis Exp*. 2019; 145:e58879. doi:10.3791/58879.

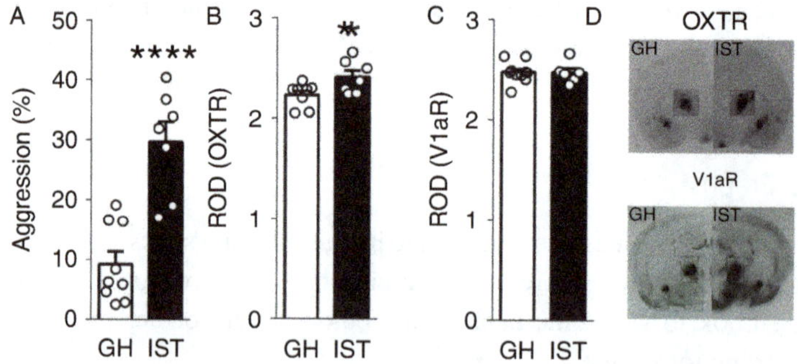

Figure 5.14 Results of an autoradiography experiment. Source: Oliveira VEM, de Jong TR, Neumann ID. Synthetic oxytocin and vasopressin act within the central amygdala to exacerbate aggression in female wistar rats. *Front Neurosci.* 2022; 16:906617. DOI: 10.3389/fnins.2022.906617 http://creativecommons.org/licenses/by/4.0/.

Summary

This chapter describes the many techniques used to observe and quantify molecules commonly found in and used by neurons and glia. *In situ* hybridization can help us identify the location of mRNA, while RNA-seq strategies help us determine which transcripts are being made in a population of neurons. Other strategies are geared toward understanding proteins. For example, using antibodies raised against certain proteins can identify the location of those proteins, while ribbon diagrams can illustrate protein structure. Still more techniques are useful for looking at interactions between proteins, such as affinity capture and receptor binding assays.

Some molecular scale techniques, particularly RNA-seq and ribbon diagrams, produce data that are more descriptive than experimental. However, the findings from these results may help other researchers develop hypotheses that can be tested in an experimental fashion using other techniques. Also, the spatial resolution of these techniques is still limited by the imaging tools: even if an antibody binds only to a presynaptic protein, a fluorescence microscope would have a difficult time determining whether that protein is pre- or postsynaptic.

A wide range of genetically encoded fluorescent biosensors can inform us about the molecular state of cells in real time, for example showing whether ion concentrations change over the course of milliseconds. However, before the development of these biosensors, researchers used electrophysiological strategies to study neuronal activity in real time. The following chapter describes the techniques used by electrophysiologists to understand the nervous system.

Key Terms

- accession number
- affinity capture
- antibody
- antisense probe
- band

- calcium imaging
- central dogma of molecular biology
- coexpression
- colocalization
- dimer
- DNA
- domain
- fluorescence *in situ* hybridization (FISH)
- gel electrophoresis
- genetically encoded calcium indicator (GECI)
- genetically encoded fluorescent biosensor
- genetically encoded voltage indicator (GEVI)
- heteromer
- homomer
- housekeeping protein
- immunochemistry
- *in situ* hybridization
- ladder
- motif
- mRNA
- optical electrophysiology
- phosphorylation
- primary antibody
- primary structure
- protein
- pull-down assay
- quaternary structure
- radioligand
- receptor binding assay
- ribbon diagram
- RNA
- RNA-sequencing
- secondary antibody
- secondary structure
- sense probe
- tertiary structure
- tetramer
- transcription
- transcriptomic
- translation
- tRNA
- Western blot

CHAPTER SIX

Electrophysiology and Electrochemistry

6.1 Introduction to Electrophysiology and Electrochemistry

Electrophysiology (informally **e-phys**) refers to research techniques involving tools that can detect or change the electrical properties of the nervous system. Since neurons are sensitive to changes in their electrical properties, manipulating and observing these differences can provide information about the way ion channels open and close, connections between cells, or changes in response to a disease condition.

A related technique is **electrochemistry**. It uses similar sets of data collection equipment to understand the chemical processes of the nervous system. **Amperometry** and **fast scan cyclic voltammetry** are two of the more common electrochemistry methods used in neuroscience research.

Learning Objectives

By the end of this chapter, you will be able to:

- Explain the theories behind electrophysiology and electrochemistry experiments, including the principles of physics, the ways biological material can be prepared for electrophysiology, the different electrode configurations, and the tools that are used for collecting these data.
- Describe the graphs used to present electrophysiological and electrochemical data, including passive and active membrane properties, synaptic communication, and current-voltage relationships.

6.1.1 Neurons as Electrical Circuits

Electrophysiological methods rely on the premise that neurons can be modeled using principles from physics. The separation of charge-carrying ions – namely sodium (Na^+), potassium (K^+), chloride (Cl^-), and calcium (Ca^{2+}) – functions as a **battery**. Each battery represents the electrical potential for that ion. An ion enters or exits the cell through ion channels or transporters, which are akin to **resistors** in the circuit. A third component of the circuit is the cell membrane, a nonconductive substance that separates charges: the definition of a **capacitor**. Named after two early electrophysiologists, the Hodgkin and Huxley model in Figure 6.1 shows a neuron as an electrical circuit, containing a capacitor (C), resistors (g), and batteries (V).

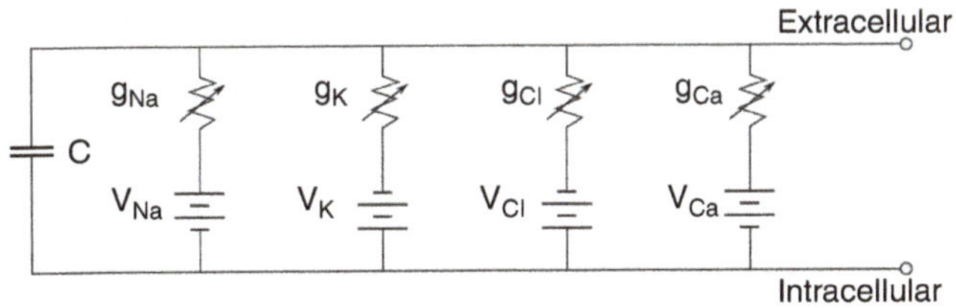

Figure 6.1 Theoretical organization of a neuron as an electrical circuit. Source: 2022, December 13. Wikimedia Commons, the free media repository. Retrieved 20:44, 13 February 2023 from https://commons.wikimedia.org/w/index.php?title=File:Cell_membrane_equivalent_circuit.svg&oldid=714643100. https://creativecommons.org/licenses/by-sa/3.0/deed.en.

Neurons, like electrical circuits, are sensitive to changes to the system. **Current** refers to the movement of charge. Current is measured in amperes (informally: amps). Amps are abbreviated as I (for "intensity"). In neurons, current is typically on the order of pico- or nanoamps (pA or nA). **Voltage** measures potential chemical energy in volts, abbreviated as V, and in neurons is usually on the order of millivolts (mV) or tens of millivolts. The terms "voltage" and "**potential**" may be used interchangeably. **Resistance** is measured in ohms, and is abbreviated by the capital Greek letter omega (Ω). Neuronal resistance is typically on the order of megaohms (MΩ).

A major principle of physics used in electrophysiological techniques is **Ohm's law**, the observation that voltage and current are directly proportional across the same resistance. It can be summarized by the relationship $V = I \times R$. Many electrophysiology strategies require that one variable is controlled, a procedure called **clamping**. With one variable held constant, the experimenter can gain data about the other variables. **Voltage clamp** (or **VC**) refers to recordings where voltage is kept steady and current is measured; **current clamp** (or **IC**) is when the current is kept steady and voltage is measured.

In voltage clamp, when voltage is injected negative to the resting membrane potential, these are **hyperpolarizing** manipulations; voltages more positive are **depolarizing**. Traces often plot current on the *y*-axis, typically measured in amperes. On the lower end, current is measured in picoamps (pA). The current moving through a single ion channel may be on the order of less than a picoamp. The upper end of current measurements may be tens of nanoamps (nA), which is the expected charge driven by the movement of ions during an action potential. By modern standard conventions, downward current deflections represent **inward** currents (positive charge moving into the neuron) while upward current deflections represent **outward** currents.

While recording in current clamp, potential is plotted on the *y*-axis. By convention, upward (more positive) deflections represent depolarization; downward (more negative) deflections represent hyperpolarization.

Additional Resources

Guo L. Equivalent circuit models of neurons. In *Principles of Electrical Neural Interfacing*. Cham: Springer; 2022.

6.1.2 Electrophysiological Preparations

Electrophysiological methods can be used to study the nervous system at several levels, from the whole organism down to single ion channels. Different ways of isolating parts of the nervous system for study are referred to as **preparations** (informally, **preps**). Different preps may change the basic electrophysiological properties of neurons: neurons that spontaneously fire action potentials in the whole animal may be silent in a brain slice preparation.

- ***In vivo*** means "in life," and *in vivo* experiments are conducted while the organism is completely intact. Some *in vivo* recordings can be performed while the animal is performing behavioral tasks (**awake and behaving**), such as feeding or playing, while neurons are being recorded from or activated. Another *in vivo* prep involves recording electrical activity while the animal is anesthetized.
- ***Ex vivo*** preparations are used when a section of living tissue is separated from the organism. The tissue will be introduced to an environment similar to that of the intact organism to keep the cells as healthy as possible. Control over this environment also allows for experimental manipulations. A common *ex vivo* preparation is the **acute slice**. Usually taken from the brain, these sections are 200–300 microns thin, and neurons can be identified under a microscope for recording. Acute slices have a limit on their viability on the order of hours. An **organotypic slice** is also a thin section cut from the animal, but it is collected under aseptic conditions and incubated in growth media. An organotypic slice can be kept alive for months in a culture dish.

  Other sections of the nervous system can also be isolated and studied, such as individual nerves. This was done by Hodgkin and Huxley in the 1930s when they isolated the giant axon from the Atlantic squid (*Loligo pealei*). This axon was selected because of its large axonal diameter (1 mm), making it easy to perform manipulations such as extruding the cytoplasm for chemical analysis and inserting electrodes. A similar modern *ex vivo* preparation is an isolated rodent sciatic nerve.
- ***In vitro*** means "in glass," and *in vitro* electrophysiological experiments study the properties of cells in a culture dish. Cells living in a culture dish need to be bathed in a nutrient-rich solution called **media**. Some applications of *in vitro* electrophysiological experiments include:

  - **Primary dissociated cultures**, where tissue from young animals (maybe three days after birth, or **postnatal day 3**, abbreviated as **P3**) is acutely dissected and the cells are isolated and dispersed across the bottom of a dish, a process called **plating**. After getting adjusted to the dish, the electrical activity of these neurons can be recorded.
  - Human-derived **induced pluripotent stem cells** (IPSCs; not to be confused with inhibitory postsynaptic currents) are cells (such as fibroblasts) taken from a person, de-differentiated back to a stem cell, and then converted to a cell type of interest, such as a cholinergic neuron or a retinal neuron. These are powerful tools because the properties of human neurons can be studied without the need to harvest brain cells.

- **Heterologous expression systems** are "blank cells" into which the researcher can inject genetic material (usually cDNA or cRNA). The recipient cell then produces protein products of that genetic material using its own ribosomes. Typically, ion channels, receptors, and transporters might be used in this experimental paradigm. These systems might be useful for understanding the cellular conditions that cause ion channels to open and close, or for characterizing the pharmacological binding properties of new compounds. Common cell **lines** (strains of origins) include **HEK 293 cells** (derived from human embryonic kidney), **CHO cells** (Chinese hamster ovary), the unfertilized egg cells of the African clawed toad *Xenopus laevis* (commonly called ***Xenopus* oocytes**), and **HeLa cells** (an immortalized cervical-cancer-derived cell; the original was taken from a patient named Henrietta Lacks).

Figure 6.2 represents a sample flow of IPSC culture creation after de-differentiation. Exposing an IPSC to different chemical signals (listed in boxes) will lead that cell to develop in a specific way. In this example, a motor neuron can be converted to a variety of spinal cord motor neurons (such as a median motor column, MMC, or a lateral motor column, LMC) by exposing it to specific signaling molecules.

6.1.3 Recording Configurations

Recording configurations are the placement of the **electrodes** (or informally, pipettes), the electrosensitive parts of the recording tools, in relation to the cells. The diameter of these electrodes may be a micron or smaller, but diameter is usually represented in terms of resistance (measured in megaohms, MΩ; higher resistance means a smaller-diameter tip). To conduct electrical signals, these electrodes are filled with an electrolyte solution, such as one that mimics the concentration of molecules inside a typical neuron (sometimes called an **internal**).

- In **extracellular recordings**, the electrode is placed in the space adjacent to neurons. Because less precision is needed for this configuration, electrodes can sometimes be placed into the tissue without needing a microscope. Extracellular recordings preserve cell integrity the best, but they can only provide information about action potential firing from a single neuron or large-scale changes in electrical properties of several neurons (a **field recording**, or a **local field potential**, or **LFP**).
- **Intracellular recordings** require the use of electrodes that pierce the cell. Because this requires precision on the order of tens of microns for mammalian cells, these experiments are typically performed under a microscope. A technique called **two electrode voltage clamp** (**TEVC**) may be used in *Xenopus* oocytes, which uses two intracellular electrodes to impale the large (1 mm diameter) oocytes.
- In **patch clamp recordings**, the electrode is placed on the neuronal cell membrane. From here, additional manipulations may be performed.
  - A **cell attached** (or **loose patch**) **recording** is an extracellular recording that isolates the signal for the patched neuron. Cell attached recordings are suitable for observing differences in spontaneous action potential firing or in response to manipulations, but they

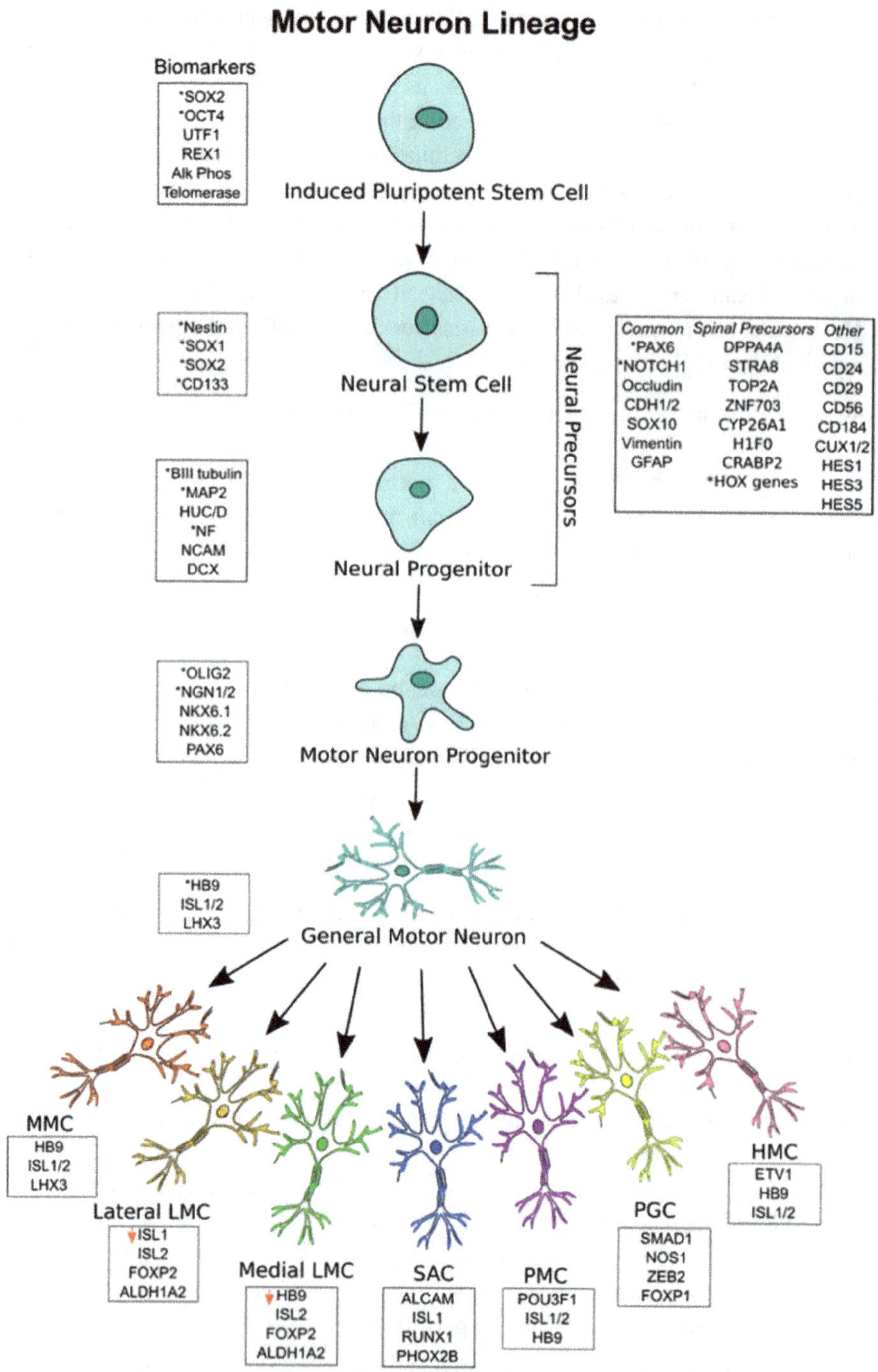

Figure 6.2 Cartoon of stem cell differentiation. Source: Trawczynski M, Liu G, David BT, Fessler RG. Restoring motor neurons in spinal cord injury with induced pluripotent stem cells. *Front Cell Neurosci.* 2019; 13:369. http://creativecommons.org/licenses/by/4.0/.

cannot provide information about membrane potential, synaptic connections, or amplitudes of synaptic inputs.

- In **whole cell recordings**, a brief suction is done to rupture the cell membrane. The solution inside the pipette is now continuous with the cytosol, which is called **gaining access**. Unlike in cell attached recordings, whole cell access provides information about membrane potential and synaptic inputs. A loose piece of membrane may interfere with the electrical access through changing **access resistance (R_a**; also called **series resistance, R_s**), so an ideal whole cell recording will have a stable R_a throughout the duration of the recording. Sometimes these values are plotted, and you expect this value to be 20 MΩ or lower with no slope over time. Another consideration of whole cell recordings is that intracellular molecules may dialyze into the pipette, which has a nearly infinite volume compared to the volume of the cell. This loss of intracellular molecules may change the intrinsic properties of the cell and could lead eventually to neuron death (informally called **rundown**).
- In **perforated patch** experiments, the electrode is filled with an internal solution containing a substance such as the antifungal amphotericin B or the antibiotic gramicidin. When placed against the surface of the cell membrane, these agents punch holes in it, allowing ions to flow between the pipette and the cell. Perforated patch recordings provide the same degree of information as whole cell but are more stable, since the intracellular molecules do not dialyze.
- **Excised patches** are preparations performed by removing a tiny patch of membrane from the cell, allowing study of transmembrane proteins in isolation of the whole neuron. An **inside-out patch** has the inside of the cell membrane on the outside of the pipette, while the **outside-out patch** has the outside of the membrane facing out of the pipette.

Figure 6.3 illustrates the different recording configurations in electrophysiology using an electrode against a cell.

Additional Resources

Graziane N, Dong Y. Extracellular and intracellular recordings. In *Electrophysiological Analysis of Synaptic Transmission*. Neuromethods, vol. 112. New York, NY: Humana Press; 2016.

6.1.4 Tools of Electrophysiological Experiments

All the equipment needed to perform electrophysiology is informally called a **rig**. The rig is typically made up of four sets of components.

1. **Optics** are tools used to visualize the sample: most commonly, microscopes. Special optics may not be necessary for extracellular recordings from whole organisms, such as an *in vivo* single-unit or arrays of cortically implanted electrodes. A dissecting microscope (up to 10× magnification) may be sufficient for some samples, such as in Hodgkin and Huxley's squid giant axon preparation. For intracellular and patch clamp recordings

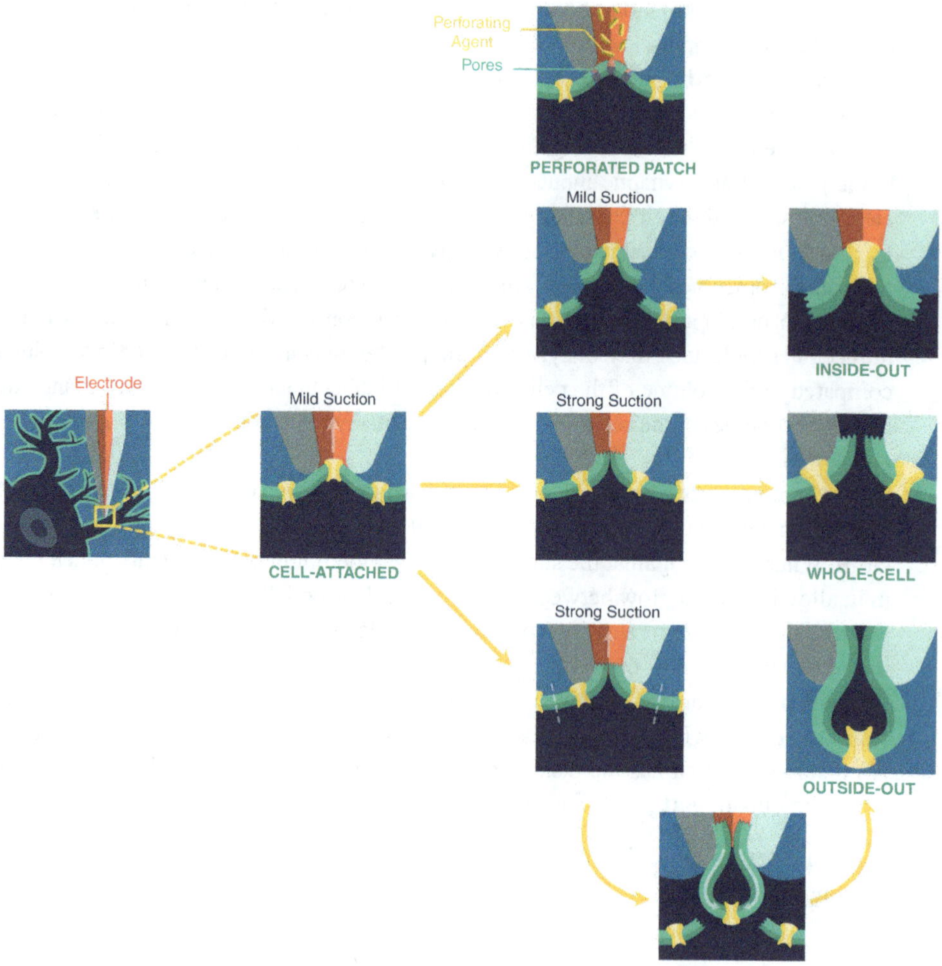

Figure 6.3 Cartoon of different recording configurations. Source: https://med.libretexts.org/Bookshelves/Pharmacology_and_Neuroscience/Neuroscience_(Ju)/03%3A_Fundamental_Neuroscience_Techniques/3.02%3A_Patch-Clamp_Electrophysiology. https://creativecommons.org/licenses/by/4.0/.

on mammalian neurons, higher magnification power is usually needed for accurate electrode placement. **Immersion lenses** are those that can be submerged directly into a solution, and they offer higher magnification power, up to 40× or 63×.

2. **Sample** refers to tools involved with the cells being recorded from, or those used to maximize the health of those cells.

   - For *in vivo* preparations, the sample elements include the intact animal along with tethers allowing for free movement (awake and behaving) or to minimize movement (anesthetized prep), and tools to deliver and maintain anesthesia or to help the animal regulate body temperature.

- *Ex vivo* preps require the use of several tools to maintain an environment that closely mimics the surroundings in the intact animal, such as a bath perfusion system to keep oxygenated, pH regulated, and temperature-controlled liquid (usually **artificial cerebrospinal fluid** or **aCSF**) flowing over the prep.
- *In vitro* experiments use a similar bath perfusion system to keep close control over the solution that surrounds the cells.

3. **Mechanics** are the tools used to control the location and placement of the electrodes. They are often **micromanipulators**, which allow for controlled movement of the electrode in three dimensions and can provide precise measurements about electrode location.
4. **Electronics** are the tools that capture or process electrical signals from the electrodes. The **headstage** connects directly with the pipette and is the first component to detect signals. These signals are compared to a ground electrode, which is placed in the extracellular space. The headstage is connected to the **amplifier** (informally, **amp**, not to be confused with ampere, the unit of current measurement), which increases the output of the signal. The amplifier is connected to the **digitizer** (or an **A to D converter**, which stands for analog to digital). In older electrophysiology rigs, the digitizer would run the signal into an **oscilloscope** (informally, **o-scope**), which is a monitor that allows for visualization of the observed signal. Speakers may also be connected to transmit signals. However, modern rigs send the digitized signal into the computer, which functions as both the oscilloscope and the speaker.

Figure 6.4 is a photograph of some equipment used to maintain a healthy brain slice in an *ex vivo* preparation. Inlets show how the flow of artificial cerebrospinal fluid bathes over and under the slice, which allows for the delivery of oxygen and nutrients to the preparation. Note the immersion microscope lens at the top of the image.

Usually, electrophysiological equipment has tremendous temporal resolution, collecting data points in excess of tens of kilohertz (kHz; 10,000+ times per second). The measure of how often data are collected is called the **sampling rate**.

Noise (also called hum) is the most common complaint among electrophysiologists. Because electrical signals being detected are very small and must be amplified several times by the electronics, it is common to detect unrelated background signals. Noise may be

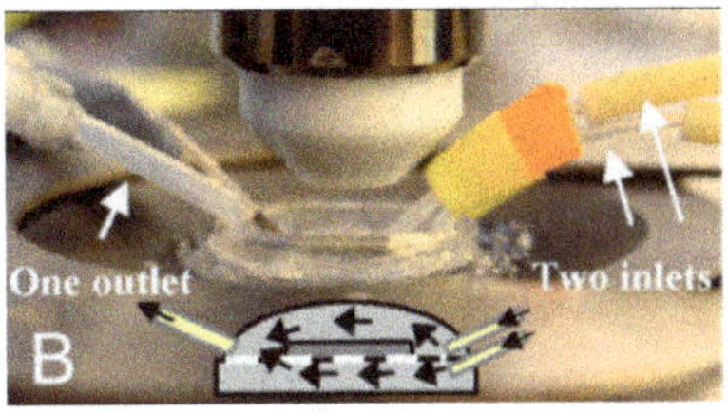

Figure 6.4 Equipment used to maintain healthy slices. Source: Hájos N, Mody I. Establishing a physiological environment for visualized in vitro brain slice recordings by increasing oxygen supply and modifying aCSF content. *J Neurosci Methods.* 2009 Oct 15 ;183(2):107–113. http://creativecommons.org/licenses/by/3.0/. Image cropped.

nonbiological: for example, interference from outside sources of radiation such as microwaves and cell phones. Current traveling through the electrical wires in the walls and electrical outlets produces a characteristic 60 Hz noise (60 cycle).

Most electrophysiological software is capable of storing several **protocols**, which are complex patterns of manipulations that are delivered by the electrode to the sample (this use of "protocol" is not to be confused with a protocol that might be submitted to and approved by a regulatory board such as IACUC or IRB). For example, one protocol might deliver a 50 picoamp step for 1 second while recording the cellular response. Another protocol might deliver a series of 100 action potentials in a second once every minute, and yet another protocol might trigger the flashing of an LED for optogenetics experiments or the activation of a bipolar stimulating electrode. When applicable, protocols are plotted on graphs alongside the response. Usually, a plot of the stimuli delivered by the electronics will appear "cleaner" with no noise, since it is nonbiological. These plots do not normally have curves (except in dynamic clamp).

A **sweep** is a single recording of an event in a time-locked fashion, such as the response of a neuron after a depolarizing current injection. In the same protocol, identical sweeps may be repeated which allows for averaging the data. Sweeps may also differ within a protocol, such as a series of progressively larger depolarizing current steps. Sometimes, data from multiple sweeps are represented on the same plot. Sweeps are short in duration (seconds to tens of seconds).

A **gapfree** recording is a continuous recording of cell activity not locked to a specific event in time. Recording of spontaneous action potential firing or the spontaneous release of neurotransmitter quanta may be done in a gapfree recording. Manipulations can also be performed during a gapfree recording to observe changes in these variables. Depending on the frequency of events being observed, gapfree recordings are long in duration (minutes to hundreds of minutes).

6.2 Passive (or Intrinsic) Neuronal Properties

The passive properties of neurons refers to features of the neurons without activation of voltage-gated ion channels (when not engaged in action potential firing). While there are many intrinsic differences in characteristics between neurons, two of the more commonly reported measures include **resting membrane potential** (RMP) and **membrane resistance** (R_m). These properties may be helpful for distinguishing unique populations of neurons and can be presented in descriptive studies.

Both require some degree of electrical access to the interior of the intact cell, so neither RPM nor membrane resistance can be observed using an extracellular configuration.

6.2.1 Resting Membrane Potential (RMP)

Background Information

The resting membrane potential (RMP, sometimes abbreviated Vrest or just Vr) is an intrinsic characteristic of every cell. The concentration of ions inside the cell differs from that outside the cell, and this difference in charged molecules causes the cell to have a net electrical charge. RMP is measured in millivolts (mV) and typical values range from −90 mV to −40 mV. Even within the same cellular population, RMP may differ among cells by as much as 10 mV.

Spontaneous neurotransmitter release might influence the membrane potential, so RMP may be reported while the preparation is bathed in a cocktail of fast synaptic inhibitors. Commonly blocked conductances (and their inhibitors) include voltage-gated sodium channels (TTX), AMPA-type (DNQX or CNQX) and NMDA-type (APV, also called AP-5) glutamate receptors, and GABAA (bicuculline, picrotoxin, or GABAzine) receptors. This measurement is especially critical when studying neurons with spontaneous action potential firing, which are never at "rest". This manipulation is only appropriate in *ex vivo* and *in vitro* preparations since these inhibitors may be deadly to the intact animal.

Reading the Graphs

Most commonly, RMP is reported in a group comparison that plots averages.

Sometimes, the RMP may be illustrated over time on a sample current clamp trace, plotting time on the *x*-axis (milliseconds to minutes) and membrane voltage in millivolts (mV) on the *y*-axis. In these graphs, the value of the RMP may be denoted by a horizontal line that runs along the trace, maybe accompanied by the numerical value. This value can be illustrated before and after manipulations, such as bath exposure to chemicals.

Interpreting the Data

Neurons with a relatively depolarized RMP (less negative values) may be more excitable, since this means that the cell rests closer to the action potential threshold and will fire in response to a smaller depolarization.

A manipulation that causes a shift in resting membrane potential may suggest a change in synaptic transmission. More excitatory (glutamatergic, possibly) or less inhibitory (GABAergic, possibly) synaptic communication may cause a depolarizing shift in the RMP. These observations can be tested with antagonist bath application.

Manipulations that change ionic permeabilities or ion distribution across the cell membrane may shift the RMP.

However, a neuron with a steadily depolarizing RMP might indicate cell **rundown**, as the cell can no longer maintain its electrochemical gradient due to low ATP. This change in RMP happens because the sodium-potassium ATP-ase, which generates part of the negative charge of the cell, stops functioning.

On the left of Figure 6.5, the RMP is due partly to the separation of charged ions across the cell membrane. On the right are representative traces from retinal ganglion cells before and after a bath application of 10 μM CIM, an agonist at the cation channel TRPM8. This cell shows spontaneous action potential activity, which are the large spikes that appear in the trace. At the top are changes in fluorescence as detected by 2 photon calcium imaging, showing a CIM-dependent influx of calcium. At the bottom is a whole cell current clamp recording of that same neuron during CIM application, showing that CIM causes a depolarization of the RMP as the

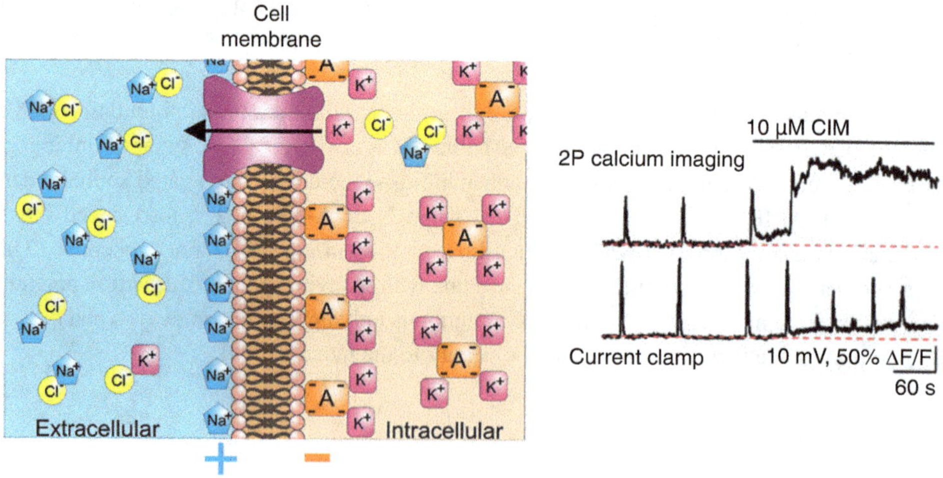

Figure 6.5 The resting membrane potential. Source of left image: Synaptidude. https://creativecommons.org/licenses/by/3.0/deed.en. Image cropped and some text removed. Source of right image: Webster CM, Tworig J, Caval-Holme F, Morgans CW, Feller MB. The impact of steroid activation of TRPM3 on spontaneous activity in the developing retina. *eNeuro*. 2020; 7(2):ENEURO.0175-19.2020. DOI: 10.1523/ENEURO.0175-19.2020 http://creativecommons.org/licenses/by/4.0/. Image cropped.

baseline shifts upwards. The authors of the study conclude that CIM opens TRPM8 channels, which allows for movement of positively charged cations including calcium into the cell.

Additional Resources

Cardozo D. An intuitive approach to understanding the resting membrane potential. *Adv Physiol Educ*. 2016 Dec; 40(4):543–547.

6.2.2 Membrane Resistance

Background Information

Membrane resistance (R_m) is a measure of how strongly incoming currents can influence cell membrane potential. In terms of cellular biology, a decrease in membrane resistance results from increased conductance of charge-carrying ions across the cell membrane, which is most often due to ion channel opening. Membrane resistance is usually on the order of hundreds of megaohms (MΩ) and is sometimes reported as a group average or a value in a table.

Also reported may be the **input resistance (R_i)** or the **total resistance**. The input resistance is the sum of the Rm and the access (pipette) resistance. R_i is always larger than R_m. The access resistance is usually only on the order of tens of megaohms but is nearly constant in a good recording (recordings where access resistance changes too much or exceeds 20 MΩ are excluded).

Interpreting the Data

Cells with a high R_m will have a larger-voltage response to changes in current. This observation can be reasoned through Ohm's law, $V = IR$: when R is big, even small changes in current I will cause big changes in V.

R_m is also important for understanding how signals move across distances. For example, when a cell receives excitatory synaptic inputs onto the dendrites, that depolarized change in membrane voltage travels from the dendrites toward the cell body. Cells with a higher R_m will see less signal loss at the soma, while cells with a lower R_m will "leak" more depolarization along the route. High R_m means the cell can more reliably pass the signal forward.

Myelination can influence membrane resistance. Myelin wraps around axons, therefore blocking the underlying ion channels and increasing R_m.

6.3 Action Potential (AP) Analysis

Background Information

The action potential is the main communicative unit of the nervous system. An action potential is a temporary depolarization on the order of ~100 millivolts of the neuron's axonal membrane potential, which results in bulk release of neurotransmitter. The action potential is an all-or-nothing phenomenon.

The action potential has a predictable and reliable shape with three distinct phases. The **depolarization phase** (or **rising phase**, or **upswing**) is driven by the mass entry of the positively charged sodium ions into the neuron through voltage-gated sodium channels. This drives the membrane potential to more positive values. The **repolarization phase** (or **falling phase**) results from the exit of positively charged potassium ions, bringing the membrane potential back toward negative potentials. Finally, the **afterhyperpolarization (AHP) phase** (or **undershoot phase**), when the membrane potential is more negative than the resting membrane potential, happens because of continued efflux of potassium with the combined slow closing of the voltage-gated potassium channels, until the cell returns to its resting membrane potential.

A current clamp configuration is the most meaningful way to measure action potentials, since this configuration detects changes in voltage. This is also the most common way action potentials are presented in figures. However, it is possible to detect action currents in a voltage clamp configuration, which measures changes in current due to ion flow during an action potential and may be used during an extracellular configuration.

Many different features of the shape of a cell's average action potential may be analyzed and reported. Sometimes, representative average action potentials may be overlaid to better illustrate differences in action potential shape. More often, the measures are reported just as a group average or in a table.

Most of these features can only be observed in an intracellular or patch clamp configuration; extracellular recordings may not reliably provide some of these data observations.

Commonly reported measures include the following:

- **AP amplitude** (or **action potential height**) is the difference between the RMP and the peak membrane voltage reached during the depolarization phase. These values are measured in millivolts (mV) and may be in the range of +40 to +90 mV. Relatedly, the AP **overshoot** measures the amount of depolarization greater than 0 mV at the peak amplitude. Overshoot does not depend on differences in RMP.
- **Maximum depolarization slope** is a measure of the fastest depolarization during the rising phase of the action potential. This value may be calculated by finding the peak of the first derivative of the membrane voltage over time, usually written out as dV/dt.
- **AP duration** is the time between the rising phase and the falling phase at some voltage (maybe 5% of total depolarization) depolarized from the RMP. Relatedly, **AP half-width** (or **half-duration**) refers to the duration of the action potential measured at halfway between the beginning of the rising phase and the moment when the potential returns to the resting membrane potential. These values are measurements of time, usually tenths of milliseconds to milliseconds (ms). The gating properties of the voltage-gated potassium channels and voltage-gated sodium channels are involved in determining AP duration and half-width. Shorter AP duration or half-width may suggest a faster firing rate.
- The **AP threshold** is the membrane voltage (Vm) at which the all-or-nothing depolarization phase of the action potential initiates. The AP threshold represents the voltage needed to cause several voltage-gated sodium channels to open, triggering a positive feedback loop that causes more sodium influx and depolarization. The AP threshold is expected to be within a range of −55 to −40 millivolts (mV). The AP threshold is always more positive than the RMP. One possible criterion for determining AP threshold is the membrane voltage when the change in potential (slope, measured in mV per millisecond; dVm/dt) first exceeds 10 mV/ms.
- **Afterhyperpolarization (AHP) amplitude (trough**, or **undershoot)** is the amplitude in millivolts from the RMP to the lowest point of the afterhyperpolarization, and is generally on the order of tens of millivolts. **AHP duration** is a measurement of time after repolarization until the RMP is restored. A combination of amplitude and duration may be presented as **AHP area**, which is the area above the curve and below the RMP line. Features of the afterhyperpolarization are determined by the properties of the voltage-gated potassium channels. Because the AHP is part of the refractory period, it contributes to how rapidly action potentials can be fired.

Figure 6.6 represents an experiment in which researchers were curious to see whether some of the basic properties of action potentials are affected by temperature. On the left, representative traces show an overlay of action potentials observed under three different temperatures. The bar graphs present group summary data showing that features such as AP width, amplitude, and latency to AP threshold are all increased at colder temperatures, while AP threshold is unchanged.

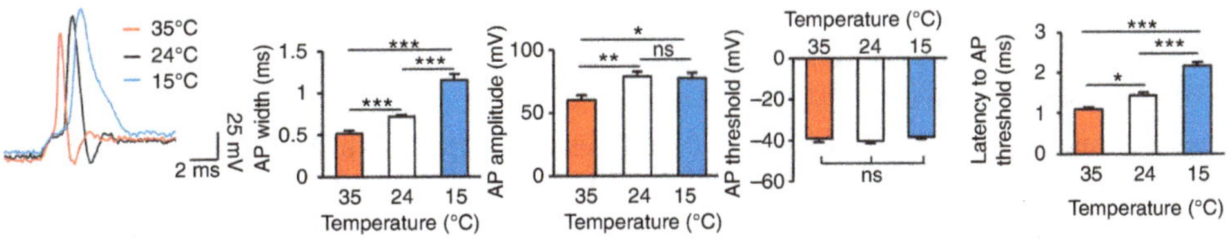

Figure 6.6 Results of an action potential experiment. Source: Kanda H, Tonomura S, Gu JG. Effects of cooling temperatures via thermal K2P channels on regeneration of high-frequency action potentials at nodes of Ranvier of rat Aβ-afferent nerves. *eNeuro*. 2021; 8(5):ENEURO.0308-21.2021. doi:10.1523/ENEURO.0308-21.2021. http://creativecommons.org/licenses/by/4.0/. Panels have been reorganized and cropped, and text labels removed.

Interpreting the Data

Some of these traits may be helpful in cell identification, since different cell types may have unique action potential characteristics. For example, midbrain dopamine neurons have been classically identified by their broad action potentials lasting longer than 2 milliseconds.

Features of the action potential are sensitive to some genetic mutations, especially genes that code for voltage-gated ion channels. For example, mutations to the $Na_v1.7$ protein shift the action potential threshold. $Na_v1.7$ is a voltage-gated sodium channel expressed on pain-sensing neurons in the peripheral nervous system. A higher action potential threshold has been implicated as the mechanism underlying a condition called congenital insensitivity to pain, where a person cannot feel pain.

Several drugs are known to modify the shape of the action potential. Apamin, a key ingredient of honeybee venom, decreases peak AHP amplitude and duration.

Additional Resources

Bean BP. The action potential in mammalian central neurons. *Nat Rev Neurosci*. 2007 Jun; 8(6):451–465. DOI: 10.1038/nrn2148. PMID: 17514198.

6.3.1 Spontaneous (and Evoked) Firing Rate

Background Information

Some neurons have network connections or intrinsic molecular properties that cause them to fire action potentials spontaneously. Measuring the action potential **firing rate** (FR; not to be confused with fixed ratio, a paradigm used in self-administration behavioral studies) can provide information about these elements.

Spontaneous firing rate is a measure of the cell's intrinsic action potential firing. These data are captured in long recordings (longer than tens of seconds) and are usually done in a gapfree protocol. **Evoked firing rate** is the change in action potential firing after some time-locked component, such as firing during injection of current, external stimulus presentation, or depolarization of synaptic inputs. These are short recordings captured in protocols using sweeps.

Detecting action potentials is also possible using calcium indicator dyes. A genetically encoded indicator such as GCaMP offers the ability to observe the activity of several (tens or hundreds) neurons simultaneously in real time. These methods are less invasive than electrophysiological manipulations, but they require the use of imaging tools.

Spontaneous activity can be measured in both current clamp and voltage clamp and can be observed in recording configurations where the cells are intact. But the activity profile of a neuron may depend on the preparation and configuration. For example, neurons that fire spontaneously *in vivo* may not fire in an *ex vivo* slice, and some neurons stop their spontaneous activity after going whole cell. Firing rate data is mostly collected from nonhuman samples but can also be collected from humans undergoing awake brain surgery.

Reading the Graphs

In recordings from single neurons, sample traces and group average data may both be shown. Sample traces may plot time (up to minutes) on the *x*-axis and membrane potential (abbreviated V_m) on the *y*-axis in millivolts (mV) when in current clamp.

Data from different manipulations or groups are likely to be plotted across the *x*-axis and frequency of firing (or **discharge rate**) on the *y*-axis, usually in hertz (events per second, abbreviated Hz; also written as spikes s^{-1}). Frequencies of spontaneous action potential firing range from 0 to upwards of a few hundred Hz, but most fire in the 0–20 Hz range. Measuring firing rate frequency is most appropriate for **pacemaker** neurons, which fire spontaneous action potentials at regular intervals.

Frequency data may also be presented as an **interspike interval (ISI**; sometimes also called **interevent interval**, or **IEI**, not to be confused with interstimulus interval), which represents an average time that has elapsed between two sequential action potentials and is expressed in units of time. Plots of these data are likely to be histograms showing ISI across the *x*-axis and number of observations on the *y*-axis. The range of ISIs will depend on the frequency of activity, and higher frequency means the ISIs will be smaller. Bins may be in the range of milliseconds or tens of milliseconds. ISI histograms tend to have a long right tail, since the refractory period limits how quickly action potentials fire in succession.

Sometimes, a **coefficient of variation (CV)** may be plotted alongside firing rate data. The CV is calculated mathematically based on each ISI and is a quantification of how unpredictable the timing of each event is. A larger CV indicates that the spiking pattern is less regular.

Some techniques allow for simultaneous observations from multiple neurons, such as an array of extracellular probes or all-optical electrophysiology using a genetically encoded voltage sensor. In these types of recordings, the data may be represented in a **raster plot**. This plots time across the *x*-axis, usually over the course of several seconds. Each row represents a single neuron that is being observed, and each vertical hash mark represents an action potential.

Evoked firing rate data can be plotted using a raster plot (multiple cells) or with a **peristimulus time histogram**. These graphs are histograms that center their focus on the instance where the stimulus was applied. Negative time gives information about baseline firing activity and time 0 indicates the onset of the stimulus. A bar or arrow indicates how long the stimulus was applied for.

In the study represented in Figure 6.7, a human stem cell line is induced into becoming neurons on a high-density microelectrode array, allowing for the electrophysiological observation of several neurons simultaneously. On the left, sample traces from a single neuron show action potentials as deflections from the baseline on the order of around 50 μV. Traces from top to bottom represent a longer time following induction into neurons (days post induction, dpi). Early on, action potentials are rarer and more sporadic. Around 63 dpi, the neurons changed their firing pattern to bursts of activity. On the right are action potentials of several neurons from each time point over time. Neuronal firing has been sorted with a raster plot based on activity. Here, each row represents an individual cell and each dot represents a single action potential. As days go by after neuronal differentiation, the cells begin to start firing more synchronously as if connected in a network.

Interpreting the Data

There are several mechanisms that may explain why neuronal firing rate changes. Ultimately, changes in ion conductances lead to increases in firing rate, such as greater Na^+/Ca^{2+} conductance or smaller K^+/Cl^- conductance.

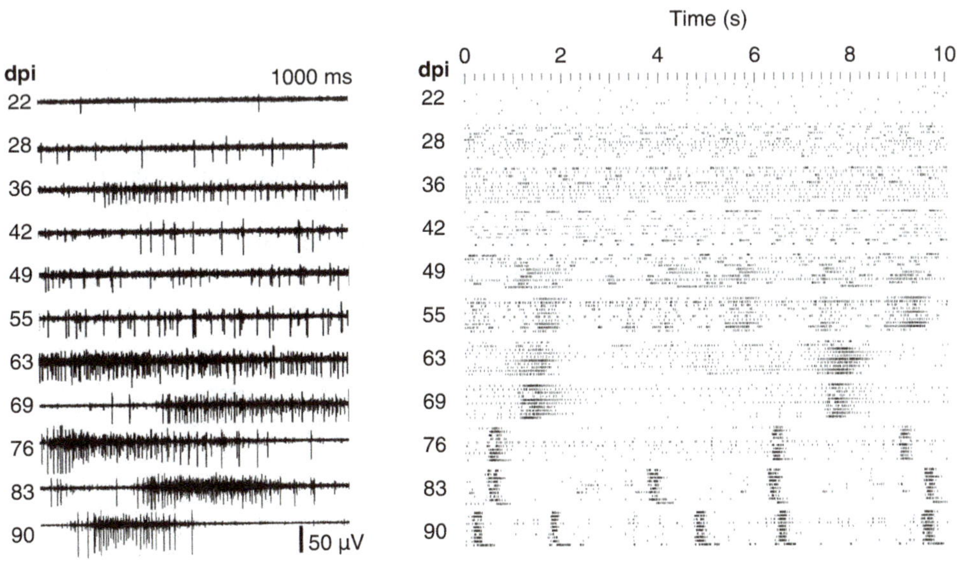

Figure 6.7 Analysis of action potential firing over days. Source: Habibey R, Striebel J, Schmieder F, Czarske J, Busskamp V. Long-term morphological and functional dynamics of human stem cell-derived neuronal networks on high-density micro-electrode arrays. *Front Neurosci.* 2022; 16:951964. doi: 10.3389/fnins.2022.951964. http://creativecommons.org/licenses/by/4.0/. Image cropped and text labels removed.

The main molecular driver of the depolarization phase is the **voltage-gated sodium channel** (**VGSC**, or $\mathbf{Na_V}$ are two names for the same proteins; **SCN** are the genes that code for those proteins). These channels are more likely to open during depolarization. Exposing these channels to antagonists such as tetrodotoxin will cause action potentials to stop firing.

Modifications of **voltage-gated potassium channels** (**VGKC** or $\mathbf{K_V}$ are the names of the proteins; **KCN** are the genes that code for the proteins) typically affect the afterhyperpolarization and therefore the refractory period. Shortened refractory periods, as brought on by the bee venom apamin for example, lead to increased action potential firing rate.

Figure 6.8 represents current clamp recordings that show the effect of the drug TGOT, an oxytocin receptor agonist, on evoked action potential firing. Oxytocin receptor activation has many cellular effects, including the inhibition of potassium conductance. Traces are overlays showing results of several current steps at different amplitudes, starting with a −200 pA step and increasing by 40 pA per step. The negative current steps cause a hyperpolarization (downward deflections), while positive steps cause depolarization (upward deflections). On the left, ACSF is the baseline experiment. Under these conditions, only two action potentials were evoked, and this was only at a strong injection of depolarizing current. They also report the resting membrane potential as −71 mV. In the middle, TGOT is added to the neurons. Here, there is an increase in excitability as more action potentials were evoked. Also, these was a depolarizing shift in resting membrane potential to −60 mV. On the right, the TGOT is removed from the solution by washing the preparation with ACSF for 25 minutes. This experiment shows a partial return to baseline, as few action potentials were initiated and the RMP became hyperpolarized to −66 mV.

Genetic mutations of these proteins contribute to differences in firing rates.

Some potential mechanisms upstream of changes to ion conductance include:

- Activation of ligand-gated ion channels by endogenous neurotransmitters or by exogenously applied ligands. For example, electrical (or optogenetic) stimulation can cause axonal fibers to depolarize, which may release glutamate onto the AMPA type glutamate receptors, which are sodium channels (increasing action potential firing). In another experiment, bath-applying exogenous GABA to an *ex vivo* slice preparation activates GABA receptors, some of which are chloride channels (decreasing action potential firing).
- Changes in intracellular signaling molecules. In a whole cell patch clamp experiment, exogenous chemicals may be included in the internal solution and may dialyze into the

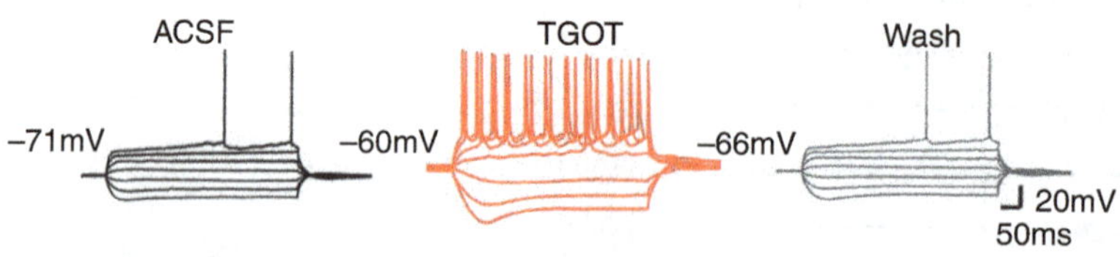

Figure 6.8 Results of another action potential experiment. Source: Liu JJ, Eyring KW, König GM, Kostenis E, Tsien RW. Oxytocin-modulated ion channel ensemble controls depolarization, integration and burst firing in CA2 pyramidal neurons. *J Neurosci.* 2022 Oct 12; 42(41):7707–7720. https://creativecommons.org/licenses/by/4.0/. Image cropped and text labels removed.

cells; conversely, intracellular signaling molecules may also dialyze into the pipette. Intracellular signaling molecules are also changed in response to metabotropic receptor activation. For example, the signaling molecule cyclic GMP (cGMP) can bind to and activate receptors called cyclic nucleotide-gated channels which increase action potential firing.
- Intrinsic differences in cellular properties. For example, for cells with a relatively depolarized resting membrane potential, less depolarization might be needed to reach threshold and initiate an action potential which can lead to increased baseline firing rate.

In representative traces of action potentials, the direction of the event depends on the recording configuration. Whole cell current clamp recordings produce the prototypical action potential shape with a positive (upward) deflection, while the same neuron recorded in voltage clamp will produce a downward deflection, which is caused by the inward current driven by sodium movement into neurons.

In measuring firing rate, the amplitude of the events also does not carry much information. For example, in extracellular recordings, the amplitude is indicative of how close the electrode is placed next to the cell, and in perforated patch, amplitude provides information about how thoroughly the cell membrane has been perforated. Action potential amplitude cannot be measured meaningfully in these circumstances.

In looking at ISI data, an ISI of 1 second means there is an average of 1 second between action potentials, which corresponds to a firing rate of 1 Hz. A decrease in firing rate is reflected by an increase in the ISI.

Frequency may not accurately represent all the subtlety of action potential firing. For example, some neurons fire in an **irregular** pattern, where the action potentials are not spaced out evenly. Some neurons exhibit **bursting** activity, short windows of time when the neuron fires several action potentials interspersed with periods of relative silence. In evoked action potential recordings, some neurons may show **spike accommodation** (or **spike adaptation**), which is a gradual slowing of action potential firing after current injection.

Different firing patterns may be presented by plotting measures other than frequency. For example, a histogram might plot ISI on the x-axis and number of events on the y-axis. Typical firing patterns and their appearance on a histogram include the following:

- Pacemaker neurons exhibit regular and predictable firing with equally spaced ISIs. On a histogram, a pacemaker neuron will show a single, narrow peak. These cells may be meaningfully represented by firing rate (in Hz).
- Cells that fire action potentials at irregular intervals may have the same average frequency as a pacemaker neuron. But a histogram of the frequency will have a single, broad peak: the flatter the curve, the more irregular the activity. The coefficient of variation may also be plotted for cells with irregular firing patterns. The higher the CV, the more irregular the activity. A cell with perfectly timed pacemaker activity (all ISIs are equally spaced) will have a CV of 0; CV will rarely exceed 3. CV is unitless.
- Cells that show accommodation decrease firing activity after several action potentials. The frequency histogram may look like one with irregular firing (a single, broad peak). To differentiate the types of firing patterns, a **spike adaptation ratio** might be plotted. This can be calculated by dividing the ISI between the last and second-to-last action

potential by the ISI between the first and second action potential. In this formula, a larger spike adaptation ratio indicates more accommodation; a cell with no accommodation will have a ratio of 1. This value is unitless.

- A cell that fires in bursts will produce an ISI histogram with a bimodal distribution, usually with the larger peak at shorter ISIs and a second smaller peak around a longer ISI. For plotting data from bursting neurons, additional observations such as **number of spikes per burst**, **duration of burst**, or **time between bursts** may be reported.

Figure 6.9 represents current clamp recordings showing spontaneous action potential firing in the subthalamic nucleus (STN), a region in the basal ganglia. Of the 88 cells recorded, neurons had one of three firing patterns: irregular (top), regular pacemaker (middle), or burst (bottom). These recordings were single-unit extracellular recordings. The amplitudes of the action potentials are small under this recording configuration.

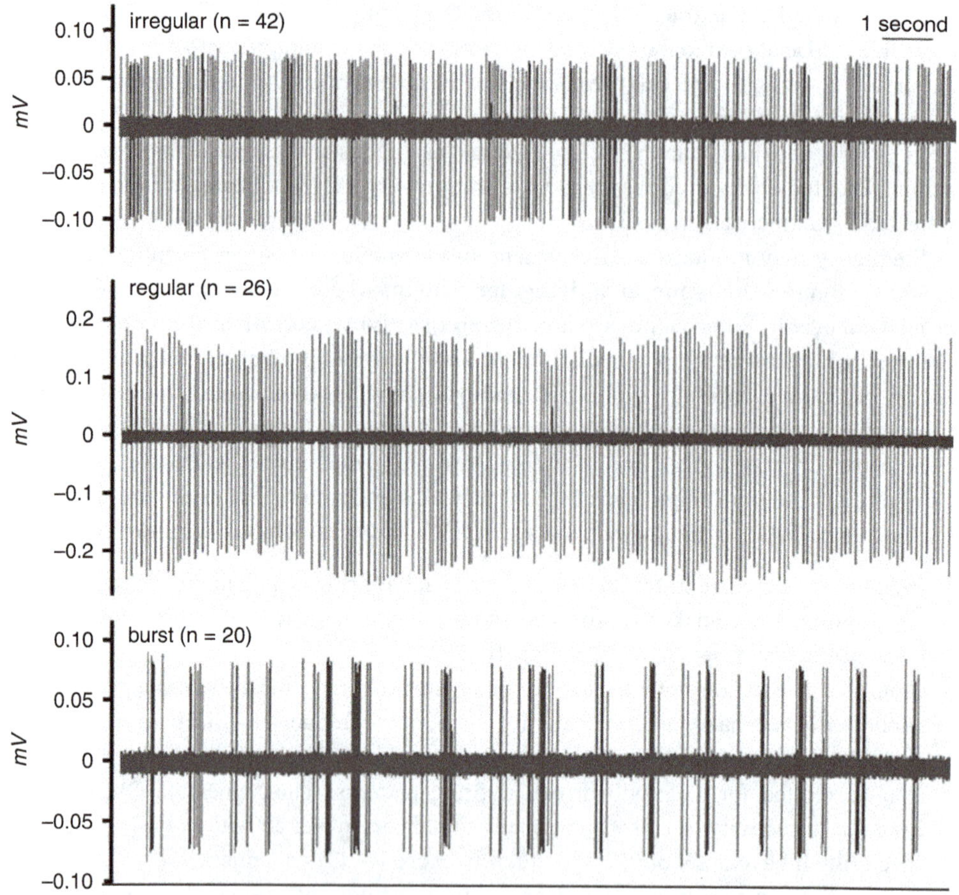

Figure 6.9 Sample patterns of action potential activity. Source: Pautrat A, Rolland M, Barthelemy M, et al. Revealing a novel nociceptive network that links the subthalamic nucleus to pain processing. *Elife*. 2018 Aug 28; 7:e36607. http://creativecommons.org/licenses/by/4.0/. Image cropped.

Additional Resources

Tomar R. Review: Methods of firing rate estimation. *Biosystems*. 2019 Sep; 183:103980. DOI: 10.1016/j.biosystems.2019.103980. Epub 2019 Jun 1. PMID: 31163197.

6.3.2 Rheobase (Current Threshold)

Background Information

Rheobase current is the minimum threshold current that needs to be delivered to evoke one action potential in a neuron. Rheobase gives us an idea about the excitability profile of the cells: neurons with a low rheobase are more excitable. Conditions that change neural excitability may be observed as a shift in rheobase. For example, differences in expression or function of voltage-gated sodium channels as seen in chronic pain or epilepsy will result in a shift in rheobase.

Collecting rheobase data requires electrical access to the intact neuron, so it can only be done in current clamp using whole cell or perforated patch recording configurations. Cells are usually from an *ex vivo* or *in vitro* preparation.

Reading the Graphs

Sample traces may show two graphs, one on top of the other: the current delivered to the cell (input) and the cell's response (output). Both graphs share the *x*-axis, which shows time, usually spanning hundreds of milliseconds (ms).

1. The input plots current amplitude being delivered on the *y*-axis. Typically, the current needed to evoke an action potential is on the order of tens or hundreds of picoamps (pA). This current can be delivered in **steps**. Usually, multiple steps of different amplitudes will be delivered. When plotted, these graphs may be overlays of multiple current injections, but technically only two current steps are needed to identify the rheobase. The injection of current can also be delivered via a **ramp** protocol. In ramp protocols, greater current is progressively injected over the course of tens or hundreds of milliseconds.
2. The other graph of sample traces are recordings of the neuron response, which plot membrane voltage on the *y*-axis, measured in tens or hundreds of millivolts (mV).

A group average graph alongside the sample traces will show different manipulations across the *x*-axis and rheobase on the *y*-axis, which is usually on the order of tens or hundreds of picoamps.

Figure 6.10 represents a rheobase experiment using a current ramp. At the top is a trace showing the current delivered to the cell. The *x*-axis represents time and the *y*-axis represents current injected. The slope (120 pA/s) and peak current injection (480 pA) are shown. In the middle, sample traces show the neuronal response where the *x*-axis represents time and the *y*-axis represents membrane potential. Compared to the control condition (vehicle, black trace), cells exposed to low-dose TTX (red trace) fire action potentials only after more depolarizing current has been injected (the first action potential peak is seen farther to the right).

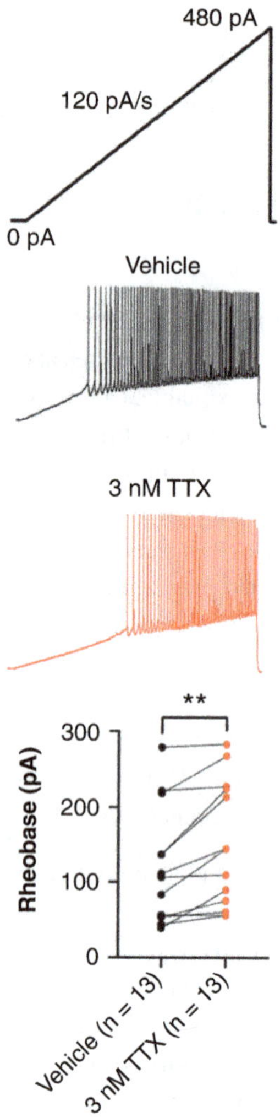

Figure 6.10 Results of a rheobase experiment. Source: Thouta S, Waldbrook MG, Lin S, et al. Pharmacological determination of the fractional block of Nav channels required to impair neuronal excitability and *ex vivo* seizures. *Front Cell Neurosci.* 2022; 16:964691. DOI: 10.3389/fncel.2022.964691. http://creativecommons.org/licenses/by/4.0/. Image cropped, panels rearranged, and text labels removed.

This suggests that TTX produces an upward shift of rheobase. At the bottom is a quantification and summary of group data in a within-cell plot, meaning that the rheobase of each data point is compared to itself before exposure to TTX.

Interpreting the Data

Lower rheobase indicates a more excitable cell: a cell with a lower rheobase will have an action potential in response to a smaller step than one with a higher rheobase.

An important control experiment to perform alongside rheobase is to demonstrate no significant difference in resting membrane potential. Cells with depolarized resting potentials may already be closer to the action potential firing threshold potential, and therefore require less current injection to reach that threshold.

6.4 Synaptic Events

When a neuron fires an action potential, that depolarization allows for Ca^{2+} entry at the axon terminal, in turn allowing neurotransmitter release. From there, the molecules may diffuse across the synapse and activate receptors, which can cause a change in postsynaptic membrane properties. These changes are described in this section on synaptic events.

Most synaptic events described in the literature are postsynaptic changes caused by glutamate (usually excitatory) or GABA (usually inhibitory). There are two changes described in figures:

1. Postsynaptic membrane potential, which is plotted on the *y*-axis. A depolarizing event will have a positive deflection, while a hyperpolarizing event will have a negative deflection. These experiments are done in current clamp.
2. Postsynaptic current, which is on the *y*-axis. By convention, inward current (movement of positive charges such as Na^+ into the cell, or negative charges such as Cl^- out) will have a downward deflection, and outward current will have an upward deflection. These experiments are done in voltage clamp. However, it is possible to change the ion concentration inside the cell, which may change the direction of the synaptic currents. The most common manipulation is to increase the intracellular concentration of chloride, which will reverse the direction of chloride current. High intracellular chloride might improve the stability of the recording. The concentration of ions used in the intracellular solution is usually written in the methods section of the research reporting.

6.4.1 Spontaneous (or Miniature) Synaptic Events

Background Information

A spontaneous **excitatory postsynaptic current** (**sEPSC**) measurement is a voltage clamp recording that detects movement of charged ions after the release of glutamate. The related measure, spontaneous **inhibitory postsynaptic current** (**sIPSC**), detects ion movement after GABA release.

On the other hand, in a current clamp recording, changes in voltage resulting from synaptic neurotransmitter release can also be measured. Depolarization is measured in spontaneous **excitatory postsynaptic potential** (**sEPSP**) recordings, while hyperpolarization is measured in spontaneous **inhibitory postsynaptic potential** (**sIPSP**) recordings.

Spontaneous events are recorded with ordinary aCSF in the extracellular bath. **Miniature** events (informally, **minis**) are synaptic events recorded in the presence of antagonists, such as **tetrodotoxin** (**TTX**), an antagonist for voltage-gated sodium channels, which block spontaneous action potential firing. Antagonists are also added to pharmacologically isolate the neurotransmitter of interest. For recording mEPSCs, a GABA antagonist such as bicuculline or GABAzine may be included in the bath. For recording mIPSCs, glutamate antagonists such as DNQX and APV might be used. On average, miniature events are smaller and less frequent than spontaneous events.

These recordings are often done in a gapfree recording protocol. Generally, data from several minutes is analyzed, depending on the frequency of events. Typically, more than 100 events should be analyzed.

These experiments are usually done in *ex vivo* or culture preparations. Similar observations can be made looking at the neuromuscular junction; these may be called **miniature end plate potentials (mEPPs)**.

Reading the Graphs

Even though there may be several different measures that can be described, the graphical representation of the data is essentially the same.

Sample traces often depict hundreds of milliseconds (or longer) of the recordings on the *x*-axis, and measures of current or voltage on the *y*-axis. For example, when measuring ePSCs in voltage clamp, downward deflections represent inward current, which is usually Na^+ or Ca^{2+} movement into the cell (however, with a high intracellular chloride internal solution, Cl^- moving out of the cell creates an inward current).

Many pieces of information can be collected from recording these events.

- **Frequency** of events, the measurement of how often the event is observed, usually measured in hertz (Hz), the number of events per second.
- **Amplitude** of events, a measurement of how large the event is. Most synaptic events have a current amplitude in the range of tens to hundreds of picoamps (pA), and a voltage amplitude on the order of millivolts (mV).
- **Kinetics** of events, observations related to the shape and time course of the event. The word "peak" refers to either the maximum value or, confusingly, a minimum value (although **trough** is sometimes used). Differences in kinetics may be illustrated by overlaying representative events on top of one another to see how the events differ. Commonly reported kinetics measurements include:
    - **Rise time** – the time elapsed from the onset of the event to the peak. A **10–90% rise time** may be reported, which represents how long it takes for the event to go from 10% of maximum value to 90% maximum. These values are typically on the order of milliseconds or faster. The word "rise" might be confusing here since the word is used even in an event with a downward direction.
    - **Decay time** (abbreviated as τ) – the **time constant**, the duration of time that passes before the measurement returns to ~37% of the peak value. Synaptic decay times are usually shorter than hundreds of milliseconds.
    - **Area under the curve** – a combined measure of amplitude, rise time, and decay time. As with "rise", the word "under" may be confusing, since this measures the area

between the curve and baseline, regardless of direction. In measures of current, area under the curve has units in pA*ms.

Frequency and amplitude are the most often summarized pieces of information. One may plot interevent interval (IEI) on the *x*-axis, which is related to frequency. This scale will range from a low of 0 (even though no data points will have 0 IEI) to the maximum time between events, which may be on the order of seconds. The second graph will plot amplitude on the *x*-axis.

The *y*-axis may plot **cumulative probability**. These values range from 0 to 1 and are unitless. Cumulative probability indicates the fraction of events that are at that specific value on the *x*-axis. On the IEI cumulative probability graph, a higher curve indicates increased frequency of events. On the amplitude graph, a higher curve indicates smaller events.

Frequency and amplitude information may also be presented as a percentage change from baseline, which is common for showing how a drug affects synaptic release events.

Histograms or group average data may also be shown to plot these data.

Figure 6.11 shows the results of miniature excitatory postsynaptic current (mEPSC) recordings from cerebellar Purkinje neurons of larval zebrafish. Researchers were curious to see how the Gjd2b gene is involved with formation of excitatory glutamatergic synapses, so they compared wild type mice (control, black) with Gjd2b-KOs (experimental, red). On the left are representative gapfree traces. Each mEPSC is a line that extends below the baseline. Here, knockouts had a decrease in event frequency but an increase in the amplitude. In the middle is a zoom-in on an average of several mEPSCs from each of the genotypes, showing that the knockouts had larger events. The inlaid graph normalizes the average event to the amplitude, which allows for a comparison of kinetics. Here, there is a shortening of the decay kinetics in the knockouts (narrower event width). On the right is a cumulative probability plot showing quantification of the frequency of events. In this plot, because the knockouts had fewer events, they had a lower curve.

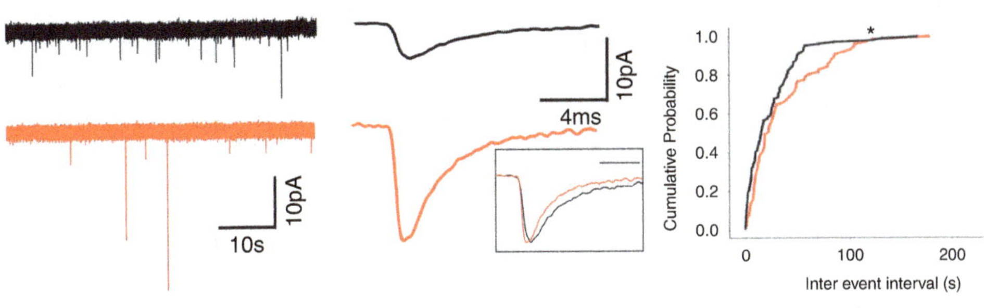

Figure 6.11 Results of an mEPSC experiment. Source: Sitaraman S, Yadav G, Agarwal V, Jabeen S, Verma S, Jadhav M, Thirumalai V. Gjd2b-mediated gap junctions promote glutamatergic synapse formation and dendritic elaboration in Purkinje neurons. *eLife*. 2021; 10:e68124. http://creativecommons.org/licenses/by/4.0/. Image cropped, panels rearranged, text labels and inset graphs removed.

Interpreting the Data

A change in frequency represents a difference in the presynaptic component. How often events occur is related to the ability of the presynaptic terminal to release neurotransmitter. For example, inhibiting the presynaptic terminal by CB1 receptor activation decreases the frequency of events.

On the other hand, a change in the amplitude of events represents a difference at the postsynaptic component. After the neurotransmitter has been released into the synapse, the postsynaptic membrane detects that signal. For example, increases in receptor expression or function will lead to a larger mEPSC amplitude.

Changes in kinetics properties may be interpreted in several ways. Faster rise times may be more related to synchronized vesicular fusion and release. Changes in decay time may involve clearance of neurotransmitter mediated by transporter proteins or astrocytes.

Additional Resources

Kavalali ET. The mechanisms and functions of spontaneous neurotransmitter release. *Nat Rev Neurosci*. 2015 Jan; 16(1):5–16. DOI: 10.1038/nrn3875. PMID: 25524119.

6.4.2 Evoked Synaptic Events

Background Information

These synaptic events are those where the experimenter delivers precisely timed stimulation which activates some number of presynaptic terminals. This stimulation can be performed by placing an electrode directly into the brain area, or by flashing light onto light-sensitive excitatory ion channels expressed on cells. These stimulations cause neurotransmitter release. Then, a corresponding change in excitatory or inhibitory potential (or inward or outward current) of the postsynaptic cells is recorded.

The letter "e" (for evoked) may be added in front of one of the abbreviations used in Section 6.4.1 to clarify exactly what is being recorded: an **eEPSP** is an evoked excitatory postsynaptic potential, for example. These measures can be performed while recording individually from neurons in an intracellular or patch clamp configuration. When recording from several neurons at once in a slice using electrodes placed extracellularly, this is a **field EPSP (fEPSP)**.

Evoked synaptic measurements demonstrate that the cell or brain area receives incoming projections and that the cell or brain area is sensitive to neurotransmitter release (the relevant receptors for the receptor are functional). The experiment can also be performed in conjunction with other electrophysiological tests, such as paired pulse ratio or measures of long-term potentiation/depression.

Interpreting the Data

On sample traces, time is on the x-axis, typically milliseconds to tens of milliseconds (ms). A millisecond or two is usually established as the baseline measurement before delivery of the stimulation. Then, the moment the stimulation is delivered will be identified.

A **stimulation artifact** may also be observed at this moment. These artifacts are produced by the electrical components that are used to deliver the stimulus. They are often the largest event in the trace, with a very sharp appearance. Because stimulation artifacts are not biological in nature, they can be safely ignored.

Following the stimulation, there is often a 1–3 ms delay before the onset of the event of interest. This delay represents the time needed for the depolarization of the axon terminal, entry of presynaptic calcium, vesicle fusion, release of neurotransmitter, diffusion across the synapse, and postsynaptic receptor binding. Finally, the sample trace should extend long enough until the event decays and returns to baseline.

For measurements of potentials, slope or peak amplitude (voltage) is on the *y*-axis. When peak amplitude is measured, it is generally on the order of tenths of millivolts or millivolts (mV). In fEPSP recordings, slope is a more accurate measurement than peak amplitude, since it represents the effect of only the first synaptic event, while the peak amplitude could be the result of many synapses activated sequentially, thereby diluting the effect of the first excitatory connection. The slope of these events is usually measured in mV/ms and is usually between 0 and 1. In intracellular recordings or in patch clamp, excitatory events are upward deflections from baseline (depolarization). In extracellular recordings, such as in an fEPSP, the event may be a negative deflection, since this recording detects the movement of positive charges going away from the electrode and into neurons during an excitatory event.

In measuring currents, peak amplitude is on the *y*-axis. Typically, peak current is on the order of tens of picoamps (pA) to nanoamps (nA). The modern convention shows inward currents, the movement of positive charges into the neuron, as downward or negative deflections from baseline. On the other hand, outward currents, the movement of positive charges out of the neuron, are depicted as upward or positive deflections. Therefore, eEPSCs are downward, while eIPSCs are upward.

Instead of using a single stimulation intensity and comparing the response between experimental conditions, some experiments may use a range of intensities and observe the different responses. These are called **input/output curves**, and they show the relationship between stimulation intensity (input) and postsynaptic response (output). Representative traces are similar to that of a single stimulation, but there may be multiple traces overlaid on the same image.

In a group average graph of input/output curves, stimulation intensity is plotted along the *x*-axis. When electrical stimulation is used, these units are usually in tenths of milliamps (mA), but with optogenetic stimulation, units may be in luminance in milliwatts (mW) or lumens. The response, either slope or peak amplitude, is plotted on the *y*-axis. An upward-shifted curve indicates increased signaling across that synapse or connection, while a downward-shifted curve indicates decreased signaling. Input/output curves may be analyzed using a linear regression analysis to calculate the slope. Groups with a greater positive slope are more excitable. (Input/output curves can also be generated with action potentials as the measured output instead of a synaptic response.)

Figure 6.12 represents evoked EPSC amplitudes measured under voltage clamp in response to progressively stronger electrical stimulations. Researchers were curious

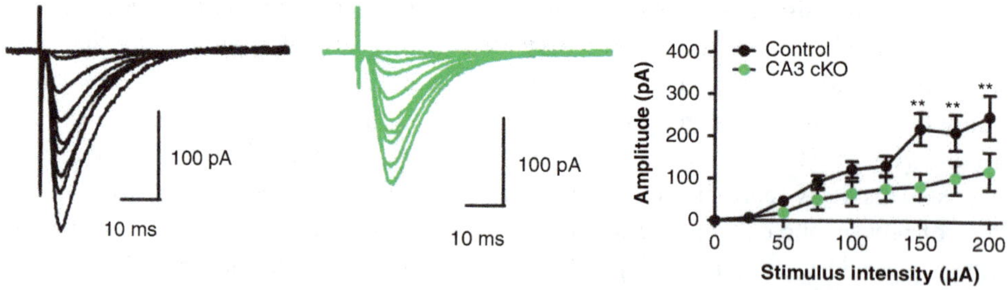

Figure 6.12 Results of an evoked EPSC experiment. Source: Glasgow SD, Wong EW, Thompson-Steckel G, et al. Pre- and post-synaptic roles for DCC in memory consolidation in the adult mouse hippocampus. *Mol Brain.* 2020 Apr 7; 13(1):56. DOI: 10.1186/s13041-020-00597-2. PMID: 32264905; PMCID: PMC7137442. http://creativecommons.org/licenses/by/4.0/. Images have been rearranged and text labels removed.

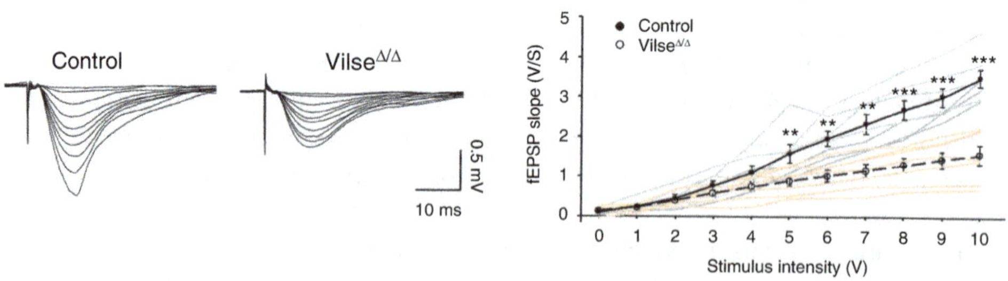

Figure 6.13 Results of an fEPSP experiment. Source: Lee JY, Lee LJ, Fan CC, et al. Important roles of Vilse in dendritic architecture and synaptic plasticity. *Sci Rep.* 2017; 7:45646. http://creativecommons.org/licenses/by/4.0/. Text labels removed.

about the role of the DCC protein in synaptic strength of the hippocampus, so they compared cells from wild type mice (black, Control) with a knockout mouse (green, CA3 cKO) that can have the protein knocked out conditionally. On the left, representative traces show overlays of several EPSCs from two animal models. The data of relevance are the slow downward curve; the sharp upward and downward spike near the beginning is a stimulation artifact. On the right is an input/output curve summarizing group data. The researchers' data show that the amplitude of the evoked EPSC is smaller in the CA3 KO animals at higher stimulus intensities, suggesting that, when the DCC gene is removed, synaptic communication is weakened.

Figure 6.13 represents an fEPSP experiment. Researchers identified a protein called Vilse and were curious about its role in hippocampal plasticity, so they developed knockout mice (Vilse $^{\Delta/\Delta}$). Then, they took *ex vivo* brain slices to perform extracellular field recordings. On the left are representative traces showing responses after progressively larger stimulations. The sharp spike is a stimulation artifact. Note that here, downward deflections indicate excitatory currents since the electrode is placed in the extracellular space. On the right, a summary of group data is represented as an input–output curve. Regardless of phenotype, higher stimulation intensities cause a greater fEPSP slope. At higher stimulation intensities, Vilse knockout mice (white circles, dashed line) had a lower fEPSP slope compared to control mice (black circles, solid lines). Individual recordings are shown by the faint lines (orange for Vilse knockouts, gray for control).

As with spontaneous events, the kinetics of evoked events, including the rising phase, decay phase, and tau, may also be analyzed and reported (keep in mind that, even if the deflection is negative-going, as in an fEPSP recording or recording inward currents, the first portion of the event is still called the rising phase). A steeper rising phase (greater slope) may indicate a greater number of axonal fibers being activated, greater release of neurotransmitter, or increased number or function of postsynaptic receptors. Increases in the speed of the decay phase, which is related to tau, could indicate an increase in neurotransmitter clearance from the synapse.

Typically, the kinetics of the rising and decay phases are fitted by exponential formulas. In comparing kinetics, the event peaks may be normalized so that they have the same amplitude. The rising phase will always have faster kinetics than the decay phase, since the release events are synchronized over several axons, while the clearance of neurotransmitter is not.

6.4.3 Paired Pulse Ratio (PPR)

Background Information

A paired pulse ratio (PPR) is a measurement of the probability of neurotransmitter release at a synapse. It is done by delivering two evoked stimulations of the same intensity separated by tens of milliseconds to hundreds of milliseconds while recording the postsynaptic current. The PPR is calculated by dividing the amplitude of the second event (P2) by the amplitude of the first event (P1). PPR is unitless.

The time delay between the two pulses is the **paired pulse interval** (**PPI**, abbreviated as Δt; not to be confused with prepulse inhibition, a behavioral test). The PPR is generally done in the whole cell voltage clamp configuration.

Typically, only the PPR of synapses with ionotropic receptors can be assessed, so many PPR studies look at glutamate (EPSC) or GABA (IPSC) release.

Reading the Graphs

Sample traces generally show inward currents. As with evoked events, the *x*-axis plots time and the *y*-axis plots current. There will be two large stimulation artifacts, which tell us about when the stimuli were delivered, allowing for calculation of the PPI. The amplitude of the artifacts can be ignored.

Since PPR is done at several PPIs, these sample traces may also be shown. They may be arranged in order of ascending paired pulse intervals or may all be overlaid on a single trace. Overlays of multiple sample traces should also display the moments of stimulation, generally indicated above the traces.

The group average graph displays PPRs across increasing intervals. The duration of the paired pulse interval is plotted on the *x*-axis and the PPR on the *y*-axis. Since values of PPR are greater than or less than 1, the intersection of the x-axis corresponds to a PPR of 1, indicating there is no difference between the amplitudes of P1 and P2.

Figure 6.14 presents results from a PPR experiment showing changes in release probability dependent on receptor expression. Three different mouse populations were used: wild type controls (black), a conditional double knockout of the BMP receptor types 1a and 1b (red), and a single knockout of 1b (blue). The left three images show representative traces from the three genotypes. The top traces show the action potential evoked presynaptically with a 20 ms PPI. The middle sample traces show overlays of several eIPSCs. Note here that the experimenters used a high-chloride internal solution, so chloride currents appear as inward currents (downward deflections). The bottom traces show the average of those eIPSCs. The dotted line indicates the amplitude of P1, which allows for a visualization of whether P2 is larger. On the right is a bar graph summarizing group data. The researchers report that cells from the double knockout mice (red) show a decrease in PPR compared to the control, suggesting an increase in release probability inhibitory synapses. X represents individual data points.

Interpreting the Data

When comparing between groups, differences in PPR suggest that the presynaptic component has changed since PPR depends on the probability of vesicle release more than receptor changes. Changes to PPR are a form of short-term plasticity at the presynaptic axon terminals.

Presynaptic vesicles can be divided into different pools. Those that are docked on the intracellular surface are called the readily releasable pool (RRP) and are the first to be exocytosed upon stimulation. When the two stimulations are close to one another in time, there may be a depletion of these vesicles after the first stimulation, so the event from the second stimulation will be smaller. This is called **paired pulse depression**, and the PPR will be smaller than 1.

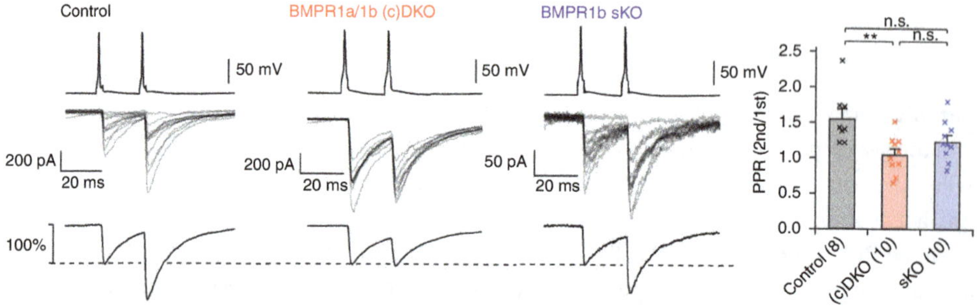

Figure 6.14 Results of a PPR experiment. Source: Vickers E, Osypenko D, Clark C, et al. LTP of inhibition at PV interneuron output synapses requires developmental BMP signaling. *Sci Rep.* 2020; 10(10047). https://doi.org/10.1038/s41598-020-66862-5. http://creativecommons.org/licenses/by/4.0/. Image cropped, panels reorganized, text labels removed.

Vesicle fusion depends on intracellular calcium concentration. At longer time intervals, there may be an accumulation of calcium following the first stimulation, so the second release event will be enhanced and the event from the second stimulation will be larger. This is **paired pulse facilitation**, and the PPR is greater than 1 in these cases. At very long time intervals approaching a second, the effect of the first stimulation will have no influence on the amplitude of the second event, so the two events will be the same amplitude and the PPR will be 1.

Additional Resources

Regehr WG. Short-term presynaptic plasticity. *Cold Spring Harb Perspect Biol.* 2012 Jul 1; 4(7):a005702. DOI: 10.1101/cshperspect.a005702. PMID: 22751149; PMCID: PMC3385958.

6.4.4 Long-Term Potentiation (LTP)/Depression (LTD)

Background Information

Long-term potentiation (LTP) and long-term depression (LTD) are forms of plasticity, a cellular correlate of learning and memory. LTP and LTD are assessed by evoking neurotransmitter release several times while observing the postsynaptic response. Then, an experimental manipulation called an **induction protocol** is delivered to the preparation. Afterwards, if there is a long-lasting (tens of minutes or longer) increase in synaptic strength, the protocol produced **long-term potentiation**. If there is a weakening, this is called **long-term depression**. LTP and LTD are usually attributed to glutamatergic synapses.

One of the classic LTP induction protocols is **high-frequency stimulation** (**HFS**) of nerve fibers using electrical or optogenetic stimulation. Such examples of HFS paradigms include **tetanic stimulation**, which is 100 stimulations at 100 Hz for 1 second in duration. A **theta burst stimulation** is less intense, consisting of multiple bursts, each 3 stimulations at 100 Hz, totaling 30 ms. Each burst is repeated at a frequency of 5 Hz, totaling 15 stimulations over the course of 1 second. The theta burst firing pattern mimics the natural changes in firing when an animal is exploring its surroundings. LTP can also be induced chemically. For example, treatment with a high Ca and low Mg CSF with tetraethylammonium induces hippocampal LTP in rats.

The evoked events are quantified as described in Section 6.4.2. Usually, LTP and LTD are done in order to look at evoked excitatory postsynaptic potentials (eEPSPs), but other measures (such as eIPSP, eEPSC, or eIPSC) can be sensitive to these plasticity phenomena. LTP and LTD can be observed in whole cell recordings, field potentials, or *in vivo* preparations.

Reading the Figures

Sample traces may be presented or overlaid on top of the time course graph. In interpreting traces, the direction of the evoked event is less important than the slope or peak amplitude, since experimental manipulations can cause eIPSCs to appear as inward currents, for example. Sample traces may appear directly on top of one another, using different colors to indicate pre- and post-LTP/LTD induction. If the events have a steeper slope or larger amplitude after the manipulation, then LTP was observed; if smaller, then LTD was observed. If the events look similar in amplitude, then neither form of plasticity was observed, or the plasticity was otherwise impaired.

In average graphs of time course, the *x*-axis shows time, usually plotted in tens of minutes. Each data point represents the response (slope or peak amplitude) following a stimulation event, which may be delivered at a low frequency (once every 20 seconds to 1 minute). Negative time, often between −5 and −30 to 0 minutes, represents the baseline for which the slopes or amplitudes of the synaptic events after the induction protocol will be compared. Time 0 represents the onset of the induction protocol, such as when the HFS paradigm is first delivered, and may be indicated with a symbol. LTP may be expected to persist for an hour or longer, so usually data points up to 60 minutes beyond the onset of the manipulation will be plotted.

The *y*-axis plots the slope or the amplitude of the evoked event as a percentage of the baseline slope or amplitude. The average event during the baseline period is the normalization factor; data points at negative time on the *x*-axis will average to 100%. Some LTP experiments may see effects as large as a 250% increase over baseline, and LTD may see decreases down to nearly 0%. If the *y*-axis values to the right of the manipulation are greater than 100%, then LTP was observed; if less than 100%, then LTD was observed. If the *y*-values remain at 100%, then no LTP or LTD was observed, or the plasticity phenomenon was otherwise blocked.

Alternatively, the *y*-axis may plot % potentiation. In these plots, the normalization factor has been set to 0. Values greater than 0 indicate LTP, while values less than 0 indicate LTD.

Figure 6.15 represents an LTP experiment. Electrically evoked EPSPs following a high-frequency stimulation (HFS) show LTP (black, control). Exposure to either chemical LET (blue) or ICI (red) block LTP, a reversal of effect. At the top are representative traces showing evoked EPSPs, which produce an upward deflection. The dotted trace shows the EPSP before HFS, while the solid trace shows the EPSP after HFS. In the control condition, the solid traces have a larger amplitude compared to the dotted traces, which is characteristic of LTP. The solid and dotted traces are similar when LET or ICI is present, showing a blockade of LTP. At the bottom is the time course of EPSPs over the course of 40 minutes of recording. Delivering the HFS at time 0 under control conditions results in an LTP lasting at least 30 minutes. That LTP is occluded in the presence of LET (blue) or ICI (red).

Figure 6.16 represents an LTD experiment. At the top is a summary of group data showing evoked IPSC amplitudes before and after a theta burst stimulation (TBS). The TBS delivered at time 6 minutes produced a long-term depression that persisted for at least 20 minutes. At the bottom are representative traces showing the IPSC amplitude before TBS (black) and after TBS (red).

Interpreting the Data

There are many potential cellular and molecular mechanisms that can explain LTP at a synapse after a high-frequency stimulation induction protocol. The classical LTP mechanism is a multi-step cascade: HFS causes massive glutamate release, activating AMPA

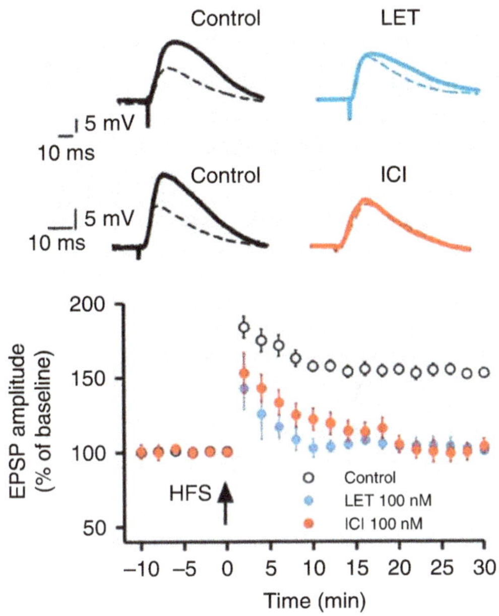

Figure 6.15 Results of an LTP experiment. Source: Tozzi A, de Iure A, Tantucci M, et al. Endogenous 17β-estradiol is required for activity-dependent long-term potentiation in the striatum: Interaction with the dopaminergic system. *Front Cell Neurosci.* 2015; 9:192. http://creativecommons.org/licenses/by/4.0/. Image cropped.

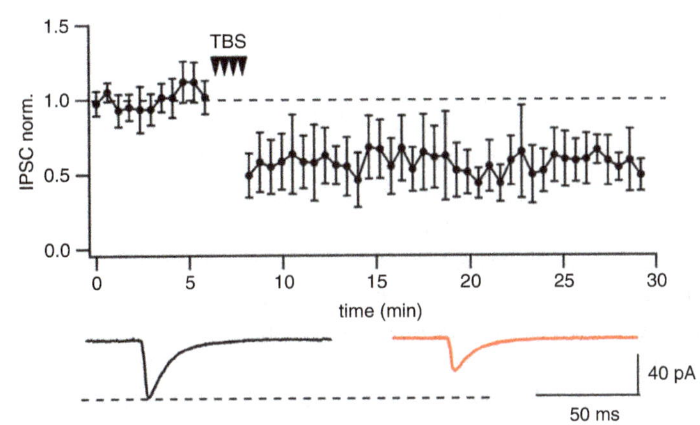

Figure 6.16 Results of an LTD experiment. Source: Jappy D, Valiullina F, Draguhn A, Rozov A. GABABR-dependent long-term depression at hippocampal synapses between CB1-positive interneurons and CA1 pyramidal cells. *Front Cell Neurosci.* 2016; 10:4. http://creativecommons.org/licenses/by/4.0/. Image cropped, text labels and dashed lines removed.

receptors, causing postsynaptic depolarization which expels a Mg^{2+} ion block at the NMDA receptor, allowing Ca^{2+} entry and activation of the enzyme CaMKII. CaMKII can then increase the number of AMPA receptors on the postsynaptic membrane and can make the AMPA receptor pass more current.

An opposing process has been offered to explain LTD. Under some circumstances, Ca^{2+} influx increases activity of the enzyme PP1, which leads to internalization of AMPA receptors, which can no longer be activated by synaptic glutamate.

Additional Resources

Citri A, Malenka R. Synaptic plasticity: Multiple forms, functions, and mechanisms. *Neuropsychopharmacol.* 2008; 33:18–41. https://doi.org/10.1038/sj.npp.1301559.

Collingridge GL, Abraham WC. Glutamate receptors and synaptic plasticity: The impact of Evans and Watkins. *Neuropharmacol.* 2022; 206:108922. doi:10.1016/j.neuropharm.2021.108922.

Lisman J, Yasuda R, Raghavachari S. Mechanisms of CaMKII action in long-term potentiation. *Nat Rev Neurosci.* 2012; 13:169–182. https://doi.org/10.1038/nrn3192.

6.4.5 Spike Timing Dependent Plasticity (STDP)

Background Information

Spike timing dependent plasticity (STDP) is a form of short-term plasticity that is dependent on the timing of a presynaptic action potential compared to a postsynaptic action potential. In the STDP literature, the words "pre" and "post" describe the physical spatial relationship to the synapse, not a time: pre usually refers to the axon terminals, while post usually refers to the dendrites or somata.

In classical STDP (also called **Hebbian STDP**), a presynaptic action potential followed shortly (within ~20 ms) by a postsynaptic action potential results in potentiation (**spike timing-dependent LTP**, or **t-LTP**) of the excitatory postsynaptic potential (EPSP) or current (EPSC). By contrast, when the postsynaptic event precedes (by ~20 ms) the presynaptic event, a depression (**t-LTD**) of the synapse is observed.

Another form of STDP is **anti-Hebbian**, which shows plasticity in the opposite direction: pre-before-post produces an t-LTD, while post-before-pre produces t-LTP.

STDP experiments can be done in a whole cell recording configuration. This observation has been observed in *in vivo* preparations, acute *ex vivo* slices, and *in vitro* cultures. However, it is controversial whether STDP is relevant *in vivo*, since high levels of spontaneous neuronal activity may block STDP.

Figure 6.17 presents results from an experiment showing classical STDP in extracellular recordings. Individual data points are shown by circles which have been fitted by two curves. Negative spike timings are post-before-pre stimulations. At long negative spike timings, there is no significant change in EPSP slope. As the two events get closer together in time (closer to 0), EPSP slopes decrease from 100%, suggesting t-LTD. Positive spike

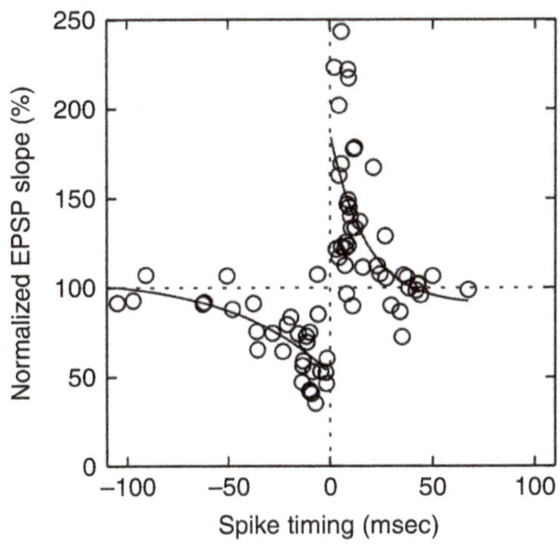

Figure 6.17 Results of an STDP experiment. Source: Froemke RC, Debanne D, Bi G-Q. Temporal modulation of spike-timing-dependent plasticity. *Front Syn Neurosci.* 2010; 2:19. Image cropped and sample stimulations removed.

timings are when the stimulation is pre-before-post. At short intervals, a strong t-LTP is observed. Then, as the delay between stimulations increases, t-LTP is no longer observed.

Reading the Graphs

Sample traces will likely show both the stimulation (with presynaptic versus postsynaptic being labeled) and the response. Other values may be reported, including:

- N, the number of pairings, which may be up to hundreds.
- **Δt** (pronounced "delta t"; also interevent interval), which is the time between the pre- and post- action potentials. Usually, Δt ranges to the hundreds of milliseconds with the strongest effect on the order of tens of milliseconds.
- Frequency in Hz, which provides information about how much time separates each pairing of stimulations.

Some graphs of STDP can be read like a standard LTP/LTD plot. The graph may show the persistence of the plasticity over the course of several minutes up to hundreds of minutes, with time on the x-axis and a measure of plasticity on the y-axis, such as EPSP slope. These graphs may show negative time prior to the onset of the induction protocol, which serves as the within-synapse control and the baseline with which to compare plasticity after induction. The duration of the induction protocol is often longer than that of other LTP measures, sometimes lasting 10 minutes. During this time, since the postsynaptic component is activated artificially, events cannot be measured so no data are plotted.

Other graphs serve to more completely describe the observed parameters that lead to STDP. In these summary graphs, the pre-post spike delay is plotted on the x-axis, representing the time between the presynaptic and postsynaptic event (Δt). These intervals are typically on the order of tens of milliseconds. This graph will have both positive and negative values with the *y*-axis crossing at the 0 time point. Usually, positive pre-post spike delay means the presynaptic event precedes the postsynaptic event, while negative *x*-values means the postsynaptic event precedes the presynaptic event.

A measure of plasticity is plotted on the *y*-axis, which might include % change in EPSC amplitude or EPSP slope. If STDP is observed, shorter time intervals between the pre and post will have nonzero values on the *y*-axis. Hebbian STDP will show LTD (negative *y*-axis) to the left of the 0 and LTP (positive *y*-axis) to the right; anti-Hebbian STDP will flip these results. At longer time elapsed between the pre-post stimuli, no plasticity is observed, and data points will hover around the *x*-axis. Individual data points may be fitted with two separate curves, one for data points to the left of the *y*-axis and one with data points to the right of the *y*-axis.

These data may also be shown as group averages, taking the values of some predetermined time window (usually tens of minutes, or when the plasticity measure reaches a plateau) after the induction protocol.

Figure 6.18 illustrates a description of a synapse that follows anti-Hebbian STDP. Panels A1 and A2 represent the stimulation paradigm being delivered to the presynaptic and postsynaptic cells (top) and a representative current clamp trace (below). A1 shows a post-before-pre stimulation. Here, the representative trace shows a large action potential spike happening at the same time as the post stimulation and a small artifact at the same time as the pre stimulation. A2 shows the pre-before-post paradigm. As in

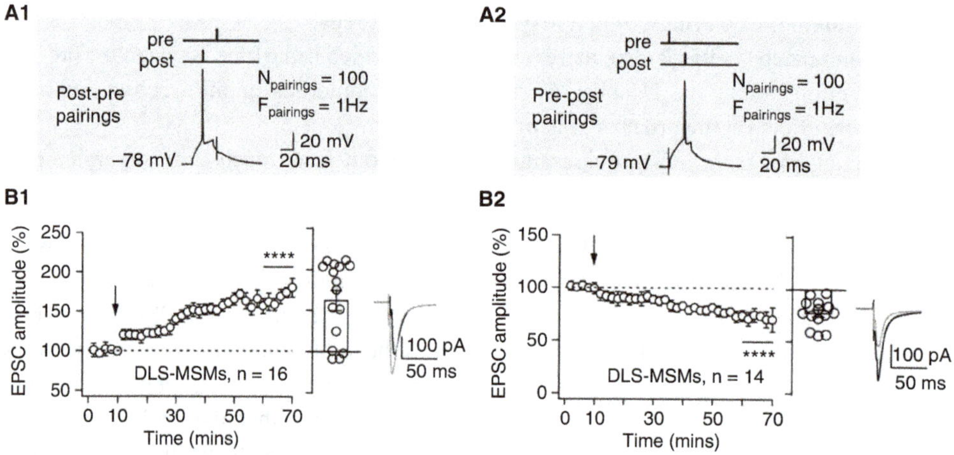

Figure 6.18 Results of another STDP experiment. Source: Perez S, Cui Y, Vignoud G, et al. Striatum expresses region-specific plasticity consistent with distinct memory abilities. *Cell Rep.* 2022 Mar 15; 38(11):110521. DOI: 10.1016/j.celrep.2022.110521. PMID: 35294877. http://creativecommons.org/licenses/by/4.0/. Image cropped and panels relabeled.

the representative trace in A1, the large spike correlates with the post stimulation and the small artifact corresponds with the pre stimulation. Panels B1 and B2 show group time course summary data of the plasticity paradigm over the course of 70 minutes. In B1, the data report that post-before-pre produces an LTP, while B2 shows that pre-before-post produces LTD. The bar graphs show group median with error bar along with circles to represent individual data points, sharing the same *y*-axis as the time course graph. Finally, the representative traces show the EPSC before the stimulation paradigm (black) and after (gray).

Interpreting the Data

Postsynaptic calcium entry is a key element of STDP. In classical Hebbian STDP with pre-before-post timing, presynaptic neurotransmitter release causes the EPSP, leading to calcium entry and subsequent LTP expression. On the other hand, in post-before-pre timing, the action potential travels from the soma retrogradely toward the dendrites (**back propagating AP**, or **bAP**), leading to calcium entry before neurotransmitter release, which may account for LTD.

Many other shapes of the STDP graph are possible, including depression only or potentiation only, regardless of pre-post or post-pre timing.

Additional Resources

Feldman DE. The spike-timing dependence of plasticity. *Neuron*. 2012 Aug 23; 75(4):556–71. DOI: 10.1016/j.neuron.2012.08.001. PMID: 22920249; PMCID: PMC3431193.

6.5 Current-Voltage Relationship (I-V Plots)

Background Information

A current-voltage relationship plot informs about the amount of current (I) that passes across the neuronal membrane under different membrane voltages (V). It can be used to show the gating properties of single ion channels. The ion of interest will be denoted as subscript after the letter I: I_{Na} refers to sodium current, I_K to potassium current, and so on. The I-V plot can also demonstrate the influence of specific neurotransmitters or different receptor populations. Here, an abbreviation may be in subscript after the letter I: for example, I_{Glu} might be used to describe the current resulting from glutamate, or I_{AMPA} to describe current through the AMPA receptor.

A typical recording protocol clamps the cell at a holding potential close to the cell's resting membrane potential, followed by three voltage steps per sweep:

1. A hyperpolarizing step, maybe as negative as −120 mV. This serves as a "reset", deactivating as many voltage-gated channels as possible and allowing them to be opened

on the next depolarizing step. This value is unchanged between sweeps and can be maintained for tens to hundreds of ms.

2. A depolarizing step is the experimental step when peak current amplitude is measured and analyzed. This value is changed between sweeps, and each sweep may increase the amount of depolarization by 20 mV intervals. This depolarization may be maintained for 100 ms.
3. A step to return to the holding potential.

A delay of seconds between sweeps is common.

I-V plots are generated in voltage clamp using whole cell, inside-out, and outside-out patch clamp, or intracellular recording configurations. These experiments can be performed in cultured cells or in Xenopus oocytes, which may be modified to express a much higher density of receptors than in the natural condition.

Reading the Graphs

Sometimes, stimulation paradigms are plotted. These show time on the *x*-axis in milliseconds up to minutes, and changes in holding potential on the *y*-axis in millivolts.

Sample traces of observations often share the x-axis scale but will plot current on the *y*-axis. In whole cell recordings, several sample traces are often overlaid on top of each other. These traces are often curves, but only the plateau current after several milliseconds is recorded for each voltage step.

In excised patch preparation examining single ion channels, sample traces will have a boxy, step-like shape, since ion channels can either pass current (open state) or not (closed, inactivated, or desensitized states). Many sample traces will show observed current when the membrane is held at different potentials. The amplitude of the current ("height of the step") may vary depending on the ion channel properties. Information about ion channel state transitions (closed to open, for example) are not considered when collecting information for I-V relationships.

The data from several traces are summarized on the I-V plot. These graphs plot voltage along the *x*-axis. The range of voltage values may run from −80 mV to +80 mV (strong depolarizing voltages may damage the cell). Peak or plateau current observed at each voltage step is plotted on the *y*-axis. Current is measured in amps, usually on the order of tens of picoamps to nanoamps, although cultured cells often produce larger currents on the order of microamps.

A closely related *y*-axis measurement is current density, which normalizes against cell membrane capacitance and has units of pA/pF (picofarad).

Alternatively, the *y*-axis may also plot **conductance** (abbreviated G_m), which is a measure of amperes passed for each volt applied to the membrane. Conductance has units of siemens (S) and is always positive. These values may also be normalized to maximum conductance, in which case they are plotted as G_m /Gmax.

Figure 6.19 illustrates a current-voltage relationship in HEK cells transfected with sodium leak channels. In panel A, representative traces show current in response to

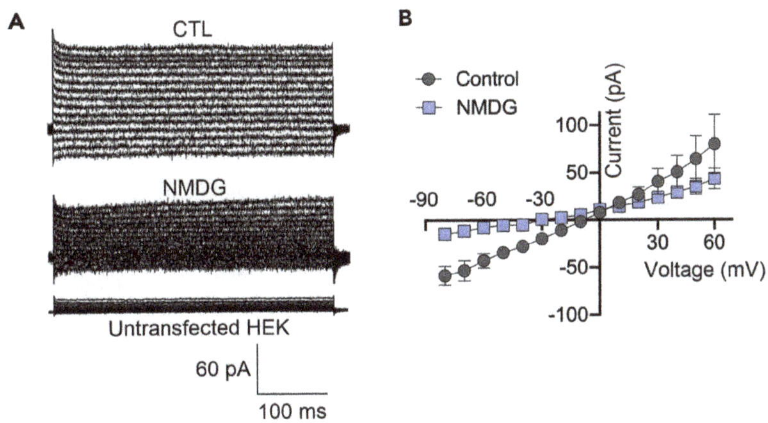

Figure 6.19 Results of a current-voltage relationship. Source: Ou M, Zhao W, Liu J, et al. The general anesthetic isoflurane bilaterally modulates neuronal excitability. *iScience*. 2020 Jan 24; 23(1):100760. DOI: 10.1016/j.isci.2019.100760. Epub 2019 Dec 10. PMID: 31926429; PMCID: PMC6956953. http://creative commons.org/licenses/by/4.0/. Image cropped.

a series of hyperpolarizing and depolarizing steps. The control cells (CTL) show that current passes both inwards and outwards. When the sodium has been replaced with NMDG, less current passes. The untransfected HEK is a negative control, and no current is expected to pass because these cells do not express sodium channels. In panel B, the I–V plot of group data shows that, across a range of voltages, less current is passed in both inward and outward direction when NMDG replaces sodium (purple squares).

Interpreting the Data

I-V plots are useful for showing a phenomenon called **rectification**. Rectifying channels are those that pass more current at certain potentials than others. Their I-V plots are not symmetrical from left to right.

An **inwardly rectifying channel** passes more inward current than outward and has been well described among many classes of potassium channels. At positive potentials, intracellular molecules with positive charge may block the channels from the intracellular side, leading to decreased outward current. On an I-V plot, inwardly rectifying channels have large values on the left and small values on the right.

An **outwardly rectifying channel** passes more outward current than inward. These channels can be identified on an I-V plot by the small values on the left and large values on the right. An example of an outwardly rectifying channel is voltage-gated potassium channels that open after the action potential, passing outward current to depolarize the cell.

The I-V diagram of the NMDA type glutamate receptor has a distinctive shape. At very negative potentials, the channels do not pass current because of pore blockade by extracellular Mg^{2+} ions. As voltage increases, current begins to pass through the channel as Mg^{2+} ions are

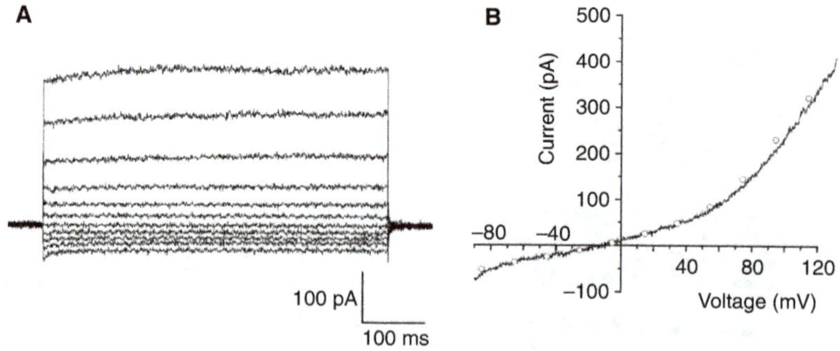

Figure 6.20 Results of another current-voltage relationship. Source: Jiang X, Newell EW, Schlichter LC. Regulation of a TRPM7-like current in rat brain microglia. *J Biol Chem*. 2003 Oct 31; 278(44):42867–42876. DOI: 10.1074/jbc.M304487200. Epub 2003 Aug 6. PMID: 12904301. http://creativecommons.org/licenses/by/4.0/. Image cropped and text labels removed.

repelled by the positive potential of the membrane. At positive potentials, the Mg^{2+} block is completely relieved, and outward current is passed linearly proportional to voltage.

Figure 6.20 shows an outwardly rectifying cation channel from cultured microglia. Panel A shows representative traces in response to equally spaced 20 mV steps. Hyperpolarizing voltage steps produce a small inward current (downward deflections), but depolarizing voltage steps produce large outward currents (upward deflections), which suggests the channel of interest is outwardly rectifying. Panel B shows an I-V plot which summarizes the data from the cell recorded from in Panel A.

Additional Resources

Nowak L, Bregestovski P, Ascher P, Herbet A, Prochiantz A. Magnesium gates glutamate-activated channels in mouse central neurones. *Nature*. 1984 Feb 2–8; 307 (5950):462–465. DOI: 10.1038/307462a0. PMID: 6320006.

6.6 Electrochemistry

Background Information

In neuroscience, electrochemistry is used to measure regional changes in the levels of certain neurotransmitters. Electrochemistry relies on understanding the chemical properties of neurotransmitters, particularly the voltages necessary for the molecule to undergo **oxidation** and **reduction**, which produce electrical currents that can be detected.

A thin carbon fiber microelectrode (CFME, or just CFE) is typically made by the experimenter. These are usually made of glass forming a tight seal encasing the carbon fiber. The electrode is placed directly into the region of interest extracellularly. Carbon fiber is a potent conductor, so changes in voltage can be applied to the electrode. In addition to the carbon fiber electrode, a **ground electrode** is placed in the bath. This is what the voltage application is compared with. A silver-plated or silver-chloride-plated (Ag/AgCl) reference electrode is the most common.

Electrochemistry is very limited as to which neurotransmitters can be measured. Table 6.1 lists electrochemically sensitive neurotransmitters and their characteristics.

A similar technique is microdialysis, which answers the same types of questions ("Are there changes in neurotransmitter levels in a brain area?"). Electrochemistry, however, offers two distinct advantages.

1. Superior temporal resolution on the order of tens of milliseconds (ms), compared to seconds with microdialysis.
2. A smaller probe, and therefore less damage to the tissue with a lessened inflammatory response. FSCV electrodes can be as small as 7 microns (μm) in diameter, compared to the microdialysis probe which might be hundreds of microns in diameter.

However, electrochemistry cannot give an accurate reading of baseline neurotransmitter levels, only changes in release under different conditions. For accurately measuring the concentration of a neurotransmitter and for measuring nonelectroactive neurotransmitter levels such as glutamate and GABA, microdialysis is more appropriate.

Electrochemistry is often done in *ex vivo* acute tissue preparations and in behaving *in vivo* preparations. In the *ex vivo* preparation, neurotransmitter release is usually evoked by a separate stimulating electrode placed or optogenetic activation of the area upstream of the carbon fiber. In the behaving *in vivo* preparation, neurotransmitter release happens in a more naturalistic setting, such as when presenting the animal with reward-related cues or a painful stimulus. Common animal models for electrochemistry include rats and mice, but it has been done in humans and primates, as well as in zebrafish and drosophila.

Table 6.1 Types of electrochemically sensitive neurotransmitters

Neurotransmitter	Oxidation potential(s)	Reduction potential	Oxidative byproduct
Dopamine	+0.6 V	−0.1 V	Dopamine-o-quinone (DOQ)
Serotonin	+0.5 V	−0.2 V	4,5-diketotryptamine (4,5-DKT)
Norepinephrine	+0.67 V	−0.2 V	Norepinephrine-o-quinone
Adenosine	+1.4 V (big peak), +1 V (little peak)		
Histamine	+ 0.8 V		

6.6.1 Fast Scan Cyclic Voltammetry (FSCV)

Background Information

Fast scan cyclic voltammetry (FSCV) is an extension of an analytic chemistry method called cyclic voltammetry, but on a time scale that is orders of magnitude faster: traditional cyclic voltammetry offers temporal resolution on the order of 20 seconds, while fast scan cyclic voltammetry measures currents on the order of hundreds of milliseconds.

In FSCV, a ramping change in voltage from negative potentials to positive and then back down is applied to the electrode. The peak positive voltage is called the **switching potential**, since it represents the potential where the voltage ramp switches direction. The voltage change causes molecules of neurotransmitter in the region to oxidize and reduce, producing a current that can be measured by the electrode. The amplitude of this current is linearly proportional to the number of molecules in that region. Finally, an estimation of the concentration of the molecule may be made by doing a calibration against the current produced by known concentrations of that molecule.

Reading the Graphs

The applied voltage ramp may be illustrated in a figure alongside the results. These graphs will have straight lines, since they are not measurements and have no biological noise. In diagrams showing the ramp protocol, time is on the *x*-axis, usually in hundreds of milliseconds. The time between ramps gives information about the sampling rate: 10 hertz (10 Hz; 10 times per second) is a common sampling rate.

Voltage delivered to the carbon fiber electrode is plotted on the *y*-axis. Ramping protocols vary depending on the neurochemical of interest. The speed (slope) of the ramp is also listed, usually measured in volts per second. Because these ramp protocols can be described meaningfully in text, they may instead be written in the methods section of the research reporting.

Representative data collected using FSCV are usually presented as a cyclic voltammogram or a pseudocolor plot.

In a **cyclic voltammogram**, the *x*-axis shows voltage applied to the CFE, with the potential at the start of the ramp at the far left and the switching potential on the far right. These units will be in volts (V), and common ranges may run from −0.6 V to 1.4 V. The *y*-axis plots current recorded, typically in nanoamps (nA). These graphs produce a loop, since the ramp increases and decreases in potential. In order of increasing time, the loop can be read from the bottom left to right, then at the switching potential, upward and to the left.

Sometimes, graphs of total current may be shown, which have the appearance of a large loop. There will be two traces overlaid on each other in these graphs, one representing current at baseline and one after the experimental condition.

However, the absolute value of the current does not carry much meaning, since the resultant current depends on the surface area of the electrode (larger electrodes = larger current). To eliminate this variable, cyclic voltammograms may show subtracted results: the

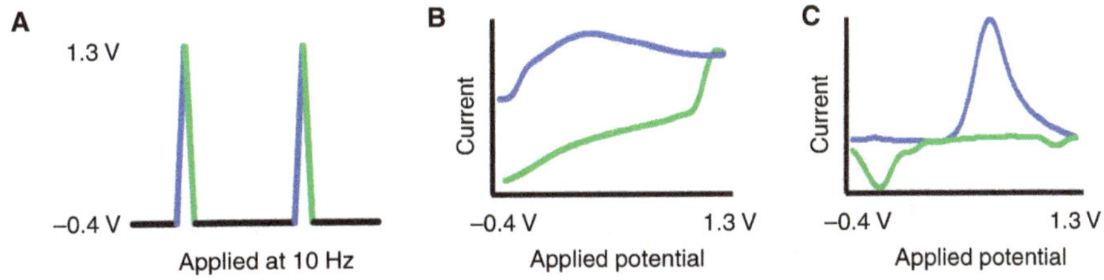

Figure 6.21 Example traces of an FSCV experiment. Source: Robinson DL, Zitzman DL, Williams SK. Mesolimbic dopamine transients in motivated behaviors: Focus on maternal behavior. *Front Psychiatry.* 2011; 2:23. http://creativecommons.org/licenses/by/4.0/. Image cropped.

current produced by the experimental condition minus the baseline current. These are more often small loops with bumps at the oxidation and reduction potentials.

Figure 6.21 represents an FSCV experiment. In panel A, an example triangle waveform protocol is applied to the electrode to measure extracellular dopamine. Here, it ramps up from −0.4 V to 1.3 V (blue) and back down (green) at 400 V/s 10 times a second. Panel B is the cyclic voltammogram showing the total current that is observed after a single sweep. The blue shows the changes in current during the ascending part of the triangle waveform and the green shows current changes during the descending part. Panel C shows a background subtracted voltammogram. In these traces, only differences in current relevant to the manipulation appear as peaks. The blue represents the oxidation peak and the green represents the reduction peak.

Pseudocolor plots can also be used to illustrate currents detected by FSCV. On the x-axis is time on the scale of seconds or tens of seconds, which represents hundreds of voltage ramp applications. Negative time may be shown, which represents the baseline before some behavior or a manipulation. The onset of the behavior or manipulation may otherwise be noted by an arrow or a horizontal bar.

The y-axis plots the voltage applied to the electrode in V, from the negative most potential at the top, the switching potential in the middle, and back down the ramp at the bottom.

The current produced by neurotransmitter oxidation and reduction are shown as color changes. The color schemes used here are arbitrary and sometimes unintuitive, but a commonly used spectrum is dark yellowish orange to blues and greens.

Figure 6.22 shows a pseudocolor plot from an *in vivo* FSCV experiment measuring dopamine release under three conditions. The x-axis represents time in seconds. The small black bar at the bottom left of each plot indicates duration of stimulation of upstream neural circuits. Baseline dopamine release (left) resulted in the same amplitude current as when saline was injected (middle image), which is shown by the same color pattern on the plot. When cocaine is injected, dopamine release produced a larger current (right image; more greens at the oxidation peak and more blues at the reduction peak), supporting the idea that cocaine increases extracellular dopamine.

Alternatively, data collected from the FSCV may simply be presented in group averages as peak concentration, denoted by square brackets. For example, the concentration of

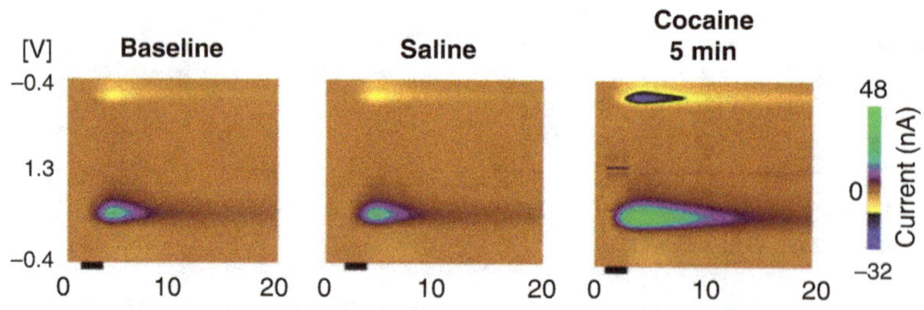

Figure 6.22 Results of an FSCV experiment. Source: Yuen J, Goyal A, Rusheen AE, et al. Cocaine-induced changes in tonic dopamine concentrations measured using multiple-cyclic square wave voltammetry in vivo. *Front Pharmacol.* 2021; 12:705254. DOI: 10.3389/fphar.2021.705254. http://creativecommons.org/licenses/by/4.0/. Images have been cropped.

dopamine (DA) would be abbreviated as [DA]o. Naturalistic concentrations of neurotransmitter are typically smaller than a micromolar (μM), but these values can reach micromolar concentrations with artificial stimulation. These data may also be plotted over a timescale of minutes following various manipulations.

Interpreting the Data

The output measure in FSCV is a current, and larger currents correspond to a greater concentration of neurotransmitter in the probe location (biological) or greater surface area of the carbon fiber electrode (artifact of the technique). Therefore, calibrating the electrodes to known concentrations of neurotransmitter allows for a more meaningful interpretation of the data.

Drugs that influence neurotransmitter reuptake or release will influence the shape of a concentration versus time plot. For example, cocaine, which inhibits reuptake of dopamine, will widen the peak, since the neurotransmitter is not cleared out of the extracellular space as quickly and can therefore produce an oxidation current over a longer time window.

Additional Resources

John CE, Jones SR. Fast scan cyclic voltammetry of dopamine and serotonin in mouse brain slices. In Michael AC, Borland LM, editors. *Electrochemical Methods for Neuroscience*. Boca Raton, FL: CRC Press/Taylor & Francis; 2007. Chapter 4. https://www.ncbi.nlm.nih.gov/books/NBK2579/.

Maina FK, Khalid M, Apawu AK, Mathews TA. Presynaptic dopamine dynamics in striatal brain slices with fast-scan cyclic voltammetry. *J Vis Exp*. 2012 Jan 12; 59:3464. doi: 10.3791/3464. PMID: 22270035; PMCID: PMC3462558.

Venton BJ, Cao Q. Fundamentals of fast-scan cyclic voltammetry for dopamine detection. *Anal*. 2020 Feb 17; 145(4):1158–1168. doi: 10.1039/c9an01586h. PMID: 31922176; PMCID: PMC7028514.

6.6.2 Amperometry

Background Information

Fixed-potential (or **continuous**, or **constant potential**) amperometry is a method to detect rapid changes in the concentration of certain neurochemicals in a specific area of the nervous system. In amperometry, a steady potential is delivered to the carbon fiber microelectrode placed in the region of interest. The voltage causes any chemical in the surrounding space to become oxidized, producing a current that is detected by the electrode.

Amperometry offers higher temporal resolution than FSCV, capable of sampling at 10,000 Hz. Amperometry can also be performed at the level of single cells. By measuring the amount of current produced after release of individual vesicles, amperometry offers high spatial and temporal resolution. However, by only holding at one potential, amperometry has a hard time differentiating molecules.

Reading the Graphs

In amperometry, sample traces are positive deflections over a stable baseline. The x-axis plots time, while the y-axis may plot current. It is also common to calibrate electrodes to fixed concentrations, and then to present the data as concentration on the y-axis. At short timescales (milliseconds), these graphs show neurotransmitter release events, perhaps as evoked by electrical stimulation or naturalistic stimuli in an *in vivo* preparation.

At longer timescales (tens of minutes), these graphs can demonstrate plasticity phenomena such as LTP (enhancement of signal) or LTD (decrease of signal).

Because of the superior temporal resolution of amperometry, parameters of neurotransmitter release other than peak current (or concentration) can be quantified, which may include kinetics measurements such as half-height duration or decay. These may be represented on group average graphs.

Figure 6.23 represents an amperometry experiment showing the influence of DHPG application on extracellular dopamine levels. Release of dopamine was triggered by local electrical stimulation. At the top is a time course summary graph. Each point represents an average normalized amount of current produced by oxidation of extracellular dopamine. Here, the researchers report a reduction of current amplitude after DHPG application that persists for at least 60 minutes, suggesting long-term depression of synaptic dopamine release. At the bottom of the figure, representative traces show the oxidation amplitude peaks at three different time points – before (a), immediately after (b), and 60 minutes after (c) DHPG application – along with an overlay trace.

Additional Resources

Fathali H, Cans AS. Amperometry methods for monitoring vesicular quantal size and regulation of exocytosis release. *Pflugers Arch*. 2018 Jan; 470(1):125–134. DOI: 10.1007/s00424-017-2069-9. Epub 2017 Sep 27. PMID: 28951968; PMCID: PMC5748430.

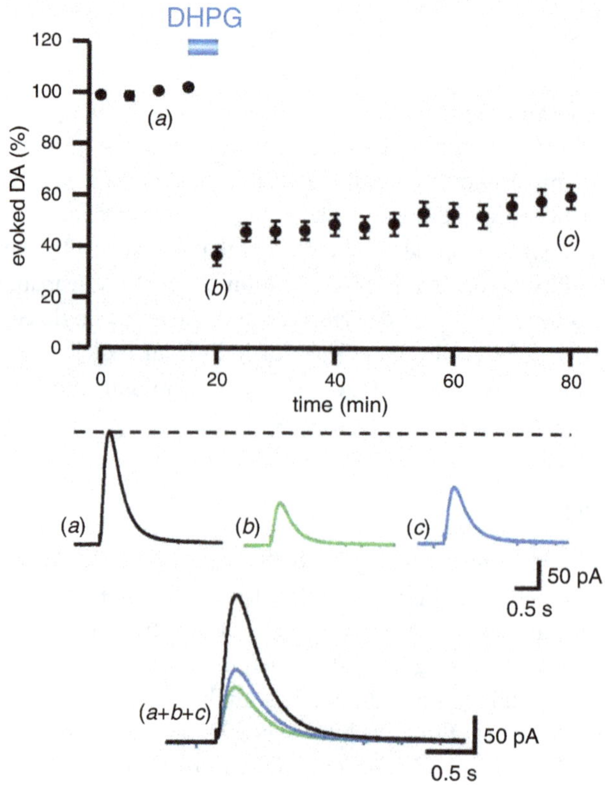

Figure 6.23 Results of a fixed potential amperometry experiment. Source: Mercuri NB, Federici M, Rizzo FR, et al. Long-term depression of striatal DA release induced by mGluRs via sustained hyperactivity of local cholinergic interneurons. *Front Cell Neurosci.* 2021; 15:798464. DOI: 10.3389/fncel.2021.798464. http://creativecommons.org/licenses/by/4.0/.

Summary

This chapter has described the wide breadth of techniques used by electrophysiologists and electrochemists to understand the electrical properties of neurons. First, we described the basic principles of these techniques: the observation that neurons can be modeled as electrical circuits, the ways the samples can be prepared, the different ways recording electrodes can be positioned relative to the neurons, and the tools that are used for collecting these data.

Next, we covered the figures that are used to represent features of individual neurons, both when they are passive and while firing action potentials. Several different figures were used to illustrate synaptic responses, some of which can be used for demonstrating plasticity. Then, current-voltage relationships were described. The chapter concluded with a discussion about electrochemistry techniques used in neuroscience research, such as fast scan cyclic voltametry and fixed potential amperometry.

Chapter 7 describes some of the techniques related to analysis of genetics questions across all scales, from molecular genetics all the way to evolutionary genetics.

Key Terms

- accommodation
- acute slice
- afterhyperpolarization phase
- amperometry
- amplifier
- anti-Hebbian spike timing dependent plasticity (STDP)
- artificial cerebrospinal fluid (aCSF)
- awake and behaving
- cell attached recording
- conductance
- cumulative probability
- current
- current clamp
- current-voltage relationship (I-V plot)
- cyclic voltammogram
- decay time
- depolarization phase
- depolarize
- digitizer
- electrochemistry
- electrode
- electrophysiology
- evoked firing rate
- excised patch
- extracellular recording
- *ex vivo*
- fast scan cyclic voltammetry (FSCV)
- field EPSP (fEPSP)
- field recording
- gapfree
- headstage
- Hebbian spike timing dependent plasticity (Hebbian STDP)
- heterologous expression system
- high-frequency stimulation (HFS)
- hyperpolarize
- induced pluripotent stem cell (IPSC)
- induction protocol
- input resistance
- input/output curve
- inside-out patch
- interspike interval (ISI)
- intracellular recording

- irregular firing
- long-term depression (LTD)
- long-term potentiation (LTP)
- membrane resistance (R_m)
- miniature end plate potential (mEPP)
- miniature postsynaptic current/voltage
- noise
- Ohm's law
- organotypic slice
- outside-out patch
- pacemaker neuron
- paired pulse depression
- paired pulse facilitation
- paired pulse interval
- paired pulse ratio (PPR)
- patch clamp
- perforated patch
- peristimulus time histogram
- preparation
- primary dissociated culture
- raster plot
- rectification
- repolarization phase
- resistance
- resting membrane potential (RMP)
- rheobase
- rig
- rise time
- rundown
- spike timing dependent plasticity
- spontaneous firing rate
- spontaneous postsynaptic current/voltage
- stimulation artifact
- sweep
- switching potential
- tetanic stimulation
- theta burst stimulation
- time constant
- two electrode voltage clamp (TEVC)
- voltage
- voltage clamp
- whole cell recording

CHAPTER SEVEN

Genetics

7.1 Introduction to Genetics

This chapter describes analysis methods related to some aspect of genetics. The field of genetics answers questions at many scales, and this chapter discusses methods from "small to large," starting with molecular genetics techniques, going on to single-organism techniques, and finally looking at techniques involving multiple organisms or research participants.

Many of these analysis methods are done in conjunction with techniques described in previous chapters. For example, transgene construct schematics are shown alongside optogenetic and chemogenetic strategies, which are among the first steps in modern behavioral or electrophysiological experiments. On the other end of the spectrum of scale, sometimes case studies with clinical brain scans may have a family pedigree showing which related family members are also affected by a rare condition.

Learning Objectives

By the end of this chapter, you will be able to:

- Describe the foundations of genetics, such as the principles of base pairing and gene and protein mutations.
- Describe the methods used in the study of molecular genetics, genetic association studies, and analyses of genetic differences in and across populations.
- Describe the figures that illustrate these data.

Genetic material is stored by molecules of DNA, which has the shape of a double helix (akin to a ladder with a twist). The smallest component of DNA is made up of a phosphate backbone, a ribose sugar, and one of four **nucleotide** molecules: **adenine** (abbreviated **A**), **thymine (T)**, **guanine** (G), or **cytosine (C)**. Each "rung" of the ladder is made by a combination of two of these molecules according to the rule that A always pairs with T, and G always pairs with C. Each of these is called a **base pair**. Due to this pairing rule, if you know one of the base pairs, you will know the other.

The sequence of DNA is almost always read in the five prime to three prime (denoted as 5′ to 3′) direction.

A set of three nucleotides of mRNA corresponds to a particular **amino acid**, which are the building blocks of all proteins. All people (except for identical twins) have differences in their genetic code; a difference in one particular nucleotide is called a **single nucleotide polymorphism** (or **SNP**). SNPs are typically identified in a study by the letters **rs** followed by a number, up to ten digits long. The letters "rs" stands for "reference SNP", while the number corresponds to an entry in the Single Nucleotide Polymorphism Database run by the USA's National Center for Biotechnology Information. The values are arbitrary and are used for convenience, but they can be cross-referenced with the database for further interpretation.

Mutations in the DNA can be denoted by a convention called human genome variation sequence (HGVs). For example, in c.547G>T, the base pair at position 547 is changed from a G into a T. The "c." at the beginning of the mutation notation stands for "coding DNA," since only the exons are counted.

When that section of DNA gets translated into protein, the protein will have a different primary structure (sequence of amino acids). A difference in the protein sequence may be denoted by the amino acid (a one- or three-letter abbreviation for that amino acid) followed by a number (its position in the amino acid sequence). For example, p.Arg158 is a protein that has an arginine amino acid residue as the 158th amino acid. The "p." in this notation stands for protein.

Since mutations in DNA may cause mutations in protein, a similar convention is used. For example, p.Glu41Lys indicates the protein at position 41 is mutated from Glu into Lys. These may also be written as a single-letter abbreviation. For example, a mutation might read H452T, which indicates that the "normal" amino acid at position 452 was a histidine (H) which has been mutated into a threonine (T).

A **gene** is the smallest unit of DNA information. In the literature, genes are usually identified by a series of capital letters and numbers. However, their protein products are usually italicized and contain both capital and lowercase letters. Oftentimes, proteins may end in the suffix -in. Some example gene–protein pairs relevant to the neuroscience of disease include the gene APOE and the protein apolipoprotein E (Alzheimer's disease); the PARK2 gene, which codes for the parkin protein (Parkinson's disease); and the gene GRN, which codes for progranulin (amyotrophic lateral sclerosis).

Figure 7.1 shows the many observed mutations in the SPG7 gene that lead to a genetic disorder called spastic paraplegia.

Additional Resources

Ogino S, Gulley ML, den Dunnen JT, Wilson RB, Association for Molecular Pathology Training and Education Committee. Standard mutation nomenclature in molecular diagnostics: Practical and educational challenges. *J Mol Diagn*. 2007 Feb; 9(1):1–6. DOI: 10.2353/jmoldx.2007.060081. Erratum in *J Mol Diagn*. 2009 Sep 1; 11(5):494. PMID: 17251329; PMCID: PMC1867422.

7.2 Transgene Construct Schematics

Background Information

A major advantage of understanding animal genomes is the ability to use tools to manipulate their genomes, producing **transgenic animals**. Transgenic animals are very common in neuroscience research because of the flexibility in experiments you can perform with them.

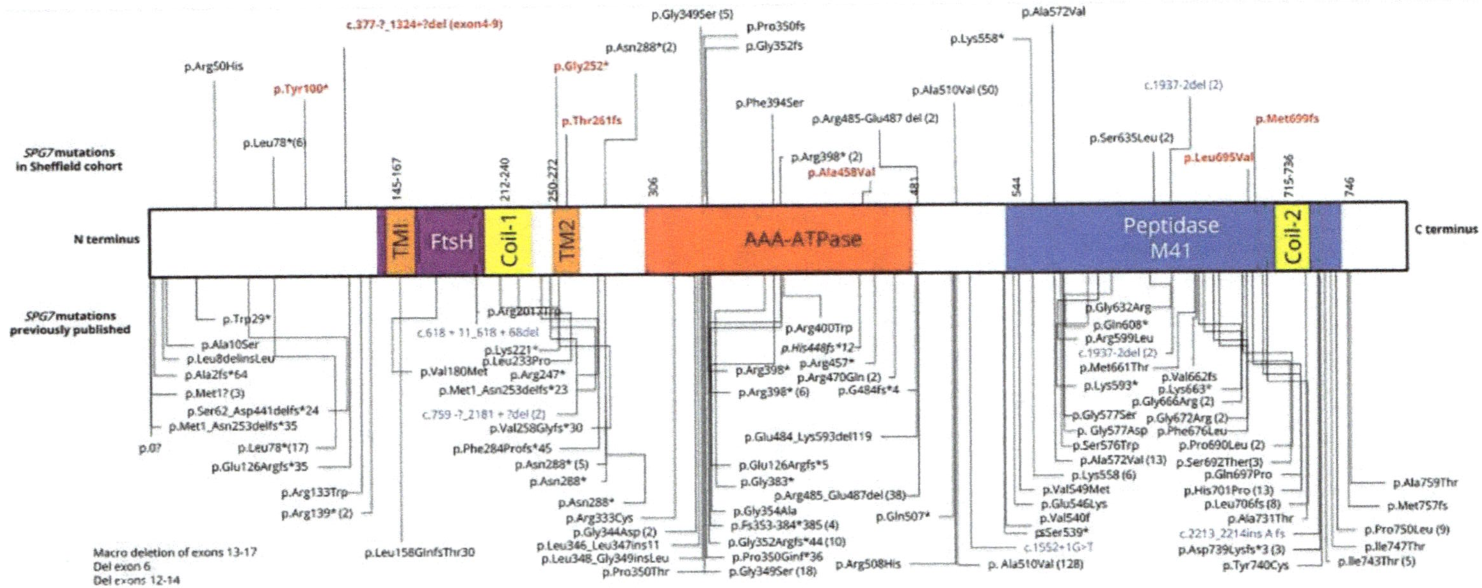

Figure 7.1 Gene schematic and mutations. Source: Hewamadduma CA, Hoggard N, O'Malley R, et al. Novel genotype-phenotype and MRI correlations in a large cohort of patients with *SPG7* mutations. *Neurol Genet.* 2018; 4(6):e279. https://doi.org/10.1212/NXG.0000000000000279. https://creativecommons.org/licenses/by/4.0/.

For example, there are transgenic mice with fluorescent molecules restricted to certain cell types, which allows an electrophysiologist to target only that specific cell type while patch clamping. As another example, researchers can create transgenic fruit flies with human genes, allowing for high-throughput screening of novel therapeutic chemicals on human receptors.

Transgenic animals can be created in at least two different ways. A **transfection** approach relies on creating a gene construct and then exposing the host cells to the foreign DNA, possibly through microinjection or electroporation. Transfection strategies are less versatile, since the gene construct is delivered only in the early phases of development and does not offer cell specificity.

Transduction relies on using a virus (called the **vector**) to insert exogenous genetic material into cells. The most common viral vectors are adeno-associated viruses (AAV), lentivirus, and rabies virus. Most viral vectors are purchased from a core facility rather than made in-laboratory. Transduction is more common in recent literature because of several advantages. The virus can be microinjected using stereotaxic surgery, providing regional specificity. Using a modified mouse called a Cre line, the virus can restrict its transduction to a limited population of cells while sparing surrounding cells, and can even target organelles. Transduction can also offer temporal specificity, since the virus can be delivered at specific points during the animal's development.

Transgenic techniques are mostly applied to animals that are easy to house with short generation times and a rapid maturation rate into sexual reproductive age: this means mostly animals such as mice, flies, and worms, although commercially available transgenic rats are becoming more common. These strategies can be performed in cell cultures as well. Gene therapy strategies in humans may also take advantage of transduction.

Figure 7.2 is a cartoon representation of the process of viral-vector-mediated transduction of genetic material. In the top image, the virus is loaded into a micropipette that is surgically inserted into the region of interest. The virus is expected to spread beyond that area. The lower image illustrates how certain Cre-dependent viruses can transduce only cells with certain characteristics.

Reading the Graphs

The foreign DNA to be inserted into the host cells (called a **cassette**) may be shown in a diagram, especially in transduction experiments. These figures are mostly protocol figures; they provide specifics about the genes to be inserted, since there is a limited amount of space that can be put into a single viral vector (for example, a typical AAV can only store about 4,700 nucleotides worth of DNA).

Construct diagrams show what genes are included in the foreign DNA and are transcribed by showing the cells from left to right. Below are some of the commonly inserted genes in these experiments.

- **Inverted terminal repeat (ITR)** regions usually flank the sequence of interest, and may be essential for putting the new sequence into the viral DNA.

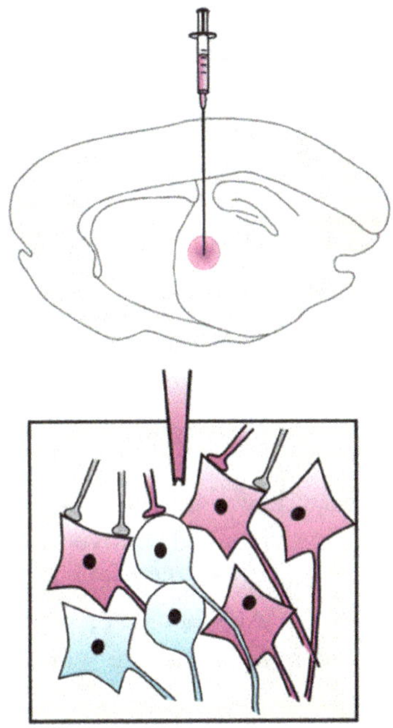

Figure 7.2 Cartoon of viral-mediated transduction. Source: Parr-Brownlie LC, Bosch-Bouju C, Schoderboeck L, et al. Lentiviral vectors as tools to understand central nervous system biology in mammalian model organisms. *Front Mol Neurosci.* 2015; 8:14. http://creativecommons.org/licenses/by/4.0/. Image cropped.

- **Regulatory regions** are "instructional" regions that guide the binding of the transcriptional machinery. The **promoter** is one such regulatory region and it determines how much of the transgene will be expressed. Some common promoters include sCAG, hSyn, hCMV, and EF1α. Promoters may be indicated by an arrow. **Enhancers** are other regulatory regions, which may increase transfection efficiency.
- **Reporter genes** code for some fluorescent proteins that are used to show which cells have been successfully transduced. These elements may be color coded based on their emission wavelength. So, a region coding for an enhanced green fluorescent protein (eGFP) may be represented by a green rectangle.
- One of many experimental genes of interest may be inserted, for example:
  - A genetically encoded calcium indicator, such as GcaMP, to allow for all-optical electrophysiological visualization of large cell populations.
  - An exogenously manipulable element, including an optogenetic protein such as channelrhodopsin or a chemogenetic protein such as a DREADD.
  - Humanized proteins to better model the human disease state, such as amyloid β to study the effects of protein aggregation in Alzheimer's pathology.

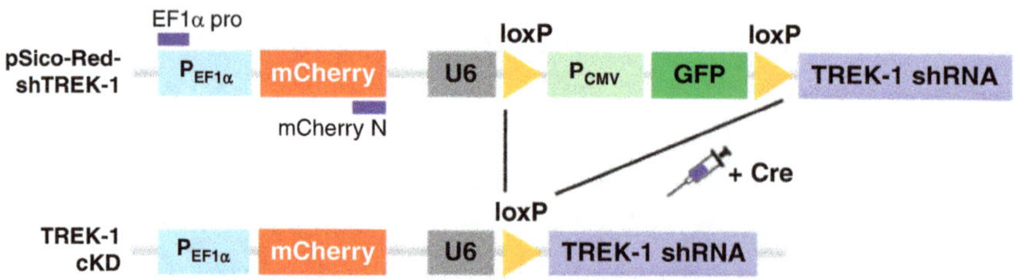

Figure 7.3 Cartoon of a gene construct. Source: Kim A, Jung H-G, Kim Y-E, et al. The knockdown of TREK-1 in hippocampal neurons attenuate lipopolysaccharide-induced depressive-like behavior in mice. *Int J Mol Sci.* 2019; 20(23):5902. https://doi.org/10.3390/ijms20235902. http://creativecommons.org/licenses/by/4.0/. Image cropped.

The information contained in these diagrams is just as often written out as a sequence, usually starting with identifying the virus and serotype followed by each of the foreign genes separated by dashes, often excluding the ITR regions. For example, a virus transduction study may report using AAV9-CAG-Tdtomato, which means they used an adeno associated virus (serotype 9) containing a cassette with a CAG promoter followed by a Tdtomato reporter gene.

Figure 7.3 shows an example gene cassette, containing elements such as EF1α and CMV promoter sequences and the reporter genes mCherry and GFP. This sequence is used to conditionally knock down the TREK-1 channel by introduction of a short hairpin RNA (shRNA).

Additional Resources

Challis RC, Ravindra Kumar S, Chen X, et al. Adeno-Associated Virus Toolkit to Target Diverse Brain Cells. *Annu Rev Neurosci.* 2022 Jul 8; 45:447–469. DOI: 10.1146/annurev-neuro-111020-100834. Epub 2022 Apr 19. PMID: 35440143.

Chen SH, Haam J, Walker M, et al. Production of *Viral Constructs for Neuroanatomy, Calcium Imaging, and Optogenetics. Curr Protoc Neurosci.* 2019 Apr; 87(1):e66. DOI: 10.1002/cpns.66. Epub 2019 Mar 18. PMID: 30883041; PMCID: PMC6530799.

Sun J, Roy S. Gene-based therapies for neurodegenerative diseases. *Nat Neurosci.* 2021 Mar; 24(3):297–311. DOI: 10.1038/s41593-020-00778-1. Epub 2021 Feb 1. PMID: 33526943;PMCID: PMC8394447.

7.3 Genome-Wide Association Study (GWAS)

Background Information

A genome-wide association study is a screen that looks at the genome of a sample population. The approach is to collect blood samples from the population and a control group (case–control design), scan the sequences for each participant, and find individual mutations (SNPs) that differ between the populations. A GWAS assesses millions of SNPs with the same blood sample. Any SNPs that are different between case and control are therefore associated with the condition.

GWAS is commonly performed in people with complex neuropsychiatric disorders. For example, GWAS has identified candidate genes associated with schizophrenia, dementia, PTSD, bipolar disorder, and many others. GWAS is minimally invasive and can be done just as easily in nonhuman animal models.

Reading the Graphs

In case–control studies, there is often also a table describing demographic information (rows) about the groups (columns). In a properly matched sample, there will be no group differences between sex, gender, ethnicity, socioeconomic status (SES), years of education, or many other factors relevant to the research question, such as a history of substance use in studies of cocaine use disorder, or family members with positive mental illness diagnosis in studies of schizophrenia.

The most common graph showing results from a GWAS is a **Manhattan plot**, named for its resemblance to the skyline of a metropolis. The *x*-axis plots different loci across the chromosomes in ascending order, with the sex chromosomes at the far right. Data from each chromosome may be presented with alternating or different colors for visual clarity. The *y*-axis plots the negative log of the *p*-value between the case and the control populations, which converts small *p*-values into a higher value so that greater statistical significance appears taller. The *y*-axis is unitless. There may also be horizontal lines to signify the cutoff for statistical significance, and data points above this line suggest an association of that gene with the condition. Each dot represents data from one individual.

A results table may also accompany the Manhattan plot. Each row of the table describes one of the candidate genes identified by the analysis. Other information provided in columns may include the specific rs number corresponding to the SNP, the *p*-value, and the proteins and corresponding mutations that SNP codes for.

GWAS data may also show a **quantile–quantile plot** (**QQ plot**). The QQ plot is also used to make predictions about data distribution, but in GWAS, it shows just how much the genes of interest deviate from the null hypothesis of "no association". The *x*-axis plots the expected negative log of the *p*-value, while the *y*-axis plots the actual observed values. A dotted line is usually drawn at the intersection of where observed equals the observed. Each dot represents an individual gene, and these are usually arranged from left to right in increasing observed $-\log(p)$.

Figure 7.4 represents the results of a GWAS of more than 1 million participants. The Manhattan plot shows 42 loci of interest among people with dyslexia. Genes with significance above the $p < 5 \times 10^{-8}$ line are denoted in red. Data points in alternating purple and green represent those with less statistical significance and are colored only to distinguish between different chromosomes.

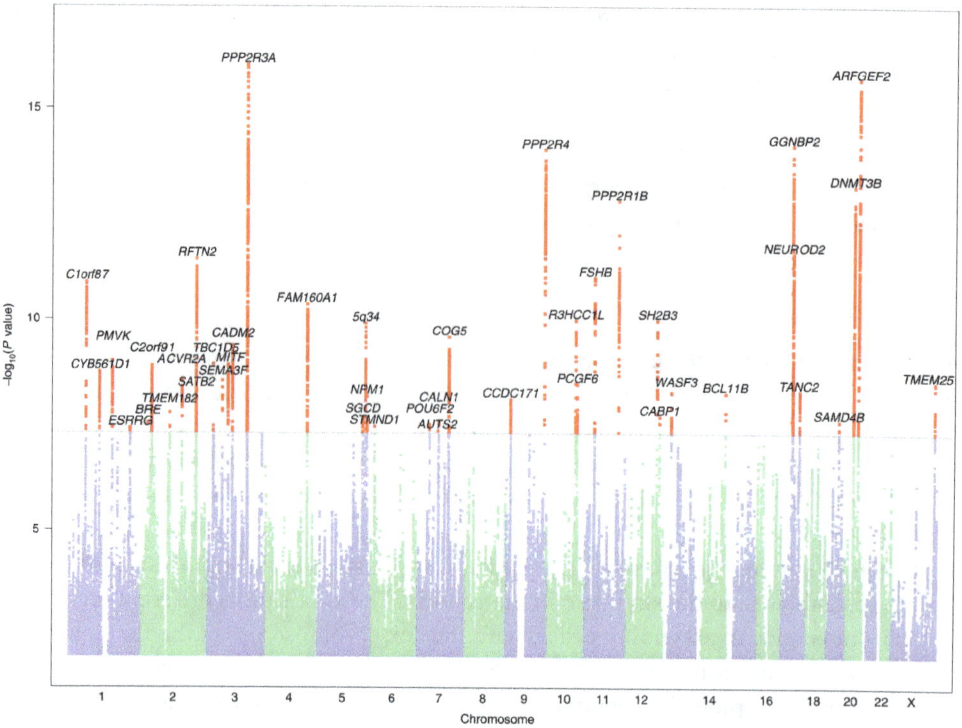

Figure 7.4 Results of a GWAS. Source: Doust C, Fontanillas P, Eising E, et al. Discovery of 42 genome-wide significant loci associated with dyslexia. *Nat Genet.* 2022; 54:1621–1629. https://doi.org/10.1038/s41588-022-01192-y.

Interpreting the Data

As the name tells us through the word "association," GWAS studies do not provide causation information, although the results can guide future experimental studies. For example, a GWAS that discovers that a SNP in the gene apolipoprotein E is associated with Alzheimer's disease might lead to an experimental hypothesis that decreasing dietary lipid intake may prevent or delay disease onset.

Because so many genes are being studied in a GWAS, the standard statistical cutoff of $p < 0.05$ leads to false positives. It is common to see threshold p-values for statistical significance on the order of $p < 5 \times 10^{-8}$. There may also be suggestive levels of significance at larger p-values, such as 10^{-5}, which increases both the number of potential candidate genes of interest and the number of false positives. The thresholds for significance values can be calculated based on the number of probes used; more probes require a lower p-value for significance. Individual gene differences may have p-values as low as 1×10^{-15}, suggesting very strong associations with the outcome.

If there are no genes of interest associated with the outcome, then the expected distribution on the QQ plot is a straight line intersecting at 1-1. The genes with the stronger associations are placed on the right, so there may be an upward slope near the right side of the curve. The taller this slope is, the stronger the association between the gene and the outcome.

Additional Resources

Uffelmann E, Huang QQ, Munung NS, et al. Genome-wide association studies. *Nat Rev Methods Primers*. 2021; 1(59). https://doi.org/10.1038/s43586-021-00056-9.

7.4 Microbiome Analyses of Populations (Bray–Curtis Dissimilarity, UniFrac)

Background Information

The bacterial colonies that are a part of the gut microbiome likely influence the brain and behavior through signaling along the **gut–brain axis**, and changes in gut flora that lead to negative health outcomes are called **dysbiosis**. It may therefore be useful to analyze the variety of the microbial species to see if there are correlations between the composition of gut flora and neuropsychiatric conditions or outcomes.

Microbiome analysis methods have been adopted from ecology, which uses similar techniques to describe how different types of forests sustain different plant species, or whether two ponds have different populations of fishes.

In neuroscience, these studies most often use case–control design. For example, samples may be analyzed between a group of participants with bipolar disorder (the case condition) and demographically matched controls without the disorder. Experimental studies can also be performed by comparing samples before and after treatment with antipsychotics, for example.

Gut microbiome is assessed noninvasively by collecting stool samples, so it is a suitable assay in both people and nonhuman animals.

Reading the Graphs

The results of these studies are presented graphically as two- or three-dimensional principal component analyses (PCoA) where each axis represents a sum of several features that have been summarized onto a single axis (dimensionality reduction). Each dot represents the microbiome composition data from each participant. Dots are often color coded to indicate case versus control. "Clouds" may be drawn around each group to more clearly highlight differences.

There are at least two statistical analysis methods that can be used to produce the principal component analysis graph.

A **Bray–Curtis dissimilarity** is a mathematical measurement to assess how different the samples are from one another. Values range from 0 to 1, with a 0 suggesting no difference between groups and a 1 meaning total dissimilarity with no overlapping species of bacteria.

The **Jaccard index** doesn't take into consideration the abundance of species, as the Bray–Curtis dissimilarity does. Instead, it only calculates the presence of species as a binary variable: the species is present, or it is not.

The **unique fraction (UniFrac)** also measures dissimilarity, but this analysis considers how closely related (taxonomically speaking) the species are from each other. If there was a large observed difference between two bacterial species of the same genus, it would carry less weight than the same difference between species of different genera.

Stacked bar charts may also be shown. On these graphs, each bar represents the data from each participant, which may be divided between cases and controls or treatment and placebo groups. The other axis plots the relative proportion of each bacterial species found in that individual's sample, and each segment of the bar indicates a species. A key summarizes which color corresponds to which bacterium.

Figure 7.5 shows results from a principal component analysis. The study represented here concluded that adenotonsillectomy in children with obstructive sleep apnea changes salivary microbiome diversity. Samples were collected before (red) and after (blue) the procedure and then analyzed through DNA extraction and bioinformatics.

Interpreting the Data

Most of these studies are performed as a case–control study and function as an exploratory screen. These designs do not provide evidence about causality, since it becomes a challenge to determine if the condition of interest affects the gut microbiome or vice versa.

Generally, the more divergent the groups appear on the principal component analysis, the stronger the correlation between gut dysbiosis and the outcome. Stacked bar charts point toward specific candidate bacterial species that may contribute to the outcome.

The gut microbiome is affected by the immune system, so gut inflammation and subsequent signaling in the nervous system may be implicated in the disorder.

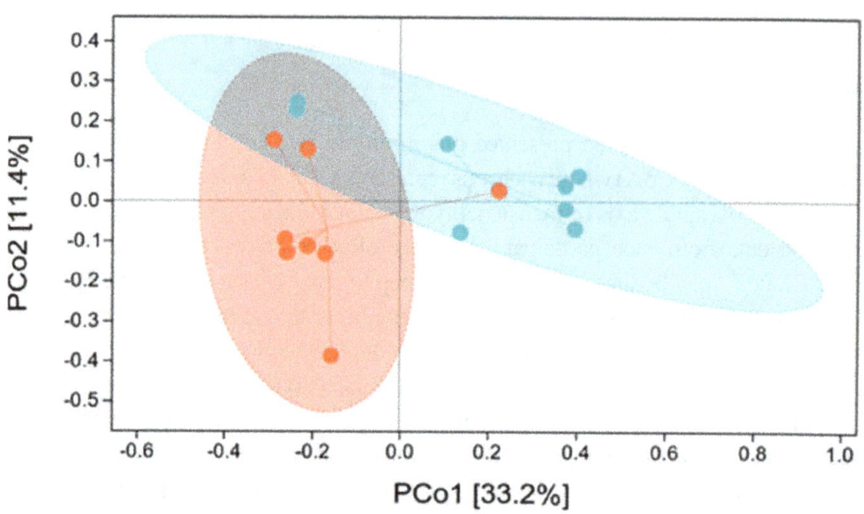

Figure 7.5 Results of a microbiome study using a principal component analysis. Source: Huang X, Chen X, Gong X, et al. Characteristics of salivary microbiota in children with obstructive sleep apnea: A prospective study with polysomnography. *Front Cell Infect Microbiol.* 2022; 12:945284. DOI: 10.3389/fcimb.2022.945284. http://creativecommons.org/licenses/by/4.0/. Image cropped.

Additional Resources

Bray JR, Curtis JT. An ordination of the upland forest communities of southern Wisconsin. *Ecological Monographs*. 1957; 27:325–349. https://doi.org/10.2307/1942268

Lozupone C, Knight R. UniFrac: A new phylogenetic method for comparing microbial communities. *Appl Environ Microbiol*. 2005 Dec; 71(12):8228–35. DOI: 10.1128/AEM.71.12.8228-8235.2005. PMID: 16332807; PMCID: PMC1317376.

7.5 Family Tree (Pedigree Map)

Background Information

Family trees are used to illustrate the passing of particular traits of individuals across generations. They provide clues about the nature of transmission of genetically inherited characteristics or diseases.

Family trees are most often shown in case studies, especially for conditions with a suspected genetic means of inheritance. The person who is described in the case study is called the **proband**. Some conditions with a strong hereditary component include Charcot-Marie-Tooth disease, color vision deficiency, dystonia, Huntington's disease, and Tourette's syndrome.

Family trees used in neuroscience nearly all depict human familial relationships and are rarely shown for nonhumans.

Reading the Graphs

In family trees, each shape represents an individual. Circles indicate women, squares indicate men, and a diamond indicates unspecified gender. A diagonal line through the shape indicates the person is deceased. An arrow may be used to identify the proband.

People affected by the condition of interest have filled-in shapes while unaffected have empty shapes. For people who are carriers for the disease (heterozygous autosomal recessive or sex-linked), their shape may be partially filled. Hollow circles inside the shape may be used to indicate cases of suspected carriers when an accurate family history is not known. Other comorbid conditions may be indicated in another color. Text may be written underneath individuals, such as the specific mutation observed in those people.

Each row represents a generation, and the most recent (youngest) generation is at the bottom. Generations may be indicated by Roman numerals at the far end of each row; younger generations are denoted by larger numbers. Individual members of each generation may be identified by Arabic numerals. The combination of the generation and individual number (Roman numeral followed by Arabic numeral) may be used to identify individuals elsewhere in the text.

When two people are connected horizontally by a line, it indicates a union. Unions connected by a double line indicate a consanguineous relationship (second cousins or closer). A vertical line extending downwards from a union indicates children, branching at right angles to indicate multiple children. Diagonal lines stemming from the union line indicate

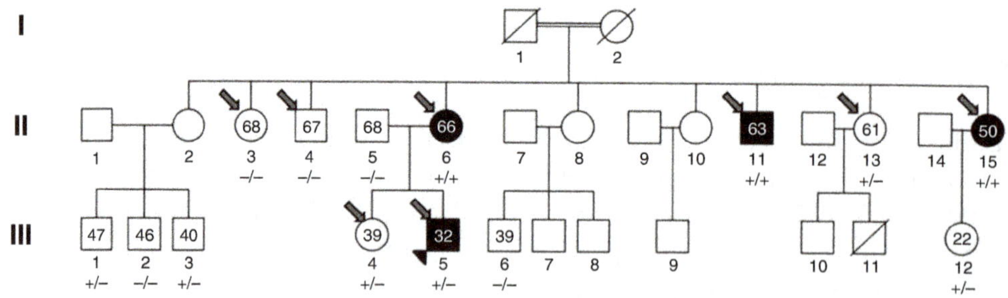

Figure 7.6 A family tree. Source: Esposito F, Osiceanu AM, Sorosina M, et al. A whole-genome sequencing study implicates GRAMD1B in multiple sclerosis susceptibility. *Genes.* 2022; 13(12):2392. https://doi.org/10.3390/genes13122392. https://creativecommons.org/licenses/by/4.0/.

twins; an intermediate horizontal line connecting the diagonals indicates monozygotic (identical) twins, while if the diagonals are not connected the twins are dizygotic (fraternal).

The family tree in Figure 7.6 hints at a genetic element to multiple sclerosis (MS) due to a mutation in the GRAMD1B gene. The arrowhead pointing to III-5 is the proband. Symbols colored in black represent people with a positive diagnosis of MS. Arrows point to the eight patients who had undergone whole genome screening. The $^{+/+}$ indicates people who are homozygous for a specific mutation of the gene, $^{+/-}$ indicates heterozygosity, and $^{-/-}$ indicates a homozygous nonmutated gene.

Interpreting the Data

Family trees are retrospective studies, and therefore do not provide experimental evidence. They are much more reliable for conditions with clear diagnostic criteria, such as epilepsy, Huntington's disease, or spinocerebellar ataxia, than for other conditions. These analyses may be less helpful for tracking mental illnesses, since complex societal-level issues influence disease diagnosis (for example, generational opinions about seeking mental health care, and shifting diagnostic criteria).

Family trees may provide clues about the method of transmission of inherited diseases. Some common inheritance patterns include the following.

- In **autosomal dominant inheritance**, the disease-causing gene is found on one of the 22 pairs of autosomes. For each affected person, at least one of their parents also must be affected. From each union with one affected person, approximately 50% of the offspring will also be affected. Both men and women are equally affected. Huntington's disease is an example of an autosomal dominant condition.
- In **sex-linked inheritance**, the gene that causes the disease is on an allosome, which are the X or Y chromosomes.
  - In **X-linked recessive inheritance**, for each affected mother, each of her sons will also be affected, while her daughters will either be carriers or noncarriers with equal

probability. However, an affected father's sons will all be unaffected, while his daughters will all be carriers. Across families, X-linked recessive traits are more common among men than women; color vision deficiency is one example.

  - In **X-linked dominant inheritance**, each affected mother's sons and daughters will be roughly 50% affected, while each affected father's daughters will all be affected with none of the sons affected. One form of Charcot-Marie-Tooth disease is passed through an X-linked dominant inheritance pattern.
  - In **Y-linked inheritance**, only males are affected. Among their offspring, only sons will be affected while all daughters are unaffected. A Y-linked gene is NLGN4Y, which codes for neuroligin, a cell adhesion molecule involved in synapse formation.

- In **mitochondrial inheritance**, all offspring of affected mothers are also affected. Leigh syndrome is one example of a genetic disorder that is passed through mitochondrial transmission.

Family trees may provide insight into the "nature vs. nurture" question: whether inherited genetic factors or environmental factors play a stronger role in the disease. This question is best studied in fraternal and identical twins, since an assumption is made that twins raised in the same household have very similar environmental influences, all the way from birth to diet and culture. Therefore, if identical twins, who have the same shared genes, have a higher rate of being affected compared to fraternal twins, who have different genes, then genetics are likely to play a stronger role than environment. Using data sets from multiple twin pairs across different families, a **concordance rate** can be calculated, which is the percentage of twins where one is affected if the other twin is affected.

Additional Resources

Genetic Alliance; New York–Mid-Atlantic Consortium for Genetic and Newborn Screening Services. *Understanding Genetics: A New York, Mid-Atlantic Guide for Patients and Health Professionals*. Washington, DC: Genetic Alliance; 2009 Jul 8.

7.6 Dendrograms

Background Information

A **dendrogram** is a graphical representation of the relationship between different things: animal species, transcriptome patterns, gene sequences, fMRI data, connectivity between brain areas, or many other potential dependent variables. Dendrograms may be used to classify a large number of observations into groups based on similarities in features.

One type of dendrogram adapted from the study of evolutionary biology is a **phylogenetic** (or **taxonomic**) **tree**, which depicts animal species. These plots show which species share a more recent common ancestor based on similarities of some feature, such as physical traits (phenotype) or genetic makeup (genotype). These are less common in neuroscience than in some other sciences, but they may be helpful when looking at the evolutionary origin of certain features. For example, a phylogenetic tree may show when along geologic time a receptor mutation that provides neurotoxin resistance evolved. Other phylogenetic trees may be useful for comparing cortex volume and shape across different species of apes.

Phylogenetic trees are useful for distinguishing **ancestors** and **descendants**. Ancestors are those animals farthest back in geologic time and are represented by a single line (akin to the trunk of the tree). There are several descendant organisms, which are represented by terminal lines called **leaves** and may be accompanied by drawings of the descendants.

A closely related figure is a **cladogram**, which plots theoretical relationships between groups of animals. Groups of animals with a shared common ancestor are called a **clade**. These graphs do not provide time information and are rare in neuroscience literature.

Reading the Figures

Dendrograms are organized from the trunk to the branches. In phylogenetic trees, this usually means that the trunk represents the organisms farthest back in geologic time, while leaves represent species which may or may not be extant.

In a dendrogram, the **root** represents the features that are shared by all of the participants (or oldest ancestor in phylogenies, where every descendant on the tree shares that ancestor in common). A **branch** is a line extending toward the descendants. In looking through evolution, the length of the line indicates approximately how many years ago (typically on the order of millions of years or longer) there was a divergence from the last common ancestor (although branches are not always to scale). A **node** is a point that separates into two or more different branches. Each node represents a biological entity, possibly some theoretical ancestor that shares features with all of the branches that extend from that node. For example, consider a phylogenetic tree of all mammals. The root would represent the most primitive warm-blooded vertebrate who feed their young with milk, a node would represent the common ancestor between marsupials and placentals, and branches may terminate in leaves with kangaroos and humans. Two descendants that are more closely related will have a node closer to the leaves.

Graphs can be linear or circular. Linear graphs may be vertical, usually with ancestors on top, or horizontal with ancestors of the left. In circular graphs, the ancestors are at the center.

Figure 7.7 is a dendrogram from a study that used mathematical modeling to examine endocranial volume, a proxy measure for brain volume, in different ape species. The data suggest that, compared to all other primates, hominins including *Homo sapiens* and *Homo neanderthalensis* had endocranial volumes that were larger than would be predicted considering their body mass.

Interpreting the Data

Since the geologic time scale may be difficult to measure, phylogenetic trees rely on approximation. Sometimes, clades (or clusters) may be highlighted by having branches labeled in different colors or having the background shaded. Species with older common

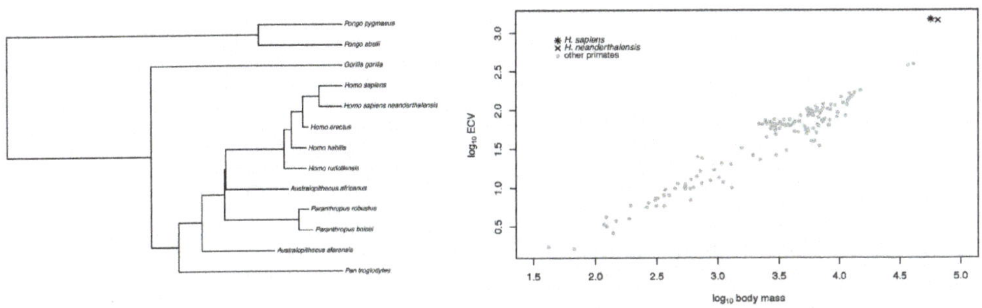

Figure 7.7 A dendrogram. Source: Miller IF, Barton RA, Nunn CL. Quantitative uniqueness of human brain evolution revealed through phylogenetic comparative analysis. *eLife.* 2019; 8:e41250. https://doi.org/10.7554/eLife.41250. http://creativecommons.org/licenses/by/4.0/. Images have been cropped and reordered, and text labels removed. Data from some species removed for clarity.

ancestors may still have characteristics more similar than species with more recent common ancestors. This is called **convergent evolution**, the observation that similar evolutionary pressures may favor a similar set of traits.

Outside of phylogenetic trees, the presentations of dendrograms provide information about commonalities of outcome variables. For example, they appear alongside RNA-seq data to show how different transcript patterns can be grouped together based on similarities.

In Figure 7.8, an unrooted phylogenetic tree shows variations of the transient receptor potential (TRP) channels found in mammals. The scale bar indicates how dissimilar the channels are from one another, with longer distances meaning more differences in point accepted mutation (PAM: single amino acid mutations). These channels have been subdivided into six categories based on primary structure similarities. TRP channels within each category are more similar to others within that category. For example, TRPC4 is most similar to TRPC5, somewhat similar to TRPC7, and highly dissimilar from TRPA1.

Additional Resources

Fitch WM, Margoliash E. Construction of phylogenetic trees. *Science*. 1967 Jan 20; 155-(3760):279–84. DOI: 10.1126/science.155.3760.279. PMID: 5334057.

Summary

This chapter has described a variety of techniques related to some element of genetics, a field that encompasses a wide range of analyses. Molecular-scale techniques such as genome manipulation are used for creating transgenic animals, which may be useful models for studying difficult complex conditions or testing theories about causality. Genome sequencing, GWAS, microbiome analyses, and pedigree maps are helpful for understanding different aspects of human diseases. Finally, dendrograms and phylogenetic trees not only offer suggestions about the evolutionary development of animals but also are useful for analyzing relationships in complex patterns.

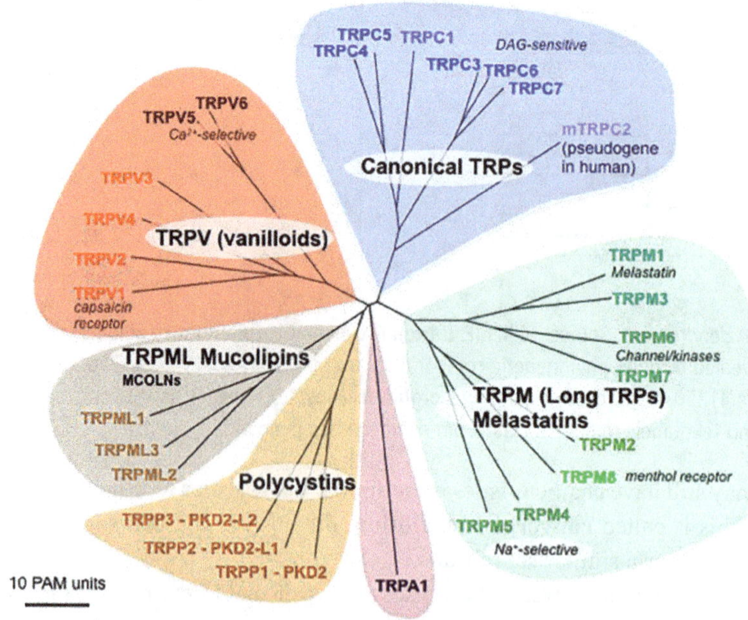

Figure 7.8 A radial dendrogram. Source: Blair NT, Caceres AI, Carvacho I, et al. Transient receptor potential channels (TRP) in GtoPdb v.2023.1. *IUPHAR/BPS Guide to Pharmacology CITE.* 2023; 2023(1). https://doi.org/10.2218/gtopdb/F78/2023.1. https://creativecommons.org/licenses/by-sa/4.0/.

The following chapter describes the figures that represent meta-analyses, a technique used in studies that use other publications as the subject of their study.

Key Terms

- adenine
- base pair
- Bray–Curtis dissimilarity
- cassette
- cladogram
- concordance rate
- convergent evolution
- cytosine
- dendrogram
- family tree
- gene
- genome-wide association study (GWAS)
- guanine
- gut–brain axis

- Manhattan plot
- microbiome analysis
- nucleotide
- proband
- promoter
- quantile–quantile plot
- reporter gene
- single nucleotide polymorphism (SNP)
- thymine
- transduction
- transfection
- transgenic animal
- vector

CHAPTER EIGHT

Meta-analysis

8.1 Introduction to Meta-analysis

A **meta-analysis** is a type of systematic review that uses statistical methods to summarize the results of several other studies. There is often methodological variance between studies, such as patient recruitment criteria, geographic location, dosing regimen, demographic characteristics, study endpoint, and outcome measurements observed, to name a few. A meta-analysis combines the results from several studies to find trends in the results despite these differences between individual studies.

In neuroscience, meta-analyses are typically used for summarizing human health-related studies. A meta-analysis may be performed to evaluate if an intervention influences outcomes, and in which direction. For example, a meta-analysis may examine if a given speech and language therapy approach affects the language capacity of stroke survivors, and whether this therapy improves or worsens language production. A different meta-analysis could be used to compile the results from several randomized clinical trials to determine if a specific anti-psychotic drug affects behaviors of patients with schizophrenia, and if the drug improves or worsens outcomes.

The nonhuman literature can also be studied with a meta-analysis. For example, a meta-analysis could be performed to examine if variability in electrophysiological properties of a neuronal population is explained by age, sex, or genetic strain.

A specific type of meta-analysis called an **activation likelihood estimation** (ALE) is used to aggregate results from different functional brain imaging methods (fMRI, PET, SPECT, and EEG, for example). The ALE meta-analysis determines patterns of brain activation in response to behaviors or conditions. For example, a meta-analysis might be used to compile results across 36 different imaging studies to discover that emotionally charged stimuli increase activity at the medial prefrontal cortex. Figures generated by an ALE meta-analysis closely resemble those produced by functional imaging methods.

Typically, two types of figures are most common in meta-analyses. **Flow charts** are a summary of the methodology of study selection, while **forest plots** are used to summarize the results. **Funnel plots** can also be presented, which visually represent the presence or absence of publication bias. We will now review these in turn.

Learning Objectives

By the end of this chapter, you will be able to:

- Explain how studies have been selected for inclusion in a meta-analysis
- Interpret the results shown in forest plots and funnel plots

Additional Resources

Hansen C, Steinmetz H, Block J. How to conduct a meta-analysis in eight steps: A practical guide. *Manag Rev Q*. 2022; 72:1–19.

Kossmeier M, Tran US, Voracek M. Charting the landscape of graphical displays for meta-analysis and systematic reviews: A comprehensive review, taxonomy, and feature analysis. *BMC Med Res Methodol*. 2020; 20:26.

Laird AR, Eickhoff SB, Kurth F, et al. ALE meta-analysis workflows via the brainmap database: Progress towards a probabilistic functional brain atlas. *Front Neuroinform*. 2009 Jul 9;3:23.

8.2 Flow Chart/PRISMA Flow Diagram

Background Information

A flow chart shows the process that the authors used in order to select studies for inclusion in their meta-analysis. Specific exclusion criteria are listed in this chart. Ideally, by following the process outlined in the flow chart, the reader will be able to pull the exact same group of studies for analysis. The flow chart is typically the first figure shown in a meta-analysis.

PRISMA, the Preferred Reporting Items of Systematic reviews and Meta Analysis, is a set of guidelines and a checklist of best practices for conducting a complete meta-analysis. Flow diagrams should follow PRISMA guidelines.

Reading the Graphs

Flow charts are a series of boxes connected by arrows, organized from top to bottom. Each box should contain brief explanatory text, for example describing the inclusion or exclusion criteria. The box also shows the number of studies included or excluded, indicated as an ***n*-value**.

The topmost box will have the most studies, and then each of the boxes below will report the number of included studies. There will also be a rightward arrow pointing to boxes that account for the excluded studies and the reason for exclusion. The bottom-most box represents the final number of studies that were included in the meta-analysis.

The main row of inclusion boxes, from top to bottom, each represent one of four stages:

1. The **identification** stage includes information about how the studies were first identified for inclusion. Overwhelmingly, study identification is done through database searches, which may include sources as varied as PubMed, Scopus, MEDLINE, Web of Science, Google Scholar, EMBASE, Science Direct, or the Cochrane Central Register of Controlled Trials. The exact search phrases (or **keywords**) may also be included in this box, along with the corresponding Boolean (AND, OR, NOT, for example) operators used in the search.

Unpublished or non-peer-reviewed data may also be identified at this stage. These studies, called the **gray literature**, can include sources such as ClinicalTrials.gov results, poster presentations or abstracts from conferences, technical reports, dissertations, informal reports to funding organizations, unfinished manuscripts, or other sources. These sources may be denoted by a box to the right of the topmost identification box, with arrows that point downwards to the next row.

2. The boxes in the row below represent the **screening stage**. Studies are checked and excluded during this stage for the following reasons:

    - Duplicate studies are identified; these are commonly found, since more than one database is searched.
    - The title and abstract is not relevant to the research question.

3. The next boxes down represent studies in the **eligibility stage**. At this stage, studies may be found to be ineligible for several reasons, and the reason and number of excluded studies are identified in a box to the right. Some general exclusion criteria include:

    - The full text of the manuscript is not accessible.
    - The manuscript is not written in a language that the meta-analysis researchers can read.
    - No data were provided, or the outcomes are not reported or are otherwise missing.
    - The study was published or conducted outside of a specific time window.
    - The study analyses an open-access data set which has been used in more than one included study (data duplication).
    - The manuscript was a meta-analysis, review paper, letter, report, commentary, editorial, or other publication category that does not present original data.

    Reasons that are more specific to the research question can also be grounds for exclusion, such as:

    - The demographic population is outside the scope of the meta-analysis (for example, in a meta-analysis of adults, a study that includes patients younger than 18 but does not analyze them separately may be excluded; in a study of disease prevalence in China, studies with patients in the US would be excluded).
    - In studies analyzing experimental interventions, quasi-experimental studies and observational studies (those lacking a control group) may be excluded.

4. Finally, the bottom-most box is the **inclusion stage**, a statement of the studies that have been included for the final analysis. It is common to include only a small percentage of studies from those identified in the first step; an inclusion rate less than 1% is common.

Meta-analyses often show a table listing the included studies along with some features of the studies, such as:

- First author and year of publication
- Number of data points reported (or the ***n*-value**)
- Type of study, some of which include retrospective studies, prospective studies, or randomized clinical trials (RCTs).

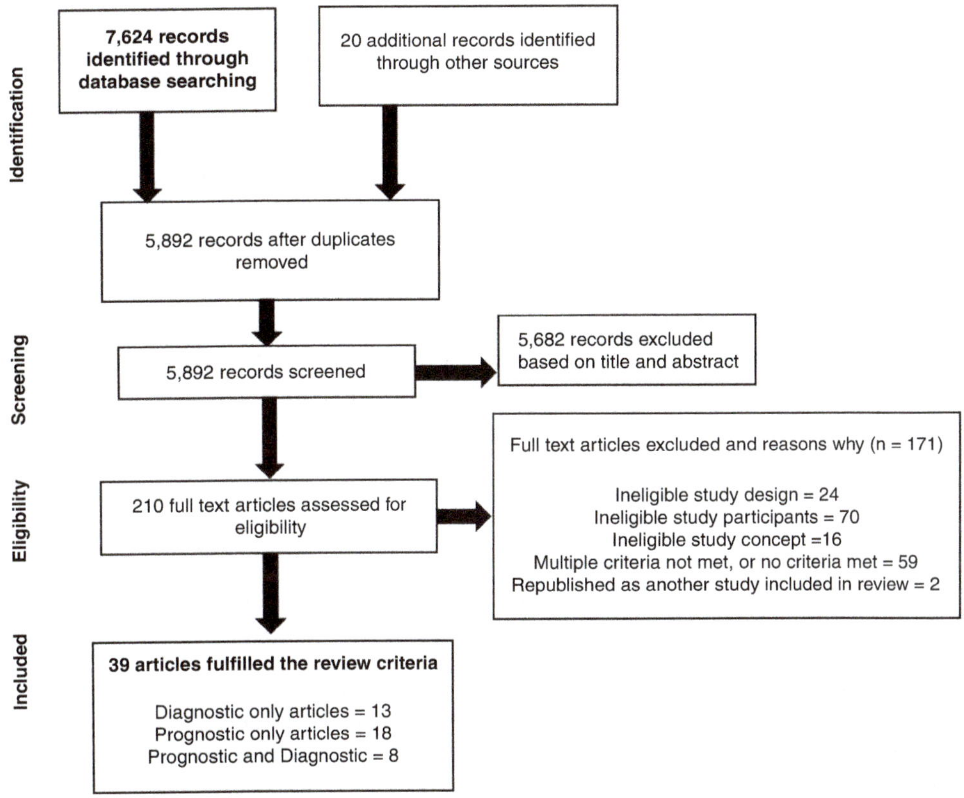

Figure 8.1 A PRISMA flow chart. Source: Sutcliffe L, Lumley H, Shaw L, et al. Surface electroencephalography (EEG) during the acute phase of stroke to assist with diagnosis and prediction of prognosis: A scoping review. *BMC Emerg Med.* 2022; 22:29. http://creativecommons.org/licenses/by/4.0/.

- Demographic information about the population. Some variables include gender (sometimes expressed as % male), location (maybe country, or site where the study recruited their patients), or age range.

In the PRISMA flowchart shown in Figure 8.1, the top boxes represent the initial articles searched (7,624 studies and 20 other sources) and the bottom left box represents the number of final articles included for analysis (39 studies). Boxes and arrows along the way indicate the reasons for why articles have been excluded.

Interpreting the Data

The information provided in the flow chart is to allow for reproducibility if others intend to perform a similar analysis of the data set. The flow chart is more similar to a figure showing the experimental paradigm than to one showing results.

Additional Resources

Preferred Reporting Items for Systematic Reviews and Meta-Analyses (PRISMA) website: https://prisma-statement.org/.

8.3 Forest Plot

Background Information

Forest plots are used to graphically summarize the results of the meta-analysis. While forest plots typically read more like a table, there is usually at least one graphical element in the plot. Only studies that have been identified by the selection criteria described in the flow chart (Section 8.1) are included in the forest plot.

Reading the Graphs

In a forest plot, each row represents a single study. Typically, a summary of all eligible studies appears in the bottom-most row, which may be labeled **overall** (or **total**).

The following columns may be presented for each row:

- **Study**, identified by lead author and year of publication.
- **Number of patients, subjects, or data points for each condition**. Sometimes, this column is labeled "total," representing the total for that given study, not the total for the whole meta-analysis.
- **Weight**, a percentage given to the study that determines how much it contributes to the overall results. The higher the percentage, the more the results from that study are valued in the calculation of the overall data. Generally, studies with larger sample sizes and smaller standard errors are given more weight.
- **Study quality**, a subjective measure that looks to see how rigorous the study was. Some features characteristic of high study quality include a well-defined research question and inclusion/exclusion criteria, few limitations of the study, and a low risk of bias.
- A graphical element, consisting of a symbol and error bars. The symbol may be a square or circle and may vary in size, with larger symbols denoting larger weight given to the results from that study. Along the x-axis is the measure of interest, such as relative risk, odds ratio, hazard ratio, or any other outcome variable. The horizontal lines extending from each point most often represent the **95% confidence interval** (or **95% CI**). A vertical line denotes the **line of no effect**, which extends from the 1 or 0 along the x-axis. The overall data may be presented as a diamond instead of a box with lines. For overall data, the points of the diamond represent the 95% CI.
- The numerical values from the graphical element may also be reported in a column next to the graph. These will often list the average and the 95% confidence interval, separated by brackets or parentheses.

The order of the columns is not always the same between graphs, but typically the study name is the farthest left and the graphical element is the farthest right.

The forest plots in Figure 8.2 represent meta-analysis results from studies of the effect of adjunctive treatment with rasagiline and levodopa for Parkinson's disease. In the top forest plot, four studies were included, and each row represents the results from one study. The meta-analysis showed that a combination of rasagiline and levodopa decreased Parkinson's disease severity as rated by a clinical rating scale compared to levadopa alone (diamond at the bottom row). All four studies found a decrease in the standardized mean difference (SMD), demonstrating that adjunctive treatment improved the Parkinson's symptoms (patients were better able to perform activities of daily life, had less severe mood changes, and had less severe motor deficits). The line of no effect is at 0, and none of the 95% confidence intervals overlaps with this line. In the bottom forest plot, six studies were included. Here, the relative risks (RR) of adverse side effects are compared when rasagiline is present. Two studies (Hattori and Parkinson Study Group) found a statistically significant increase in risk for side effects; the other four did not. In summary, the meta-analysis

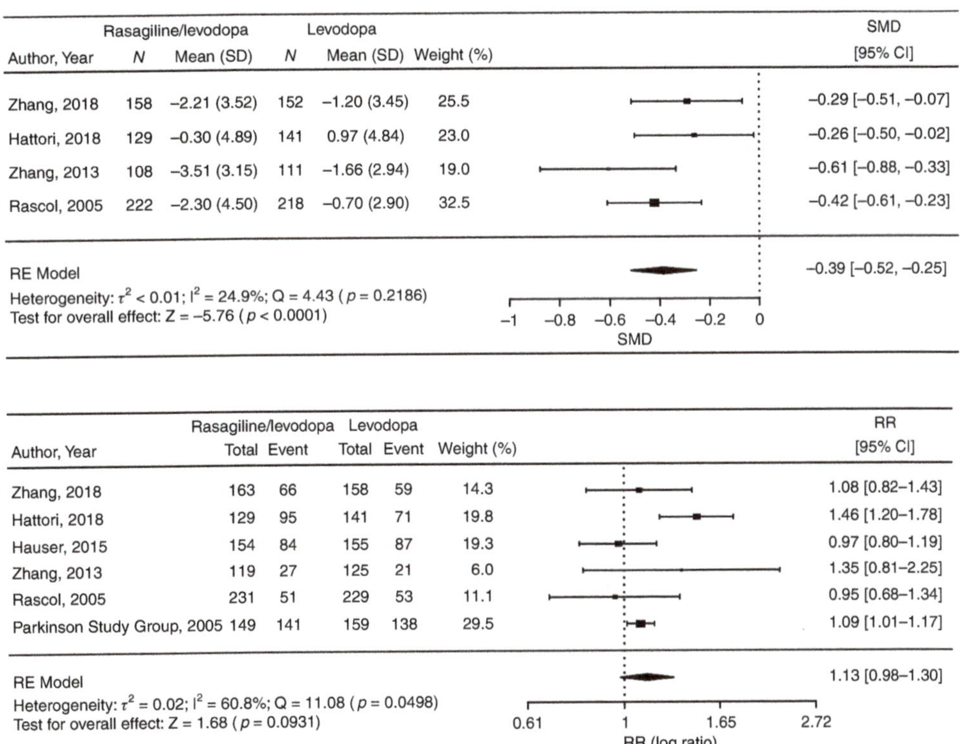

Figure 8.2 Two forest plots. Source: Kano O, Tsuda H, Hayashi A, Arai M. Rasagiline as adjunct to levodopa for treatment of Parkinson's disease: A systematic review and meta-analysis. *Parkinson's Disease*. 2022; 2022:4216452. http://creativecommons.org/licenses/by/4.0/. Images have been cropped and reorganized.

discovered no increase in risk – the summary (black diamond) overlaps with the line of no effect at 1, meaning no difference in risk. The size of each square represents the weight given to each study.

A different plot for meta-analysis results is a **Galbraith plot**. These are scatterplots with regression analysis where each point represents the results from one study. The x-axis is an indirect measure of sample size, with larger values representing studies that have a bigger sample size. These points carry more weight in the regression analysis since these have a larger sample size. The y-axis typically plots the magnitude of the effect observed. The solid line, starting at a y-axis value of 0, shows the pooled effect. When this line shows no slope, the results are not significant. The lines above and below the pooled data indicate the 95% confidence interval. In a forest plot showing the same data, the points outside of the confidence interval represent studies that do not overlap with the line of no effect and are therefore notable for their effect.

The Galbraith plot in Figure 8.3 shows the results of a meta-analysis. In this plot, each dot represents the results from a study. The blue highlighted area represents the 95% confidence interval. Dashed and dotted lines represent the expected distribution of the data if there were no significance. The positive slope of the regression suggests a positive correlation between the variables being studied.

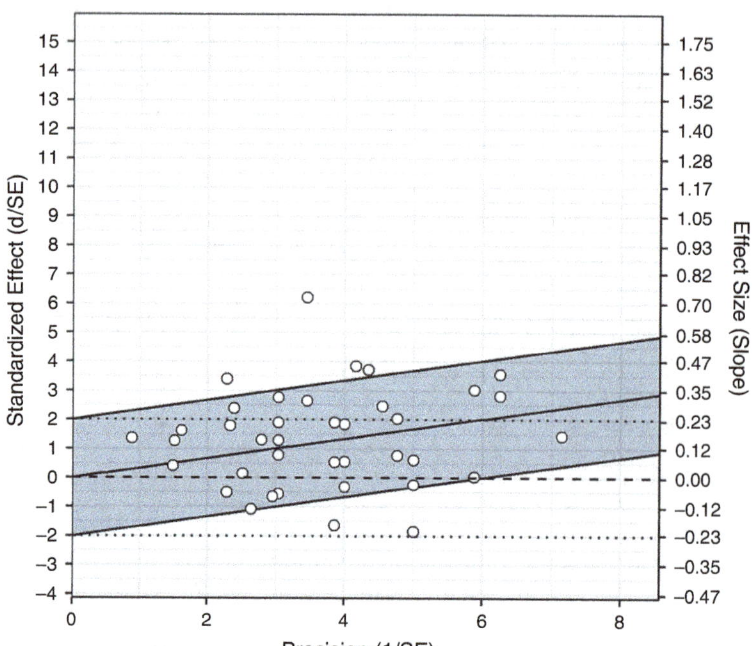

Figure 8.3 A Galbraith plot. Source: Kossmeier M, Tran US, Voracek M. Charting the landscape of graphical displays for meta-analysis and systematic reviews: A comprehensive review, taxonomy, and feature analysis. *BMC Med Res Methodol.* 2020; 20(26). http://creativecommons.org/licenses/by/4.0/. Image cropped.

Interpreting the Data

To quickly visualize the results of the meta-analysis, look for the diamond or the row labeled "total" and see if the diamond intersects with the line of no effect. If they overlap, the study found no statistically significant effect.

Results from a meta-analysis may be reported as a **relative risk (RR)**, which is an estimation of the risk that some outcome will result from the condition or manipulation. Risk values are numerically represented as relative to 1, which represents no difference in risk compared to placebo, no treatment, or the total population. When data are greater than 1, this indicates the study found an increased risk, while data points less than 1 indicate studies showing decreased risk. If the 95% confidence interval of an individual study or the diamond representing total effect intersects with the line of no effect, that study or the meta-analysis observed no statistically significant difference.

Alternatively, an **odds ratio (OR)** may be presented. Odds ratios represent the relationship between some outcome depending on the exposure or treatment. Like relative risk, the higher the odds ratio, the stronger the link between the treatment and the outcome.

Both odds ratios and risk ratios offer the same theoretical information, but they differ slightly in interpretation. An odds ratio is more meaningful for interpreting case–control studies since it represents a sample and not the entire population.

Additional Resources

Jiroutek MR, Turner JR. Relative vs absolute risk and odds: Understanding the difference. *J Clin Hypertens (Greenwich)*. 2019 Jun; 21(6):859–861. DOI: 10.1111/jch.13548. Epub 2019 Apr 25. PMID: 31020779; PMCID: PMC8030315.

8.4 Funnel Plot

Background Information

One of the issues with a meta-analysis is **publication bias**. Typically, only studies that find statistically significant results get published, while findings of **negative data** (results that show no significant difference) do not get published (this is informally called the **file drawer problem**, as negative data get stored away in a file drawer and forgotten). If the experimenter includes only studies that have been published, then the meta-analysis may be biased toward a result. This publication bias is especially present among studies that examine relationships between an intervention and outcomes.

Funnel plots are graphical representations of publication bias; however, they are not presented if there are a small number of studies (fewer than 10) included in the final analysis.

Reading the Graphs

Funnel plots put the mean difference of some measurement (commonly, odds ratio or relative risk) along the x-axis with a vertical line indicating the group average as determined by the forest plot analyses. Sometimes, the logarithm of these data is presented.

The y-axis will plot some measure of sample size. The most common variable reported here is **standard error** (abbreviated **SE**), which is inversely proportional to the square root of sample size. Smaller SE indicates larger sample size (or smaller standard deviation, or both). An SE of 0 is the theoretical smallest value and is represented at the top of the y-axis.

Alternatively, the y-axis may just plot sample size.

Each dot on the funnel plot represents the results from one of the included studies.

The general idea is that studies with large sample sizes are more likely to be close to the true average. Studies with a smaller sample size are likely to be less precise. If this distribution holds true, then the data points in the upper part of the graph will have less spread on the x-axis, while data points in the bottom part have more spread. This data point distribution forms the general shape of an upside-down funnel.

Diagonals are often drawn from the peak to the bottom of the graph. These diagonal lines represent the 95% confidence interval for the data. A **contour enhanced** funnel plot shows additional diagonal lines containing areas of different colors or shades. These represent different confidence intervals commonly used in statistical analysis, such as $p > 0.1$ or $p < 0.01$. This can help the reader identify the cause of why studies are missing. Publication bias may be present in the data set if studies are missing in areas with low statistical significance.

Figure 8.4 illustrates two funnel plots for showing publication bias. To the left is a funnel plot showing no major asymmetry across the dotted line, suggesting no publication bias in the results. To the right is a funnel plot suggesting publication bias. The studies that the researchers included in their search (black circles) are in an asymmetrical spread, with more studies finding a strong magnitude of effect (rightward on the x-axis) combined with

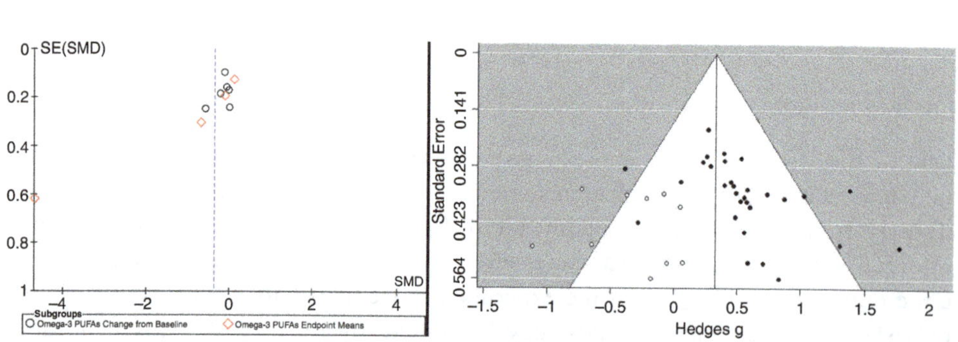

Figure 8.4 Two funnel plots. Source: Left: Kelaiditis CF, Gibson EL, Dyall SC. Effects of long-chain omega-3 polyunsaturated fatty acids on reducing anxiety and/or depression in adults: A systematic review and meta-analysis of randomised controlled trials. *Prostaglandins Leukot Essent Fatty Acids.* 2023 Apr 2; 192:102572. http://creativecommons.org/licenses/by/4.0/. Right: Mertens G, Engelhard IM. A systematic review and meta-analysis of the evidence for unaware fear conditioning. *Neurosci Biobehav Rev.* 2020; 108:254–268. http://creativecommons.org/licenses/by/4.0/.

smaller sample size (lower on the y-axis). The researchers corrected for this publication bias by including data points on the lower left quadrant of the graph (white circles).

Interpreting the Data

Visually, if more studies fall to one side of the vertical line, a publication bias may be present in the sample. Most asymmetries are found at the bottom left or bottom right quadrants of data, which may be missing if a publication bias is present.

Statistical tests are often reported alongside these data.

- **Egger's test** is a linear regression analysis that looks for an association between the effect and the standard error. It is a relatively conservative test that may detect a publication bias where other tests do not.
- **Begg's test** is a rank test that looks at effect size and variance.

In either the Egger's or Begg's tests, if the p-value for the tests is less than 0.05, a publication bias is present in the meta-analysis.

The **trim and fill method** is used to correct for publication bias by identifying when studies have not been published or have otherwise been suppressed, and then adding in those data points for the conclusion. This has the advantage of correcting for bias rather than simply detecting it.

Additional Resources

Egger M, Davey Smith G, Schneider M, Minder C. Bias in meta-analysis detected by a simple, graphical test. *Brit Med J.* 1997 Sep 13; 315(7109):629–34. DOI: 10.1136/bmj.315.7109.629. PMID: 9310563; PMCID: PMC2127453.

Lin L, Chu H. Quantifying publication bias in meta-analysis. *Biometrics*. 2018 Sep; 74 (3):785–794. DOI: 10.1111/biom.12817. Epub 2017 Nov 15. PMID: 29141096; PMCID: PMC5953768.

Shi Linyu, Lin Lifeng. The trim-and-fill method for publication bias: Practical guidelines and recommendations based on a large database of meta-analyses. *Med.* 2019 June; 98(23): e15987.

Sterne JAC, Sutton AJ, Ioannidis JPA, et al. Recommendations for examining and interpreting funnel plot asymmetry in meta-analyses of randomised controlled trials. *Brit Med J.* 2011; 343:d4002.

Summary

This chapter has described the graphs that are presented in meta-analyses, a special type of systematic review that uses strict statistical methods to examine results across several publications. Meta-analyses provide strong evidence because they look for bigger trends that underlie results across varying methodological approaches, interventions, populations, or any other differences that come up during experimental design.

Not very many figures usually appear in a meta-analysis. The forest plot shows the results of the analysis and is therefore the most important figure to understand. Flow charts show how to replicate the meta-analysis, and funnel plots show the results of statistical tests for bias.

Key Terms

- activation likelihood estimation (ALE)
- Begg's test
- Egger's test
- file drawer problem
- flow chart
- forest plot
- funnel plot
- Galbraith plot
- gray literature
- line of no effect
- meta-analysis
- odds ratio
- PRISMA
- publication bias
- relative risk
- trim and fill method

Index